The Emergence of Women into the 21st Century

Edited by

Patricia L. Munhall, ARNP, EdD, PsyA, FAAN
Professor
Associate Dean of Graduate Program
Director of the Center for Nursing Science
School of Nursing
Barry University
Miami, Florida

Virginia Macken Fitzsimons, RN, C, EdD
Professor
Chairperson
Department of Nursing
Kean College of New Jersey
Union, New Jersey

NLN Press • New York
Pub. No. 14-6622

The art on the part opener pages was created by Aide Rayas, a student at Ithaca College, Ithaca, New York.

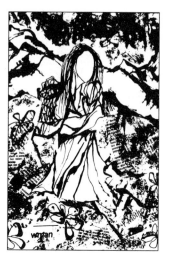

Copyright © 1995
National League for Nursing
350 Hudson Street, New York, NY 10014

The views expressed in this book reflect those of the authors and do not necessarily reflect the official views of the National League for Nursing.

Library of Congress Cataloging-in-Publication Data

The emergence of women into the 21st century / edited by Patricia L. Munhall, Virginia M. Fitzsimons.
      p.   cm.
    Includes bibliographical references.
    ISBN 0-88737-662-2
    1. Women. 2. Women—Social conditions. 3. Women—Health and hygiene. I. Munhall, Patricia L. II. Fitzsimons, Virginia Macken, 1943-
HQ1154.E454   1995
305.42′ 09′ 05—dc20   95-25518
                                                     CIP

This book was set in Garamond by Publications Development Company, Crockett, Texas. The editor and designer was Allan Graubard. The printer was Clarkwood Corp. The cover was designed by Lauren Stevens.

Printed in the United States of America.

Prologue

At the end of the meeting of the Commission on the Status of Women, the final "PrepCom" for the Fourth World Conference on Women, Secretary-General Gertrude Mongella told the gathering of representatives of governments and non-governmental organizations (NGOs) that "a revolution has begun and there is no going back. There will be no unravelling of commitments—not today's commitments, not last year commitments, and not the last decade's commitments. This revolution is too just, too long overdue. Take back the message of the Platform, and see you in Beijing" (UN NEWSLETTER, May 1995).

The message of "the platform" is described in the first piece of this book, entitled, "Women Being and Becoming: Backdrop to the U.N. Fourth World Conference on Women." We, Virginia and myself, were asked by one of the U.N. NGOs to compile a volume of readings in preparation for the conference, and to speak at the conference. That was October 1994.

Let us tell you what has happened since. All was well concerning the conference until April 1995 when the Chinese government, who was hosting the conference, decided that all U.N. NGOs were not to be allowed in Beijing, but in a smaller city 40 to 50 miles away. Reasons given for this ranged from insufficient accommodations for the 40,000 planned registrants in Beijing to the removal of NGOs to a place where there would be little media coverage and little, if not impossible, transportation to Beijing. Fear of messages being expressed by women from all over the world on human rights, women's liberation issues, education and emancipation for women, elimination of women's illiteracy, and promotion of peace and sexual equality were cited by some analysts as reasons to move these groups to a more rural and less accessible city. These analysts also considered the move as a means of suppressing the agendas of these groups.

Nonetheless, this book, *The Emergence of Women into the 21st Century,* is dedicated to any woman experiencing suppression of any type, anywhere in the world or in the home. This volume is not a history. It is a portrayal of women today as they enter the next century. That in itself is arbitrary, because time is an artificial construct and our being in time is influenced by our constructed age as well as the situated context from which we experience reality through individual perceptions. However, to ignore a turn of the century is to ignore that piece of reality. Much like New Year's Eve, we mark time. When we were younger, the year 2000 was almost considered science fiction and perhaps that is or will be part of how the next century will be constructed.

There is so much to say. A "snapshot" of a time period requires so many considerations of so many contingencies, so many of which are not included here. We are sure that other books marking this time will be forthcoming, and we hope to do a second volume of the present publication. In the meantime, if your experience is not captured or not captured well, please write to us and we will try to incorporate it elsewhere.

This work presents a post-modern perspective of women's development and potential within the theoretical constructs of "contingency" and "situated context." Such constructs guide each paper in the acknowledgement that the contingencies and situated context of living influence each person's life world. Contingencies considered important here are health, political contexts, relationships, culture, age, education, social conditions, nationality, and economic status. The situated context of space, time, body, and relationality further the post-modern perspective by addressing women's roots, level of education, environment, emotional status, and belief systems. Myths about stability and certainty are rejected in favor of an everchanging, serendipitous, multi-mind, many-things-are-simultaneously possible perspective.

For example, the year of a woman's birth, the color of her skin, her parents, childhood neighborhood, the messages she received about being a woman, her level of trust, self-esteem, cultural and religious beliefs, and even her weight, whether as a result of poverty or wealth, construct a situated context. At the same time, we are calling all such concepts into question. Critical theory, deconstruction, and revisionist theory question who establishes the beliefs, who makes the rules, who perpetuates the myths, and who controls prevailing modes of social and political discourse. In Beijing, such may appear more obvious, but women anywhere would be naive to reject this knowledge as not being critical to the advancement of women everywhere.

Women today, on the verge of entering the twenty-first century, will do so from individual perspectives and realities. Some will be teenagers, thinking the world has always been this way; others will be older, in their nineties, not believing how much the world has changed and some believing that recent changes in this last generation have been of their own creation. Yet all is evolving. Nothing is possible without what preceded it, no matter how long or short ago.

As editors and contributors, we hope the reader receives from this compilation of papers, written by wonderful writers of all backgrounds, a further enhancement of the meaning of being a woman and human being. We also hope, in some small way, to further women's search for peace, equality, and development. Your story may be here, or your sister's, friend's, or neighbors. The writers in this volume give voice to women's experience, to inspire women to reach the heights they aspire to, to suggest solutions to problems, and to bring to consciousness ways in which women can feel safe and secure in this world. In a world with many ways to live as a woman, hopefully free, and where the "multi-mind," multiplicity, and polyvocality of women are celebrated, humanity at large can only benefit. In the next century, as with all others, this, too, is where our sons and daughters will grow to mark time in their own liberated ways.

P.L.M. and V.M.F.

Preface

This book is guided by an overwhelming concern for the human condition. By focusing on women, we are more encompassing, for they are the mothers and teachers of our sons and daughters. Women have often been "given" the care-taking role and simultaneously have become one of societies oppressed groups. While care-taking, they are, in many countries as well as this country, often dependent on economic status and knowledgeable experts who exert power, make the rules, and control the discourse. Some of this is blatant, even more dangerous is the subtle; some of this is explicit, even more dangerous is the implicit.

This volume is also guided by post-modern thought or a post-modern way of being. So some assumptions should be made explicit, though not all writers in this volume are clearly, nor should they be, of the same vein. A book prospectus went to all contributors, containing the post-modern perspective guiding the writing, but that certainly was not a requirement. In fact, Virginia is a Conservative and a Republican and I (Patricia) am a Liberal and a Democrat. We do not often discuss politics, nor agree on post-modern ideas! But what of these post-modern guiding assumptions?

In a political sense, the sociopolitical context of women's lives is analyzed by critique, especially of the relationship between power and knowledge. One of the major platform issues for this U.N. World Conference on Women had to do with the advancement of education for women. A post-modern analyst would also want to know the content of that education, whose agenda is being served by that education, and what political agenda is being perpetuated within that educational content and, perhaps more important, the educational process, that is, how the process is conducted— is it by indoctrination or by critiquing and constructing the content?

Continuing through the lens of post-modernism, while the discourse of education is important, so are the silences, the ambiguities, the voices held quiet for fear of repercussion. Here in this volume's discourse are voices. We have placed them into eleven themes, comprising

42 narratives, experiential and theoretical. Because of the composition of women's lives, the individual pieces could easily be placed within a number of themes. And while the placement has a rationale, such placement is more for structure and semblance of order. Paradoxically, a post-modern perspective rejects this concept of order and readers will see the overlap and that indeed this volume is a whole with many voices.

We attempted to select papers that reflected the post-modern era of entering the twenty-first century (though some say that era has already passed). The papers reflect the simultaneity of many possibilities of living one's life depending on context and contingencies. There is an overwhelming multiplicity and "multi-mind" way of perceiving the same phenomenon. Meaning is open, individual, and not characterized by any one institution. Interpretation of an event runs the gamut and yet does not lose validity in differing interpretations. Antithetical ideas and theories can be possible and even preferable at the same time. Ambiguity makes perfect sense. The world is characterized by flux, disorder, chaos, confusion, and tension.

To argue otherwise would make this volume and the daily newspaper invalid—the world is more often dysfunctional. To think elsewise is wishful thinking. This book thus does not pretend to make sense of this, but it does offer a reading, a hearing, of the voices of women situated in this context and how they interpret the uncertainty and ambiguity of this age—which also recognizes that "laws," "truths," "theories," "assumptions," and "myths" are time-bound and have changed. Thus we know knowledge is always changing and should always be questioned within the context of the concepts of time and power.

We fool ourselves, for instance, if we do not believe that racism, sexism, homophobia, ageism, hatred, self-righteousness, and intolerance of differences are rampant. In this small volume, we see these conditions in other countries as well. How these conditions are considered and the actions that follow reflect, whether consciously or unconsciously, the wishes of those in power. So we return to the relationship of education, power, and polyvocality, many voices and many perceptions.

In the many voices herein, there are those of pain and suffering: starvation, AIDS, other health problems, homelessness, war zone, societal and domestic violence, poverty, and discrimination are among our problems as we enter the turn of the century. Yet they are not new; perhaps some progress has even been made toward their alleviation. But while one woman is being raped, or one child is starving, and another peddled for money, we cannot be content.

We also know the human spirit has been indomitable. Voices of immigrants, who have struggled and succeeded, projects supported by foundations to attempt to solve social problems, hopeful ways of treating women's health, women giving children opportunities for family life, women enjoying life and finding meaning in what is before them, young voices filled with optimism, women helping other women succeed, sharing secrets of success, and their interpretation of power, suggestions of cultural images, and the incredible importance of all our small efforts— small efforts magnified to become magnificent.

May you, as we, feel inspired, motivated, and perhaps upset enough to add another small effort, as we mark this time. In our work, toward the aim of improving the condition of fellow human beings, we will find meaning in emergence.

PATRICIA L. MUNHALL
VIRGINIA M. FITZSIMONS

September 1995

Acknowledgments

Giving voice to the emergence of the 21st Century Woman are the generous, sensitive, and involved contributors to this volume. We are deeply grateful for their commitment to this project, in the telling of their own personal stories, the sharing of their work toward the alleviation of problems, and the raising to consciousness the critical nature of conditions that women, children (and men) bear. We thank them for risking personal disclosure, for providing inspiration, for contributing to our understanding, for providing moments of tears, as well as humor.

We as co-editors and contributors wish to acknowledge the gift of friendship that has grown throughout the years and has assisted invaluably to our own emergence. Many individuals who wrote for this volume are colleagues and/or friends as well. We are very appreciative of these relationships and in the very human way they have emerged.

One contributor, Allan Graubard, is a dear friend as well as director of NLN Press. We thank him for encouraging this unexpected project and for providing the support to bring to fruition a book for an international conference on women. Nancy Marcus Land of Publications Development Company works behind the scenes, providing ideas and creativity to the production and we thank her for her dedication.

The connections in this one volume are representative of the richness of a web of relationships. We all must continue to interweave our lives to mutually assist one another, to make sure no child goes hungry, no human suffers from deprivation, no rock goes unturned in our efforts to make this world a humane place to roam about. For all our connections to human beings, we say, thank you.

P.L.M. and V.M.F.

Editors

Patricia L. Munhall, ARNP, EdD, Psy A, FAAN
Professor and Associate Dean of Graduate Program
Director of the Center for Nursing Science
School of Nursing
Barry University
Miami, Florida

Virginia Macken Fitzsimons, RN, C, EdD
Professor
Chairperson
Department of Nursing
Kean College of New Jersey
Union, New Jersey

Contributing Authors

Betty W. Barber, RN, PhD
Dean
School of Natural Science, Nursing
  and Mathematics
Kean College of New Jersey
Union, New Jersey

Barbara Stevens Barnum, RN, PhD,
  FAAN
Professor
Columbia University School of
  Nursing Division
New York, New York

Marilyn Burk, MLS
Researcher
Randolph, New Jersey

Elaine L. Cohen, RN, EdD
Assistant Vice President for
  Nursing
The General Hospital Center at
  Passaic
Passaic, New Jersey

Marcia Szmania Davis, MS, MSEd,
  RNC, WHCNP, ANP
Faculty, School of Nursing
Virginia Commonwealth University
Richmond, Virginia

Marcia Dombro
Doctoral Candidate
Florida International University
Miami, Florida

Fatemeh B. Firoz, PhD
Psychologist
Summit, New Jersey

Agnes Fleming (Pseudonym)
South Orange, New Jersey

Elizabeth J. Forbes, EdD, FAAN
Professor
Department of Nursing
College of Allied Health Sciences
Thomas Jefferson University
Philadelphia, Pennsylvania

David Anthony Forrester, RN, PhD
Professor
University of Medicine and
    Dentistry of New Jersey
School of Nursing
Newark, New Jersey

Joyce Wells-Gentry, RN, MS
Nursing Administrator Supervisor
Childbirth Educator
Nursing Clinical Instructor
Miami Dade Community College
Miami, Florida

Sandra Gibson, EdD, ARNP
Associate Professor
Nurse Practitioner Program
Barry University
Miami Shores, Florida

Simon Glynn, PhD
Associate Professor
Department of Philosophy
Florida Atlantic University
Boca Raton, Florida

Allan Graubard
Poet, Playwright, Critic
New York, New York

Pedro José Greer, Jr., MD
Medical Director
Camillus House
Assistant Dean, Poverty Medicine
University of Miami
Miami, Florida

Claudia Hauri, ARNP, EdD
Associate Professor
Director of Primary Care
    Treatment
Barry University
Miami, Florida

Lynne Hektor, RN, PhD
Assistant Professor
Florida Atlantic University
Boca Raton, Florida

Sheila J. Hopkins, MSN, ARNP
Assistant Professor of Nursing
Barry University
Miami Shores, Florida

Maureen Hreha, MS
Nurse Practitioner
Child Care
Randolph, New Jersey

Noreen O'Callaghan Jenott, MAEd
School Counselor
Briehta Elementary School
Tucson, Arizona

Myrna Morales Keklak, RN, BSN
Coordinator
Nursing Academic Support Center
Robert Wood Johnson
    Foundation, Inc.
Transcultural Leadership
    Continuum Grant
Union County College
Cranford, New Jersey

Glenda Kirkland, MBA
Executive Director
Isaiah House, Inc.
East Orange, New Jersey

Cheryl Demerath Learn, PhD, RN
Assistant Professor
College of Nursing
Health Sciences Center
University of New Mexico
Albuquerque, New Mexico

Veronica Magar
New York, New York

Mia Rene Martin
Undergraduate Student
Barry University
Miami, Florida

Judith Mathews, RN, MS
Dean
Muhlenberg Regional Medical
  Center
Schools of Nursing and Allied
  Health
Randolph, New Jersey

Patricia R. Messmer, RN, C, PhD
Director of Nursing Research
Mount Sinai Medical Center
Miami Beach, Florida

Judith Migoya
Undergraduate Student
Barry University
Miami, Florida

Jacqueline B. Mondros, DSW
Associate Dean/Professor
Barry University School of Social
  Work
Miami, Florida

Jackie Moore, RN, BS
Nurse Epidemiologist
Mount Sinai Medical Center
Miami Beach, Florida

Craig T. Munhall
Undergraduate Student
Barry University
Miami, Florida

Lynne Nelson, RN, BSN
Director of Tutorial Services
Elizabeth General Medical Center
  School of Nursing
Elizabeth, New Jersey

Kathleen Mary Nugent
Oakknoll School
Short Hills, New Jersey

Evelyn Ortner
Execituve Director
Unity House, Inc.
Shelter for Battered Women and
  Children
Summit, New Jersey

Katherine Parry, PhD, PT
Nova Southeastern University
College of Allied Health
North Miami Beach, Florida

Suzanne Rodriguez, RN, BSN,
  CCRN
Nurse Clinician/Case Manager
NICU & Nursery
Mount Sinai Medical Center
Miami Beach, Florida

Gabriella Rosetti, PhC, MFA
Director and Performing Artist
Department of Theater
CUNY Graduate Center
New York, New York

Suzanne Maguire Santoro
Seaford, New York

Amela Sapcanin
Second Secretary
Permanent Mission of the Republic
    of Bosnia and Herzegovina
United Nations in New York
New York, New York

Mahnaz Sarachi, MPH, PhD
Executive Director
International Health Awareness
    Network
United Nations in New York
New York, New York

Victoria Schoolcraft, RN, PhD
Professor and Associate Dean
Barry University School of Nursing
Miami Shores, Florida

Davida R. Schuman, PhD
Professor
Department of Communication
    Sciences and Educational
    Services
Kean College of New Jersey
Union, New Jersey

Suzanne G. Sitelman
Riverdale Country School
Riverdale, New York

Janice T. Thomas, ARNP, PhD
Professor of Nursing
Barry University
Miami, Florida

Tracy R. Thomas, JD, LLM
Washington, DC

Kathy Washburn, RNC, MSN
Nurse Manager of Pediatrics
Newborn Nursery & NICU
Mount Sinai Medical Center
Miami Beach, Florida

Ellis Quinn Youngkin, PhD, RNC,
    OGNP
Associate Professor
School of Nursing
Virginia Commonwealth University
Richmond, Virginia

Contents

Voices Four: Violence and Women

Voices Five: Women and AIDS

Voices Six: Women and Health

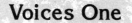

Voices One

The Fourth Decade of the Women Beijing Conference

1

Women: Being and Becoming

Mahnaz Sarachi

In Beijing, we will determine what can be done to eliminate gender discrimination and promote new partnership between women and men into the 21st century.

Gertrude Mongella
Secretary-General of the Fourth World
Conference on Women
September 4–15, 1995
Beijing, China
Action for Equality, Development, and Peace

*M*obilizing women and men to achieve equality by the 21st century is a fundamental goal of the Fourth World Conference on Women. Over the past 20 years, there have been important changes in women's rights depending on the hardships and opportunities they face.

In the post-war world, women enjoyed the right to vote in only 31 countries—the equal rights of men and women were enshrined in the Preamble of the United Nations Charter which legally established gender equality as a fundamental human right for the first time in history.

3

The Commission on the Status of Women, which has been the locus for United Nations activities to support women's struggle for equality, was one of the earliest intergovernmental committees set up by the United Nations. The Commission was established in 1946 to monitor the implementation of women's rights around the world. Later its focus shifted to the role of women in social and economic development and to equipping women with the tools to overcome centuries of discrimination.

CONFERENCE BACKGROUND

Discrimination against women, entrenched in deep-rooted cultural beliefs and traditional practices, persisted throughout much of the world. In order to draw attention to these obstacles and catalyze a swifter change in women's status, the United Nations declared 1975 as International Women's Year. It also convened the 1975 World Conference of the International Women's Year in Mexico City, the First Global Conference ever held on women.

The World Plan of Action for the attainment of the objectives of the 1975 International Women's Year aimed at narrowing the gap between the sexes by emphasizing equal opportunities for men and women, but did not question the prevailing development models or the forms of social and economic participation by individuals. Consequently, efforts were targeted toward achieving women's equitable participation in development benefits, but little was said about what type of development should be sought, and less still about the causes of discrimination and inequality. Thus, an agenda was set for future action by governments and development agencies during the United Nations Decade for Women, (1976-1985) (PAHO, p. 4).

It was in this context that the convention on the elimination of all forms of discrimination against women has been formed. A major step toward the attainment of the goal of equal rights for women was taken on December 18, 1979, when the General Assembly of the United Nations adopted the Convention. The comprehensive Convention calls for equal rights for women, regardless of their marital status, in all fields—political, economic, social, cultural, and civil. It calls for national legislation to ban discrimination; it recommends temporary special measures to speed equality, between men and women, and action to modify social and cultural patterns that perpetuate discrimination. Other measures provide for equal rights for women in political and public life; equal access to education and the same choice of curricula; nondiscrimination in employment and pay; and guarantees of job security in the event of marriage and maternity. The Convention underlines the equal responsibilities of men and women of family life. It also stresses the social services needed—especially child-care facilities—for combining family obligations with work responsibilities and participation in public life.

Additional articles of the Convention call for nondiscriminatory health services for women, including services related to family planning, and a legal capacity identical to that of men, with parties agreeing that all contracts and other private instruments that restrict the legal capacity of women "shall be deemed null and void." Special attention is given to the problems of rural women.

The Convention sets up machinery for the international supervision of the obligations accepted by States once they have ratified or acceded to it, The Committee on the Elimination of Discrimination Against Women (CEDAW), made up of 23 experts serving in their personal capacity and elected by states parties to the Convention, monitors progress made in its implementation (UN/DPI/929).

The Convention became effective on September 3, 1981 and has been ratified by over 100 nations, thereby legally binding them to implement its provisions (Women/UN).

The second Conference on Women, held in Copenhagen in 1980, adopted a program of action for the second half of the Decade for Women. This Conference gave priority to women's health needs—maternal health care, nutrition, family planning, prevention and treatment of infectious diseases. This Conference also focused on increasing women's health research, improving women's access to medical training opportunities, legislation to eliminate occupational hazards and environmental pollution, especially as effect reproductive health, maternal and infant mortality programs, health education, and prevent mutilation practices.

The third World Conference on Women was held in Nairobi, Kenya in 1985. The Forward Looking Strategies for the Advancement of Women were adopted by the Conference to Review and Appraise the Achievements of the United Nations Decade for Women: Equality, Development, and Peace.

Nairobi Forward-Looking Strategies

Paragraph 38 of this strategy indicates that "The Forward-Looking Strategies are intended to provide a practical and effective guide for global action on a long-term basis and within the context of the broader goals and objectives of a new international economic order" (UN/DPI/926).

The Nairobi Forward-Looking Strategies call for:

• Sexual equality
• Women's autonomy and power

- Recognition of women's unpaid work
- Advances in women's paid work
- Health service and family planning
- Better educational opportunities
- Promotion of peace
- Minimum targets for the year 2000:
  - enforcement of laws guaranteeing implementation of women's equality
  - an increase in the life expectancy of women to at least 65 years in all countries
  - the reduction of maternal mortality
  - the elimination of women's illiteracy
  - the expansion of employment opportunities

In 1990, the Commission on the Status of Women undertook a five-year review and appraisal of the Nairobi Forward-Looking Strategies. The results were discouraging. The Commission found that the situation of women had deteriorated in many parts of the world, especially in developing countries where economic stagnation or negative growth, continued population increases the growing burden of debt and the reduction of public expenditures for social programs had further constrained opportunities for women to improve their situation. There was also evidence of an alarming regression in the status of women in the spheres of education, employment, and health (Women/UN).

The Fourth World Conference on Women

The Fourth World Conference on Women will take place from September 4-15, 1995, in Beijing, China. It will build on the three previous women's conferences and the UN Decade for Women, the Conference will encourage the full implementation of the Nairobi Forward-Looking Strategies for the Advancement of Women to the Year 2000. It will provide the opportunity to assess how much has been achieved, to bring out women's strengths, skills, and talents, and to move on from there to achieve the goals set for the Decade. In order to attain its goal, the Conference must put in place a global policy of gender equality, development, and peace.

The Conference will take place during the 50th Anniversary of the United Nations. This will provide the opportunity to see how far the organization has come with regard to gender issues. It will be the occasion to put forward a global vision of the 21st century that fully reflects a gender perspective.

Objectives of the Conference

- To create the impetus in society for women to move forward, well-equipped to meet the challenges and demands of the 21st century for scientific, technological, economic, and political development.
- To address the question of how women can be empowered by taking part more effectively in decision making.
- To draw up a platform for action in order to ensure the completion of the unfinished work of implementing the Nairobi Forward-Looking Strategies.

At Beijing, delegates from United Nations member countries will look at recent trends affecting the status of women, with an eye to the future. They will review how women have fared in the areas of health, education, employment, family life, politics, and human rights. Despite the progress that has been made during the past 20 years, disparities between North and South, rural and urban, rich and poor, continue to concern women everywhere.

Progress has not been felt by women at all levels of society, particularly at the grass roots. The purpose of the Conference is not to emphasize the differences between countries or regions, but to use our diversity as a source of strength and unity. We are going to share our different experiences in order to take action for a better world. (Mongella/DPI/1424)

Education

In many parts of the world, girl children receive less education, less food, and less health care than boys. According to the World Health Organization (WHO), one sixth of all female infant deaths in India, Pakistan, and Bangladesh were due to neglect and discrimination (1986 figures). Nevertheless, trends in education are, for the most part, encouraging. The percentage of girls and women enrolled in primary and secondary schools as well as in graduate study programs rose 1 percentage point between 1980 and 1988, to 45 percent. However, despite a declining proportion of illiterate women—from 46.5 percent in 1970 to 33.6 percent in 1990—girls and women still represent two thirds of the world's illiterates, and they are becoming litrate at a slower rate than are men. These figures have serious implications, since children's health and child mortality rates are affected much more by a mother's schooling than by a father's.

There is concrete proof that women's education leads to fewer births, fewer infant deaths, more women in the formal labor force, and greater economic growth. Yet in some 37 of the world's poorest countries, health budgets have been halved, according to the International Fund for Agricultural Development (IFAD), largely as a result of the recession of the 1980s. The outlook is good for increased literacy, however, the United Nations Educational, Scientific, and Cultural Organization (UNESCO) predicts that only 28.2 percent of women will be illiterate by the year 2000, due to efforts by governments working in tandem with international development agencies and women's groups to come up with innovative ways of boosting female literacy.

Health

Women's health has improved substantially in some areas and worsened in others. While life expectancy is greater, and fertility and infant mortality rates have fallen, there has been little progress in reducing maternal mortality rates. Each year at least half a million women worldwide die from complications due to pregnancy, and another 100,000 as a result of unsafe abortions, according to the United Nations Children's Fund (UNICEF). The proportion of married women in developing countries who use contraception has doubled within one generation, but an estimated 300 million women worldwide still have no access to family planning; one fifth of all pregnancies in developing countries are unplanned and unwanted.

Even more disturbing, Scholar Amartya Sen reports that, based on global mortality patterns, some 100 million Asian women are estimated to be missing, attributable largely to female infanticide and the abortion of female foetuses. Even in industrialized countries like the United States, gender discrimination in health care is responsible for the deaths of thousands of women.

Women now constitute 40 percent of HIV-infected adults, and the WHO is projecting that by the year 2000, more than 13 million women will be infected with the virus and about 4 million of them will have died. Health issues will therefore figure prominently at the World Conference in Beijing, as delegates attempt to address long-term consequences and seek common ground for dealing with the challenges. As Conference Secretary-General Mongella puts it, "the problems of women are not different from country to country. They only differ in intensity."

Economic Power

Progress in the economic arena has been limited for women. Their participation in the formal labor market increased in many regions between

1970 and 1990, particularly among women with children. Women now represent 41 percent of all workers in developed countries, 34 percent worldwide. But while the wage gap may have closed somewhat, women still earn, on average, 30 to 40 percent less than men in lower paid jobs, according to the United Nations' publication, *The World's Women 1970-1990: Trends and Statistics.*

Levels of inequality vary from place to place, but the pattern is international. Men are more likely to have regular full-time work and to receive greater seniority and benefits. Nonetheless, women are definitely breaking through what has variously been called the glass ceiling, the bamboo ceiling, or the old boy's network, honing their leadership skills and abilities to command respectable salaries commensurate with their work. In the United States, for example, women earned 72 cents for each dollar earned by men in 1990. And while women are entering nontraditional occupations in increasing numbers, most still work in the informal sector, with its insecure and frequently dangerous working conditions; they also far outnumber men in this sector. Known in many parts of the world to be successful entrepreneurs and traders, women have frequently been thwarted in their attempts at financial independence by lack of access to capital and other resources, inadequate education and training, and uneven distribution of assets and responsibilities within the family. Although they usually bear the costs of setting up informal activities, they often turn over the benefits to the male members of the family. When they do work in the formal sector, women tend to be concentrated in the pink ghetto—clerical work, domestic service, subsistence agriculture, and export processing, where they account for 70 to 90 percent of all employees. Although women work longer hours than men—up to 13 hours more, in Africa and Asia—much of what they do is often unrecorded, undervalued, or not valued at all.

Women's organizations and the United Nations have been in the forefront of innovative efforts by statisticians to identify accurately the economically active population, particularly in the informal sector, and determine how to assign an economic value to women's unremunerated domestic, agricultural, and reproductive work. The Beijing Conference will showcase ongoing work to refine such statistics and ultimately to use those data to supplement the national accounts that are used in determining policy directives.

Poverty

The invisibility of women extends beyond their economic roles. Frequently living on the margin of established society, poor women, migrant women, and women refugees are even more vulnerable than men living under the same circumstances.

Poverty is one area where women's situation has taken a dramatic turn for the worse, given that women are living longer and receiving less support from families, husbands, and fathers. This is due to a general rise in male migration as well as overall unemployment trends. The number of rural women living in poverty nearly doubled over the past 20 years and today women constitute at least 60 percent of the world's 1 billion rural poor. Experts concur that extreme poverty, combined as it frequently is with discrimination, causes the deaths of millions of girls and women, especially the elderly. Poverty is also apparent in the fact that there are more and more female-headed households—about one fifth of all households worldwide—and the figure is rising. In rural areas of Africa and the Caribbean, the proportion is higher.

Political Power

Women's access to political and economic power is not commensurate with their influence in other spheres of life; they constitute a minority in the corridors of power and decision making both nationally and internationally. But world events, and the three previous United Nations conferences on women, have politicized them to an extent unprecedented in history. Largely as a result of the United Nations Decade for Women, many governments have established special offices for women's issues, included women as a key component in development policies, and taken steps to increase the numbers of women decision makers. Women activists have been acquiring the managerial and negotiating skills needed to move from the town square to the bargaining table, from the spectator's gallery to the convention center.

Again, however, the progress is uneven; the proportion of women parliamentarians worldwide dropped from 12.5 percent in 1975 to 10.1 percent in 1993. As of November 1993, there were six female heads of government, and only eight of the 184 Member States of the United Nations had women permanent Representatives. Women's representation at the cabinet level is less than half that in national legislative bodies, and close to 100 countries have no women in parliament at all (Women/UN/DPI/1424).

Surveys in recent years indicate that about a quarter of the world's women are violently abused in their own homes. Community-based surveys have yielded higher figures—up to 50 percent in Thailand, 60 percent in Papua, New Guinea and the Republic of Korea, and 80 percent in Pakistan and Chile. In the United States, domestic violence is the biggest single cause of injury to women, accounting for more hospital admissions than rape, muggings, and road accidents combined.

In more and more countries, attempts are being made to bring this problem into the open, to help the victims, and to expose the causes. Research indicates the possibility of a link between domestic violence and progress toward equality for women (as measured, for example, by the closing of the literacy gap between males and females). The suspicion is that the risk of violence rises when male partners feel that their traditional position of superiority and control is being threatened (UNICEF/1995).

CONCLUSION

The Fourth World Conference on Women will attempt to break down the overall aim of progress for women into specific goals. The experience gained in recent years should make it possible to advance doable propositions in fields such as equal opportunity legislation, women's reproductive health, equality of educational opportunity, and the widespread promotion of the kind of low-cost technologies that could be an important first step in liberating the time and the energies of many hundreds of millions of rural women in the developing world.

The effectiveness of any and all of these goals will depend on their being broken down, until the doable propositions are identified. If this can be done, then the Fourth World Conference on Women will have built the basis for a renewed international development effort in the second half of 1990s (UNICEF/1995).

REFERENCES

Pan American Health Organization. (1993). *Gender, women, and health in the Americas,* Scientific Publication No. 541.

United Nations. (1991). *Women, challenges to the year 2000.*

United Nations. (1991). *The world's women 1970-1990, trends and statistics.*

United Nations Children's Fund. (1995). *The state of the world's children 1995.* Oxford University Press.

United Nations, Dept. of Public Information. (1994). *Women,* DPI/1424. Rev. 1.

United Nations Population Fund. (1994). *The state of world population.*

Women 2000, No. 1, 1994, United Nations, Division for the Advancement of Women.

World Health Organization, Geneva. (1992). *Women's health: Across age and frontier.*

2

The Status of Women and Health under International Law

Tracy R. Thomas

While the United Nations has made great strides in recognizing the needs of women and in remedying past injustices, rights need to be recognized within a legal system, both national and international, for their meaningful definition, implementation and enforcement. Without a means for effective implementation and binding enforcement, rights may remain nothing more than declarations whose impact may never ultimately be felt, no matter how significant its goal. Therefore, while the necessity of improving women and children's health and related needs for social and economical advancement has been widely recognized, it is of the utmost importance to define these rights within a legal system for their enforcement.

THE UNITED NATIONS AND HUMAN RIGHTS

*It is essential, if man is not to be compelled to have recourse, as a last re-
sort, to rebellion against tyranny and oppression, that human rights
should be protected by the rule of law . . . .:*
  —*Preamble to the Universal Declaration of Human Rights*[1]

The modern concept of human rights has its origins in the United Nations and its Charter. Following World War II, the nations of the world decided that the promotion and protection of human rights, fundamental
individual rights which nations should have an obligation to respect, were
to be one of the principal purposes of the United Nations.[2] As stated in the
Preamble to the Charter of the United Nations "We the Peoples of the
United Nations . . . reaffirm faith in fundamental human rights, in the dignity and worth of the human person, in the equal rights of men and
women and of nations large and small, and to establish conditions under
which justice and respect for the obligations arising from treaties and
other sources of international law can be maintained, and to promote social progress and better standards of life in larger freedom. . . ."[3] To advance the implementation and protection of these fundamental rights the
United Nations created the Commission of Human Rights, the primary
human rights organ of the United Nations and a specialized commission
answerable to the Economic and Social Council. The Commission's original mandate included the formulation of an international bill of rights,
recommendations for international documents addressing civil liberties,
status of women, freedom of information, protection of minorities, prevention of discrimination based on sex, race, language or religion and matters likely to impair general welfare or friendly relations between nations.[4]
    Later international conventions expanded and elaborated upon the
Charter of the United Nation's broad concept of human rights, starting
with the Universal Declaration of Human Rights of 1948.[5] Considered the
most important human rights document,[6] the Universal Declaration provides the framework for many subsequent documents. As stated in the
preamble to the Convention on the Elimination of Discrimination against
Women: "the Universal Declaration of Human Rights affirms the principle
of the inadmissibility of discrimination and proclaims that all human beings are born free and equal in dignity and rights and that everyone is entitled to all the rights and freedoms set forth therein, without distinction
of any kind, including distinction based on sex."[7] The Declaration's thirty
articles broadly delineates many rights, including: the right to life, liberty
and security; a prohibition against slavery and torture; an individual's
legal rights; the right to privacy, freedom of movement and freedom from

persecution; the right to a nationality, marriage, family and to own property; the freedom of thought, conscience and religion; peaceful assembly, participation in government; employment; a standard of living encompassing health, food, clothing, housing, medical care, social services, and education.

Eventually a core group of documents became known as the "International Bill of Human Rights." These documents include the United Nations Charter (1945), the Universal Declaration of Human Rights (1984), the International Covenant on Civil and Political Rights (1966), its Optional Protocols, the International Covenant on Economic, Social and Cultural Rights (1966).[8] The United Nations Charter is binding on its members and establishes at least general obligations concerning human rights.[9] The Universal Declaration is a manifesto with primarily moral authority; however, certain of its standards are arguably legally binding under the principles of customary international law. The two Covenants are binding upon those nations which ratify them. Taken together, these documents represent the obligations of United Nations members to ensure the equal right of men and women to enjoy all economic, social, cultural, civil, and political rights.[10]

Growing regional interest and interest in specific groups or issues have led to further United Nations involvement through the continued establishment of human rights commissions and treaties. These include but are not limited to the Inter-American Commission on Human Rights (1960), the European Convention on Human Rights (entry into force 1953), the International Convention on the Elimination of All Forms of Racial Discrimination (entry into force 1969), the American Convention on Human Rights (1978), the Convention on the Elimination of All Forms of Discrimination against Women (1981), the Convention Against Torture and Other Cruel, Inhuman or Degrading Treatment or Punishment (entry into force 1987) and the Convention on the Rights of the Child (1989).[11] The establishment of these specialized commissions and conventions illustrates the evolution of human rights from the concepts and standards enunciated in the International Bill of Human Rights into new and more specific areas, such as the right to health, food and environment, the right to education, and the rights of women and children.[12]

THE UNITED NATIONS: IMPROVING THE STATUS OF WOMEN SINCE ITS INCEPTION

Discrimination against women shall mean any distinction, exclusion or restriction made on the basis of sex which has the effect or purpose of impairing or nullifying the recognition, enjoyment or exercise by

women, irrespective of their marital status, on a basis of equality of men and women, of human rights and fundamental freedoms in the political, economic, social, cultural, civil or any other field.
—*Convention on the Elimination of All Forms of Discrimination against Women*

The United Nations has long recognized the injustices and inequalities suffered by women: promoting the rights of women and preventing injustices against women has been one of the United Nation's purposes since its inception after World War II. The United Nations Charter[13] first noted[14] the necessity of realizing and remedying injustices against women socially and legally, while at the same time affirming women's fundamental equality within the world order. The Preamble to the Charter reaffirms "faith in fundamental human rights, in the dignity and worth of the human person, in the equal rights of men and women and of nations large and small, and to establish conditions under which justice and respect for the obligations arising from treaties and other sources of international law can be maintained. . . ." An underlying tenet of the United Nations is "to achieve international co-operation in solving international problems of an economic, social, cultural or humanitarian character, and in promoting and encouraging respect for human rights and for fundamental freedoms for all without distinction as to race, sex, language, or religion."[15] Article 55 of the Charter identifies specific goals, including health, and encourages "solutions of international economic, social, health, and related problems; and international cultural and educational cooperation; and universal respect for, and observance of, human rights and fundamental freedoms for all without distinction as to race, sex, language or religion." To meet these goals, the United Nations endowed the Economic and Social Council with the authority to initiate studies, make recommendations, prepare draft conventions, set up commissions and work with other specialized agencies with respect to "international economic, social, cultural, educational, health and related matters."[16]

In furtherance of its devotion to women and their needs, in 1946 the United Nations established the Commission on the Status of Women[17] as a subsidiary body to the Economic and Social Council.[18] The Commission's mandate[19] was to document the status of women's rights in political, economic, social, cultural, and educational fields and to make recommendations to the Council. The Commission has remained a focal point for United Nations' activities relating to women in spite of its rocky history.[20] For its first twenty-five years of existence, the Commission functioned essentially in a human rights framework, focusing its energies primarily on the recognition of equal rights for women through standard-setting, legal studies and promotional actives. During the International Women's Year

in 1975 the Commission's orientation shifted towards economic and social development, with a particular emphasis on the conceptual structure
and development of concrete policies at the national and international
levels, including the participation of women within their societies. During this time, however, the Commission gradually declined in both power
and responsibility until it reached a low point in 1980 where a proposal[21]
requesting the abolition of the Commission during a general attempt at
restructuring the economic and social sectors of the United Nations was
tabled in the General Assembly. The Commission was subsequently revi-
talized since the end of the Women's Decade in 1985. Now the focus is on
the empowerment of women and their mainstream integration. Throughout its history, the Commission has remained active in preparing the
world conferences on women and the conventions regarding the rights of
women, including the Convention on the Elimination of All Forms of Discrimination against Women.

Concerned with the continuing unequal status of women thirty years
after the formation of the Commission, in December of 1972 the General
Assembly of the United Nations declared 1975 as the International
Women's Year.[22] The highlight of the Year was the first United Nations
Conference on Women, held in Mexico City. Entitled the World Conference
for International Women's Year, the Conference adopted by consensus a
World Plan of Action, led to a declaration by the General Assembly of the
United Nations Decade for Women 1975-1985 and approved the Draft Con-
vention of the Elimination of All Forms of Discrimination Against Women.

The agenda of the Conference reflected the emphasis of the Commission on creating a structural framework for the development of social and
economic structures at the national and international level. The plan entailed a five-year program designed to improve the status of women, with
steps encompassing: an increase in literacy for women and equal access
at every level of education; legislation to provide for voting on equal
terms with men and equal opportunity and conditions for employment;
greater participation of women in policy making positions at all levels of
society; development and extensions of modern rural technology, cottage
industries, day-care centers, and coeducation technical and vocational
training in basic skills; recognition of the economic value of domestic and
other work not traditionally remunerated; establishment of national machinery to accelerate the full integration of women into national life; and
efforts to improve the research base on the status of women.[23]

Also in 1975, the United Nations General Assembly proclaimed the period of 1976-1985 as the United Nations Decade for Women, emphasizing the themes of equality, development, and peace. The Decade
included the second United Nations Conference on Women,[24] entitled

the World Conference for the Decade of Women: Equality, Development, and Peace. Held in 1980 in Copenhagen, 57 countries signed the Convention on the Elimination of All Forms of Discrimination against Women, expanded the scope of the conference to include the subthemes of employment, health and education, and finally adopted a Program of Action for the Second half of the United Nations Decade for Women.[25]

The Program of Action reviewed the progress of the first half of the decade in banishing inequality and concluded "that while governments have become more aware of the importance of integrating women more fully into all aspects of national life and some legislation has been passed, implementation and enforcement mechanisms remain far from adequate." To remedy this situation, the full Conference by consensus adopted national targets and strategies in the areas of employment, health and education, set international targets and strategies in the same areas at the global and regional levels, and called upon the United Nations family of institutions for assistance.

The highlight of the decade was the ratification of the Convention on the Elimination of All Forms of Discrimination against Women.[26] The Convention was adopted unanimously by the General Assembly in 1979, opened for signature on March 1, 1980, and was entered into force September 3, 1981. A human rights treaty, the Convention addresses the need to "ensure the universal recognition in law and in fact of the principle of equality of men and women." In its resolution accompanying the adoption of the Convention, the United Nations General Assembly stated that "discrimination against women is incompatible with human dignity and the welfare of society."

Designed to function as an international bill of rights for women, the Convention is the most comprehensive document concerning the advancement and empowerment of women. Article One broadly defines the term "discrimination against women" to mean "any distinction, exclusion or restriction made on the basis of sex which has the effect or purpose of impairing or nullifying the recognition, enjoyment or exercise by women, irrespective of their marital status, on a basis of equality of men and women, of human rights and fundamental freedoms in the political, economic, social, cultural, civil or any other field." The following fifteen articles obligate the signatory nations to eliminate discrimination in areas of primary importance to women, including an emphasis on legal status, civil rights and fundamental health and reproductive rights.

Article Two obligates states to take measures to ensure equality between men and women through state constitutions, legislation, and legal protections. The article also mandates the eradication of any discriminatory measures against women by way of public authorities and institutions

and by any person, organization, or enterprise. Finally the article calls
upon the states to take affirmative action to eliminate penal provisions,
laws, and customs which discriminate against women. Following the spirit
of Article Two, Article Three requires states to take action in "all fields" to
guarantee women equality in fundamental freedoms and human rights. Article Four encourages the adoption of temporary measures to accelerate the
attainment of women's equality; these will later be discontinued once
equality is achieved; the Article also declares that special measures protecting maternity shall not be considered discriminatory. Article Five addresses the need to modify the social and cultural practices which have
detrimental impacts upon women; accordingly, the Article directs states to
eliminate prejudicial practices "based on the idea of the inferiority or the
superiority of either of the sexes" while it promotes viewing maternity and
child rearing positively. Article Six opposes the exploitation and prostitution of women.

Articles Seven through Nine cover the political rights of women based
on a policy of equality. Article Seven requires the elimination of discrimination in national political and public life; it further ensures equality in
the right to vote, in the formulation and implementation of government
policy, the right to hold public office and to participate in political and
public organizations. Article Eight recognizes the right of women to represent their government at the international level and to participate in international organizations. Finally, Article Nine states that women shall have
equal rights as to their nationality, that marriage shall not automatically
change the status of her nationality and that both mothers and fathers will
have equal rights concerning the nationality of their children.

Article Ten promotes equality in education, including: access to education and the same curricula and teachers, career and vocational guidance, scholarships and grants, continuing education, sports and physical
education, educational information on health and family. The article also
calls for the reduction of female school drop outs. Article Eleven directs
states to ensure equality in the employment arena by recognizing the
right to work as an inalienable right, the rights to same employment opportunities, the right to free choice of employment, the right to promotion
and training, the right to equal remuneration including benefits, the right
to social security, and the right to protection of health and safety in working conditions. The article emphasizes the need to end discrimination due
to marriage and maternity by requiring states to prohibit dismissal based
upon marriage or maternity; paid maternity leave, special protection during pregnancy (when necessary due to job requirements) and supporting
services for family and child care are also mandated. Article Twelve
requires equal access to health care services, while also recognizing the

need to receive "appropriate" services during pregnancy, confinement and post-natal periods. Article Thirteen addresses the elimination of economic and social discrimination by ensuring the right to family benefits, the right to financial credit and the right to participate in all aspects of cultural life.

Article Fourteen covers the special needs of rural women, emphasizing the right to participate in development planning, access to health care facilities and family planning services, benefits from social security programs, education and training, the right to organize groups for economic employment opportunities, to participate in community activities, agrarian rights, and adequate living conditions "particularly in relation to housing, sanitation, electricity and water supply, transport and communications."

Article Fifteen directs states to accord women equal status with men under the law, including equal legal capacity, the right to contract and to administer property, the right to equal treatment within legal systems, the same rights as to movement of persons and freedom of choosing domiciles. Article Sixteen requires equality in marriage and family relations. Among the rights detailed are the right to enter into marriage, to freely choose a spouse, to marry with free and full consent, equal rights at marriage and its dissolution, equal rights in parenting, family planning, guardianship of children, as husband and wife, ownership and disposition of property.

Finally, the Convention establishes the Committee on the Elimination of Discrimination against Women[27] to monitor and supervise the implementation of the Convention. This body consists of twenty-three experts, all women elected by the state parties, and is one of five supervisory bodies of independent experts which supervise the implementation of a United Nations human rights treaty.

While the Convention is the most comprehensive document detailing the rights of women, it has been criticized[28] for allowing reservations which weaken the treaty's impact and underlying purpose. Other shortcomings include its weak enforcement mechanisms and its failure to discuss certain issues of particular importance to women, such as violence against women, discrimination against lesbians and final authority in reproductive rights.[29] The Convention also lacks a mechanism to process complaints by individuals who feel that their rights have been violated and by the states parties which feel that another state party has committed a violation.[30]

The Convention's ratification was the fastest of any existing human rights treaty; this was due in large part due to Article 28(2) which accommodates reservations which are not incompatible with the object

and purpose of the Convention. The most threatening to the effectiveness
of the Convention are the broad reservations which only accept the obligations of the major substantive articles of the Convention insofar as they are
compatible with their national law, or traditional customs and practices. So
far, many of the states parties have made less than a full commitment to the
Convention's obligations. Other states parties objecting to these reservations have pinpointed the contradiction: the treaty is designed to eliminate
all sources of discrimination against women, yet Article 28(2) severely un-
dermines this objective. Furthermore, the Convention, unlike other human
rights conventions, provides no procedure for deciding authoritatively
whether a reservation is valid apart from Article 29 which provides for a
possible reference to the International Court of Justice. However, Article
29 has been rendered almost useless due to its reservations.[31]

As its enforcement mechanism, the Convention relies upon each state
party to file reports with the Committee. However, many reports are late
and many nations, particularly developing countries, have difficulties
meeting the reporting requirements of the Convention. Often it is beyond
their finances and their structure to efficiently and accurately research
the impact of their laws and of the Convention upon the lives of women,
particularly in the domestic arena.

Following the ratification of the Convention in December of 1980, the
General Assembly voted to accept the recommendation of the Copenhagen
Conference that a World Conference to Review and Appraise the Achieve-
ments of the United Nations Decade for Women be held at the end of the
Decade in 1985. The third United Nations Conference on Women, the
Nairobi Conference adopted a plan of action entitled the Forward-Looking
Strategies. Based on the three objectives of the Decade - equality, development and peace - the Forward-Looking Strategies "provide a framework for
action at the national, regional and international levels to promote greater
equality and opportunity for women." The agenda items included a review
of progress in the attainment of the goals of the Decade, a world survey on
the role of women in development, statistics on the status of women and a
report on strategies up to the year 2000.

As a result of the Decade for Women, the Convention on the Elimination of All Forms of Discrimination Against Women came into force during September 1981, the International Research and Training Institute
for the Advancement of Women was established in 1975 for the training
and research for and on women including gathering of statistics, training for participation in international conferences, fellowships, and a
special program on women and water, and in 1976 the Voluntary Fund
for the United Nations Decade for Women was established to provide
technical and/or financial support "to assist the poorest of the world's

women in rural and urban areas of developing countries, including projects encompassing income-generating, training, development-planning
and information."[32]

The Decade for Women also saw the launching of what the World
Health Organization calls "the most optimistic statement of purpose ever
made by the world community." In September 1978, 134 nations met at
Alma Ata in the U.S.S.R. and pledged their support for a world-wide effort
to bring "health for all by the year 2000." Primary health care was to be
the key to the success of this effort. Recognizing the correlation between
the lack of clean drinking water, sanitation inadequacies and illnesses,
and also between malnutrition and disease, the Alma Ata participants realized the necessity of improving water,[33] sanitation and nutrition in conjunction with the preventative and curative medical services already
offered by primary health care workers. Once the conference focused on
the need to motivate people to change their personal living habits and to
improve the living conditions of their communities, the spotlight fell on
women and their central role in the family and the community as "cooks
and feeders of children; as fetchers of water and firewood; as custodians
of cleanliness and hygiene; as teachers of healthy habits."[34]

The Fourth World Conference on Women: Action for Equality, Development and Peace will be held in Beijing, China from September 4–15, 1995.
Not only will the Conference adopt a Platform for Action, concentrating
on key obstacles to the advancement of the majority of women of
the world, including awareness-raising, decision-making, literacy, poverty,
health, violence, national machinery, refugees and technology, but it will
also review and appraise the progress made in the advancement of women
according to the objectives defined by the 1985 Nairobi Forward-Looking
Strategies for the Advancement of Women to the Year 2000.[35]

The Conference's purpose includes the mobilization of women and men
at both the policy-making and grass roots levels to achieve the Nairobi objectives, and to determine the priorities to be followed in 1996–2001 for
implementation of the strategies within the United Nations system. The
documents to be generated by the Conference include a draft Platform for
Action, a report of the Secretary-General on the second review and
appraisal of the implementation of the Nairobi Forward-Looking Strategies
for the Advancement of Women to the Year 2000, the 1994 World Survey
on the Role of Women in Development, an updated edition of the World's
Women 1970-1990: Trends and Statistics, the outcome of regional preparatory meetings for the Conference, an updated compendium on the
implementation of the Convention on the Elimination of All Forms of Discrimination against Women and national reports to be prepared by Governments as a basis for future national action.[36]

NOTES

1. Universal Declaration of Human Rights, G. A. Res. 217 (III), U.N. GAOR 3rd Sess., U.N. Doc. A/810 (1948).

2. See generally: Hurst Hannum, *Guide to International Human Rights Practice,* (University of Pennsylvania Press, 1984).

3. Charter of the United Nations, 59 Stat. 1031, T.S. 993, 3 Bevans 1153, signed at San Francisco, June 26, 1945, entered into force on October 24, 1945.

4. Report of the Preparatory Commission of the United Nations, PC/20, chap. 3, § 4, Ps 14–16 (1945). For further information on the United Nations and its components, see The United Nations and Human Rights, A Critical Appraisal, edited by Philip Alston (Clarendon Press, Oxford, 1992).

5. Universal Declaration of Human Rights, supra note 1.

6. The Universal Declaration of Human Rights was formulated in response to articles 1, 55 and 56 of the Charter of the United Nations. Articles 1 and 55 mandate that the United Nations promote universal respect for human rights; Article 56 requires member states to take international action to promote human rights. After two years of debate, on December 10, 1948, the General Assembly approved the Universal Declaration, not as a binding treaty subject to ratification, but as a General Assembly resolution. Later the International covenant on Economic, Social and Cultural Rights (1966) and the International Covenant on Civil and Political Rights (1966) were designed to transform the principles enunciated in the Universal Declaration into international standards through binding treaty obligations.

Initially, the Universal Declaration of Human Rights was a recommendatory document, which was not legally binding upon its signatories. Now, however, at least two arguments exist concerning the enforceability of the Declaration. One argument recognizes that certain standards enunciated by the Declaration have the force of law as a source of customary international law, since many nations have accepted its standards. The second argument finds the Declaration binding upon all members of the United Nations, since the Declaration is recognized as the authoritative interpretation of the human rights commitments outlined in the Charter of the United Nations. Richard B. Bilder, *An Overview of International Human Rights Law,* in Guide to International Human Rights Practice, supra note 2, at page 11; Universal Declaration of Human Rights, supra note 1.

7. Convention on the Elimination of all Forms of Discrimination against Women, G. A. Res. 34/180, 34 U.N. GAOR Supp. (No. 46), U.N. Doc. A/34/46 (1976).

8. Charter of the United Nations, supra note 3; Universal Declaration of Human Rights, supra note 1; International Covenant on Civil and Political Rights, G. A. Res. 2200 (XI), U.N. GAOR 21st Sess., Supp. No. 16, U.N. Doc. A/63/16 (1966); International Covenant on Economic, Social and Cultural Rights, G.A. Res. 2200 (XI), U.N. GAOR 21st Sess., Supp. No. 16, U.N. Doc. A/63/16 (1966).

9. Bilder, supra note 6, at 7.

10. See note 6.

11. European Convention for the Protection of Human Rights and Fundamental Freedoms, 213 U.N.T.S. 221, E.T.S. 5; International Convention on the Elimination of All Forms of Racial discrimination, G.A. Res. 2106A, U.N. GAOR, 20th Sess., Supp. No. 14, U.N. Doc. a/60/14 (1965), entry into force January 4, 1969; American Convention on Human Rights, signed at the Inter-American Specialized Conference on Human Rights, San Jose, Costa Rica, November 22, 1969, OAS Treaty Series, No. 36, OAS Official Records, OAS/SER.A/16; Convention on the Elimination of all forms of Discrimination against Women, supra note 7; Convention against Torture and Other Cruel, Inhuman or Degrading Treatment or Punishment, Annex G.A. Res. 46 (XXXIX), 23 I.L.M. 1027 (1984), as modified, 24 I.L.M. 535 (1985); Convention on the Rights of the Child, G.A. Res. 44/25, U.N. GAOR Supp. 49, U.N. Doc. A/44/736 (1989).

12. See for general information: *Human Rights in the Twenty-first Century, A Global Challenge*, Kathleen E. Mahoney & Paul Mahoney, (Eds.), (Martinus Nijhoff Publishers, 1993).

13. Charter of the United Nations, supra note 3.

14. A United Nations publication entitled "United Nations Work for Women" discusses the activities of international organizations which dealt with the question of equal right for women before the inception of the United Nations. These organizations include the Inter-American Commission of Women of the Organization of the American States, whose first meeting took place in 1930 and which continues to this day. The League of Nations also considered the status of women in all aspects in 1935 after ten Latin American countries requested that the subject be placed on the Assembly's agenda. In 1937, the League resolved to publish a study on the legal status of women, but the only section completed before the Second World War was that on private law.

15. Charter of the United Nations, Chapter One, Article One, Paragraph 3, supra note 3.

16. The Economic and Social Council, Chapter X of the Charter of the United Nations, supra note 3.

17. For information on the Commission on the Status of Women, please read Laura Reanda, "The Commission on the Status of Women," in *The United Nations and Human Rights* (Philip Alston, ed.; Clarendon Press, Oxford, 1992).

18. As background information: "when the Economic and Social Council first met in February 1946, it set up 'nuclear' subsidiaries to recommend the type and function of expert advisory bodies in all fields of the Council's competence. One of these groups was the 'nuclear' Commission on Human Rights, under which was placed the 'nuclear' Sub-Commission on the Status of Women. All these groups met in April and May 1946, and reported to the Council's second session the following month. At this session, the Council on June 21, 1946, took the important step of establishing a full Commission on the Status of Women. Composed of 15 members (this was expanded to the present 32 members in 1967, which reflected the expanding membership of the United Nations as a whole), its function was to serve as the Council's export body. Initially the commission's major thrust was in the setting of standards, and to this end it began work on the adoption of legal instruments, such as the convention on the Political Rights of Women, because it

considered that until women shared in decision-making they would make no progress. The culmination of its work in this area was the adoption of the Convention on the Elimination of All Forms of Discrimination against Women, which encompasses the rights of women."

The information is excerpted from a publication entitled "Women at Work," a September 1984 United Nations publication prepared by the Branch for the Advancement of Women, Centre for Social Development and Humanitarian Affairs, Department of International Economic and Social Affairs, United Nations.

19. Economic and Social Council Res. 48 (IV) (1947): "The functions of the Commission shall be to prepare recommendations and reports to the Economic and Social Council on promoting women's rights in political, economic, civil, social and education fields. The Commission shall also make recommendations to the Council on urgent problems requiring immediate attention in the field of women's rights with the object of implementing the principle that men and women shall have equal rights and to develop proposals to give effect to such recommendations."

20. Reanda, supra note 17, at 266-267, 275.

21. Draft Res. A/C.2/L.20 Rev. 1 (1980).

22. The Conference was held in Mexico City from June 19 to July 2 and was headed by Secretary-General Helvi Sipila of Finland. Sources: "The State of the World's Women 1985," World Conference to Review and Appraise the Achievements of the UN Decade for Women: Equality, Development and Peace, published in conjunction with the Third World Conference at Nairobi, Kenya, July 15-26, 1985, a United Nations publication; Issues of the Eighties," published by the United Nations Association of the United States of America.

23. Issues of the 80s, supra note 22.

24. The Mid-Decade Conference was headed by Secretary-General Lucille M. Mair of Jamaica and met in Copenhagen from July 14 to 31, 1980.

25. Issues of the 80s, supra note 22, at 2.

26. Convention of the Elimination of All Forms of Discrimination against Women, supra note 7.

27. For information on the Committee on the Elimination of Discrimination against Women, see Roberta Jacobson, "The Committee on the Elimination of Discrimination against Women," in *The United Nations and Human Rights,* supra note 17.

28. For more sources, see Renee Holt, "Women's Rights and International Law: The Struggle for Recognition and Enforcement," *Columbia Journal of Gender & Law,* 1:117 (1991); Andrew C. Byrnes, "The 'Other' Human Rights Treaty Body: The Work of the Committee on the Elimination of Discrimination Against Women," *Yale Journal of International Law,* 14:1 (1989); Rebecca J. Cook, "Reservations to the Convention on the Elimination of All Forms of Discrimination Against Women," *Virginia Journal of International Law,* 30:643 (1990); Hilary Charlesworth, Christine Chinkin & Shelly Wright, "Feminist Approaches to International Law," *American Journal of International Law,* 85:613 (1991). Convention on the Elimination of All Forms of Discrimination against Women, G.A. Res. 34/180, 34 U.N. GAOR Supp. (No. 46) at 194, U.N.

Doc. A/34/46 (1979), opened for signature March 1, 1980, entered into force September 3, 1981, reprinted in 19 I.L.M. 33 (1980), *Yale Journal of International Law,* 384 (1985).

29. By its wording, Article 16(e) grants women equal rights with men "to decide freely and responsibly on the number and spacing of children . . ." This arguably fails to give women the final authority in their rights of reproduction. However, Article 5(a) could possibly be interpreted to implicitly cover these shortcomings. Article 5(a) provides that "State parties shall take all appropriate measures: To modify the social and cultural patterns of conduct of men and women, with a view to achieving the elimination of prejudices and customary and all other practices which are based on the idea of the inferiority or the superiority of either of the sexes or on stereotyped roles of men and women."

30. In the meantime, however, individuals may have an avenue for the complaints. The Human Rights committee has concluded that it has jurisdiction to adjudicate an individuals' claim based on gender based discrimination, if the claim falls under a provision of the Convention which overlaps with the Covenant on Civil and Political Rights.

31. The problems with reservations can possibly be remedied by amending the Convention to include a provision similar to other human rights treaties, which allow a reservation by a state party to be incompatible with the purpose of the treaty if two thirds of the states parties object to that particular reservation.

32. The fund was established by the General Assembly. Most of its contributions is from voluntary governmental contributions, but individuals and nongovernmental organizations have contributed a significant amount. The fund has financed more than 35 projects, averaging roughly $100,000 per project, since it began work in 1978. Issues of the 80s, supra note 22.

33. From page 13 "State of Women's Health," supra note 22: "The Decade for Women also saw the launch of another major worldwide initiative: the International Drinking Water Supply and Sanitation Decade which began in November 1980. WHO estimates that (excluding China) 25% of people in cities and 71% of those in the countryside of developing countries are without safe water to drink and 47% of town dwellers and 87% of people in rural areas have no adequate sanitation.

The consequences of being without these basic amenities are ill health for all and great hardship for women who often have to walk long distances to fetch water. A person needs around five litres of water a day for cooking and drinking and a further 25 to 45 litres to stay clean and healthy. But the most a women can carry in comfort is 15 litres. Even if she lives near a standpipe, that means about 15 journeys a day with a full bucket to keep a family of five in good health.

But some women live so far from the nearest water source that they only have time to make one journey a day. In Burkina Faso, for example, some women leave at dusk to walk to the water hole, sleep there overnight, and return at dawn to escape the harsh rays of the sun. Small wonder that an estimated eight million children die each year of diseases that might have been prevented by sufficient clean water from a nearby tap."

34. Review and Appraisal: Health and Nutrition, World Conference to Review and Appraise the Achievements of the United Nations Decade for Women: Equality, Development and Peace, Nairobi, Kenya, July 1985. A/Conf.116/5/Add.3.

35. The Nairobi Objectives identify specific areas for action by governments and international organizations to improve the status of women over the fifteen year period from 1985 to 2000; the targeted areas include education, health, employment, participation in politics and the peace process and quality of family life. According to a United Nations publication entitled "Women, Challenges to the Year 2000,": "In 1990 the Commission on the Status of Women undertook a five-year review and appraisal of the implementation of the Nairobi Forward-Looking Strategies. The results were discouraging. The Commission found that the situation of women had deteriorated in many parts of the world, especially in developing countries where economic stagnation or negative growth, continued population increases, the growing burden of debt and the reduction of public expenditures for social programmes had further constrained opportunities for women to improve their situation. There was also evidence of an alarming regression in the status of women in the spheres of education, employment and health. Too often the issue of the advancement of women had received only low priority.

Citing 'entrenched resistance,' exacerbated by the global economic crisis and the subsequent reduction in resources available for change, the Commission noted that there had been a 'loss of impetus and even stagnation' in certain areas. Although there had been some progress at the grass-roots level, the success had been largely invisible since it had not been translated into improvements in women's daily lives.

The Commission warned that the cost to societies of failure to achieve true gender equality in all realms of life would be high in terms of slowed economic and social development, misuse of human resources and reduced progress for society as a whole. It therefore urged that the pace of implementation be improved in the crucial last decade of the twentieth century." Women: Challenges to the Year 2000, a United Nations publication (United Nations, New York 1991); The United Nations: Fact Sheet #4 of October 1994 on The Fourth World Conference on Women: Action for Equality, Development and Peace.

36. The United Nations: Fact Sheet of September 1993 on The Fourth World Conference on Women: Action for Equality, Development and Peace. In preparation for the Fourth Conference, the last large United Nations conference of the century, five regional meetings took place. In the region of Asia and Pacific, a meeting in Jakarta, Indonesia was held during June 7-14, 1994, convened by the UN Economic and Social Commission for Asia and Pacific. For Latin America and the Caribbean, a meeting in Mar del Plata, Argentina was held on September 24, 1994, as convened by the UN Economic and Social Commission for Latin America and the Caribbean. For Europe and North America, a meeting in Vienna, Austria was held during October 17-21, convened by the UN Economic Commission in Europe. In Western Asia, a meeting was held in Amman, Jordan, November 6-10, as convened by the UN Economic and Social Commission for Western Asia. For Africa, a meeting was held during November 16-23 in Dakar, Senegal, convened by the UN Economic Commission for Africa.

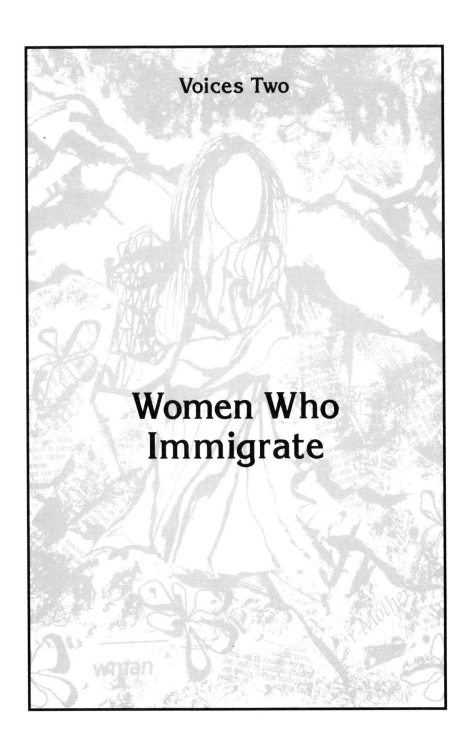

Voices Two

Women Who
Immigrate

Of Hot Dogs and Rice and Beans

Myrna Morales Keklak

*M*y search for equality, a journey which begins early in my childhood and continues to develop with my every breath, has led me to the deepest and darkest corners of my soul and accounts for much of what I have become. Equality, I have discovered, is not something you are born with or given but instead is something you allow yourself to feel and believe in and is not synonymous with sameness. For me, this realization translates into an inner peace that allows for greater acceptance and appreciation for those and that which is different.

THE ENTREE

My life began in Puerto Rico in the early 1950s. I do not remember a lot about Puerto Rico. What I do remember is how Puerto Rico felt, the sun always warm against my skin, with the rain so cool to the touch, and how great it felt to have everyone sound and look like me.

My family left Puerto Rico for the first time when I was three but returned within a year. All I remember of my stay in Texas was that it was not so different from Puerto Rico. I did not know at the time that we lived among Mexicans, in the Mexican section of the city of San Antonio.

Our final exodus from Puerto Rico came when I was six. I still remember the anticipation of leaving my friends and relatives and wondering how this new place, this "America," would look.

My mother tried to prepare us. She told us of the new language, and of the way Americans looked: tall, with light skin and hair. She told us about this white, cold powder that came down from the sky. She tried to put on a brave front for us, but we knew she was worried. At night, when she thought we were asleep, my brothers and I could hear her whisper to my father, "Will they adjust to the cold, to the school, and to this new language? You know I won't be able to help them. I am scared for them and how this new country will treat them." Though I remember hearing the words. I don't remember being scared. Me scared? Not me, for I was too busy daydreaming about the plane ride, and about these "Americans" and all of the new things that we were going to see.

Nothing in my first six years of life quite prepared me for my venture to this new world. My parents, though very different, always left me feeling cared for and well protected. We were a people of little means; we were materially poor but emotionally and culturally rich. We had music, color, and riches that couldn't just be bought at the local store. We were a family rich in heritage and in life's experiences.

ARMY RATIONS AND KP (KITCHEN PATROL)

My father was born in Jauco, a small farm town on the outskirts of Ponce, Puerto Rico, in 1922. He was the first-born of a poor farmer and his wife. At the age of 14, with both of his parents deceased, he left school and, together with his five brothers and two sisters, were placed in an orphanage. He left the orphanage the following year with the goal to work and to raise enough money to support his siblings. He found work as a farmhand, working 16-hour days, using the floor of an old shed as his bed and a bowl of rice per day as his only meal. At the age of 17, unable to continue at that pace and with four siblings still in the orphanage, he enlisted in the United States Army. The year was 1939 and though he could not produce documentation of being of the legal age of 18 he was accepted. Within months of his enlistment, all of his brothers and sisters were out of the orphanage and living with him.

Military life proved to be hard, and in some instances, even more difficult than the life he left. The demands of learning a new language and of a different way of life were difficult. The unexpected burden of dealing with racism and prejudice took its toll on him.

I am always amazed that he can talk about the injustices done to him in such a matter-of-fact manner. He was not permitted to eat in the regular mess (military dining room); he was overlooked for promotion after promotion even though he was more qualified then his white counterparts; and he endured verbal abuse and degradation for most of the many years he served.

Yet, I understand, because life is not perfect for anyone. He chooses to remember and make significant not the bad, but all the good in his life including his military experience. He often tells the following story of one of his first encounters with his new country. He tells it in a jestful manner, though to many it might seem sad:

> Our military company arrived in New York City after what seemed like hours, for most of us had never been out of Puerto Rico let alone traveled on an airplane. I can still remember the loudness of the plane's engines and how some of the guys were so afraid of the plane and of those noisy engines. The Company Commander forced the rest of us to push them into the back of the plane, screaming and all. None of us spoke English. Upon arriving, we were directed off the plane with our gear and told to stand in an area not far from where we had landed. A short while later we were each handed a large bulky package and again directed to wait. Under any other circumstances, the waiting would not have been unreasonable, except that we had landed in New York City during one of the coldest winters ever recorded. I can still feel the way the wind felt as it cut through me and my fatigues (military clothing). My hands lay frozen in my pockets. My mind raced with thoughts of fear and confusion, "Why would they bring us here and then leave us with no explanation? What were they planning for us?" After what seemed an eternity, we were called to attention by our new Company Commander, who, as he stared at us in disbelief, shouted, in Spanish, "Why are you not wearing the gear you were given?" The new Company Commander, a Puerto Rican who had been born in the United States, could not understand how we stood there freezing with coats and gloves right under arms. What he didn't understand was that we were nothing more than the sons of poor farmers with little schooling. We had never known the cold, let alone seen a coat.

That was my father's story.

ARROX CON DULCE (SWEET RICE)

My mother, when asked, says very little about her life with my father. When questioned about their experiences in the United States, the response is slow and limited. When asked if she regrets her life in the United States, she quietly answers "no." Her eyes gaze downward, and for that moment what she is really feeling remains a mystery.

Unlike my father, my mother was born in the city. Also unlike my father, she was not born in poverty but came by it as a result of her father's liking for fine wine and the ladies. As an engineer, my grandfather and his family traveled only in the finest of circles. My mother's face still lights up with pride as she recalls being the first family on her street to own a telephone. Shortly before her ninth birthday, all of this ended. Her father, in love with another woman, abandoned the family. My mother was forced to leave school and, together with her two brothers and two sisters, went to live as domestics with distant relatives.

AT THE FAMILY TABLE

How it is that my parents met and married is a mystery to my siblings and myself. It is not my family's way to talk about such things. I know they married shortly after my father returned from his two-year tour in war-torn Germany. He continued to raise his younger brothers and sisters.

As I write this it occurs to me where I get my "way." After all, I'm like most folks whose life has not always been kind; I've managed. I believe I learned from my parents, and they from theirs, that you manage and accept, or you don't survive.

Life in Puerto Rico at the time my parents married was not easy. My father, the optimist, left the military soon after his return from Germany and, with the little money he had been able to save, opened a small grocery store. Three years later, in great debt and broken after the death of his first born, a daughter, he sold the store and reenlisted in the United States Army.

The years that followed were both good and bad according to my mother. My older brother was born when my father was "missing in action" during the Korean War, I followed two years later, with my younger brother following two years later still.

MEAT AND POTATOES

In 1958, three years after my younger brother's birth, my family left Puerto Rico. At the time, I did not realize that we would never again live in Puerto Rico.

My first encounter with "Los Americanos" took place, only days after our arrival, on the grounds of the neighborhood playground. I remember the incident clearly for it was the day I discovered that I was different. I will never forget the way *they* sounded when they spoke. Nor will I forget the color of their hair, eyes, and skin, or the perplexed look in their eyes when they saw me and heard me speak. I will never forget the gestures, the pointing, and the whispers all because I was not exactly like them.

Only now is it that I realize what their behavior might have been reflective of nothing more than curiosity and simple uncertainty. But for me, a foreign child, their behavior translated into humiliation. For you see, it was at this very moment that I realized that I did not want to be whatever it was that I was, simply because I was different.

HOT DOGS VERSUS RICE AND BEANS

"Different"—what might I say about that word and how I use it so that I'm better understood? Let me begin with the *Random House College Dictionary* (1994). "Different" is defined as:

> *Differing in character or quality, not alike, dissimilar, or not identical.*
> *(p. 370)*

As I read over these definitions, I see and feel only the negatives associated with the word, but does the world around me see it this way. If so, is it fair to those like myself who are different and does it better explain why we are thought of as less? Or are we? How much of this obsession with being different has more to do with myself than with those around me? Is it, instead, that we are eyed cautiously, not because we are thought of as less, but because we are presumed to exceed in character and quality? Still I struggle to find the words *I* need to define for you this word, "different."

Perhaps, I cannot define this word "different" because it exists for me as a feeling and can only be communicated that way. Imagine, if you can, the feeling you might have when you are in clothes that don't fit. When clothes are too tight, they hold fast to the body, restricting how you move and breathe, constantly reminding you that they are there, on you, at you, over you. On the other hand, when clothes are too large, they hang on you, you are lost in them, an entity without form, a form without definition. That is what my being different is for me, much like wearing clothing that doesn't fit; always feeling tight, restricted and uncomfortable; always struggling to pretend to not be different, feeling like a non-entity, lost and shapeless.

When clothes fit, you don't even feel them. Your movements go unrestricted; your form takes shape. It is that feeling, which I equate with having made peace with being different, that I continue to strive for.

FRIED CHICKEN AND GRITS

My father's U.S. military career took us to many different parts of the United States. In 1962, we moved to Atlanta, Georgia, where I learned how different I actually was, and how bad it was to be different.

I am still surprised when people think you know just because they know. You see, I really didn't know that people had less value because they had darker colored skin. I didn't even know that skin color could dictate where you sat, what bathrooms you used, or what schools you attended. I didn't know, but I learned. Little did the citizens of the South realize how quickly a small child could learn about life by just reading the "White Only" and "Colored Only" signs over the top of the bathrooms in the "Sears & Roebuck" in downtown Atlanta.

My most vivid recollection of our stay in Atlanta is also one of my most painful childhood memories. It is not about me, only about something I saw being done to someone else.

I remember clearly that it was a Sunday. My dad always took the family for a ride in the car on Sundays. Our first stop was the local gasoline station. While at the pump, we watched an elderly black man shyly pull his car into the gasoline station only to be turned away by the attendants. I can still see the hurt in his face. Again I learned; this being different was not a good thing.

For my classmates at the Clayton County Elementary School also, it was a lesson to be learned. It seemed that I was the first individual whom they had seen who was not white, but yet was not black. "After all," they discussed among themselves, "this is a white school. They don't let niggers in here. She must not be a nigger." One little girl finally asked me why I was so brown and still had good (fine, straight) hair. I never answered her.

I was not the only member of my family to be confused about being different. I remember how my mother would sneak the next door neighbor's maid, who was black, into our kitchen and have coffee with her. This woman was afraid to be seen socializing with a white woman; at first, she was afraid to sit down in my mother's presence. It is only now that I understand my mother's motives. My mother, so fair-skinned that she could pass for a white American, needed the company of this black woman because this woman could understand what it was to be different. I hated the fact that my mother spoke to that maid. I felt embarrassed that she wanted this woman for a friend. I hated the fact that she was not ashamed of what she was or of this woman. It is only now, as I write this, that I realize what a remarkable and courageous woman my mother is.

CAFETERIA FOOD

School conferences were one of my few recollections in which I actually was not ashamed of my mother. It did not matter that she spoke very little English and, because of this, she made the sessions very difficult for my teachers. What matters was that my classmates could see her. "See she's white," I remember thinking as my classmates stared at her. My heart filled with pride at the prospect of not being so different. I found out later as an adult that the only reason we were allowed to attend the "white" people's school was because of my mother. It seems the day we were scheduled to be enrolled in school, my mother and my younger brother, who is fair-skinned like my mother, were the only ones well enough to attend.

My father came only once to the school. He had been called by the school nurse, who after I had vomited up my lunch, decided that I was too sick to stay in school. I can still feel the shame I felt when the school's secretary voiced her shock at learning that this very dark, curly-haired man was my father.

Friends are always shocked when I confide in them about some of my experiences. Many question why I did not fight back against some of the injustices that my family encountered. I am not always successful in explaining how being from a different country, with an entirely different language and way of life, envelops all that you are. Having those around you not respect this difference robs you of what you are and leaves you without the courage to hold onto your own uniqueness. I continue to wrestle with these feelings, with the battle quietly raging in me and at times leaving me with too little energy to challenge others about their attitudes and behaviors.

Most of us now recognize the dangers of prejudice and racism, but I wonder if we realize the destruction they can cause when an individual is labeled and prejudged by that which he or she has no control over, an overwhelming anger incurs. Many times this anger displays itself in violence and as militant behavior. As horrible as the outcomes of these reactions can be the most ruinous reaction of all, I believe, is that of shame, for shame has the capacity to destroy an entire people by eroding away hopes, dreams, and futures—one soul at a time. I believe that this did not happen to me because of an experience I had one late afternoon, the year I was in second grade. I can still remember that classroom like it was yesterday; cool, drafty, and full of mystery and color. Miss James, our pretty yellow-haired teacher, had been coaching the class as a whole on memorizing the numbers 1 to 100. I remember sitting in my seat, my chest tight from not letting myself breathe, as she called upon child after child. Finally it was my turn. I jumped out of my chair and began counting "1, 2, 3" and didn't stop until I hit 100. I did not pronounce all the numbers correctly but still they were recognizable. The look of amazement and admiration of my classmates faces that day has never left me. That was the day I discovered that different did not mean stupid. I sometimes wonder what would have become of my life if I had not had that experience.

EATING LIKE THE AMERICANS

I am frequently asked how it is that I lack an accent when I speak English. I usually answer that it is sheer luck. That is not entirely true. I clearly remember the feeling of loneliness as I stood on the edge of the playground wanting so much to be part of the fun and not being able to talk with the other children. I am convinced that it is these types of feelings that motivate us and that can lead to very positive outcomes. I am also convinced that it was these feelings of isolation and of being different that were responsible for my learning the English language quickly with very little accent. Although I did not realize it at the time, being different can be quite motivating.

It took only a few times of being excluded from the fun at that neighborhood playground for me to catch on to what I needed to do; I had to understand and be understood. I remember how, in the beginning, all the other children sounded the same. Little by little, the sounds they made, turned to words, and little by little, I started to understand. "Play" and "swings" were two of the first words that I learned.

Sometimes, I find myself somewhat frustrated with those who are insensitive to how difficult it is to learn a new language. In the first grade, I remember learning the words "walked" and "talked" and knowing their meanings, yet it would take until the end of second grade before I could say them correctly. I did not understand that you did not pronounce the ending "ed" exactly as it looked. The children in my neighborhood never told me that I was saying those words incorrectly. After all, by now I had proven myself to be quite good at baseball and jump rope. No one cared about how I sounded or how I looked.

SANDWICHES ARE NOT REAL FOOD

For my mother, learning the language proved to be more difficult. This was not due to a lack of motivation. Each day she would listen to the radio and television, pick up new words, and try them out on us. I must admit we were not terribly patient or helpful, after all we were learning it, too, why couldn't she? It would not be until twenty years later that we realized how much she understood and had taught herself. My mother, who had always dreamed of returning to school, convinced my older brother to enroll her in the nearby high school adult education program. My brother, who was at that time a high-ranking administrator for the state office of adult education, called upon one of his colleagues to humor my mother by testing her reading ability in Spanish. Shortly after my mother was tested, my brother received a phone call from his colleague requesting that they meet. It seems that my mother had refused to be tested in Spanish and had insisted that she be administered the reading comprehension exams in English. My brother still gets choked up when he recalls seeing my mother's exam results, which indicated that she was reading at above the 12th-grade level and more than capable of sitting for the high school equivalency exam which she took in English and passed four months later. To this day, he wonders how someone with less than four years of formal education and who calls meat loaf, "loaf meat," could have done so well.

"Loaf meat"—what memories that brings back! Preparing meat loaf was one of my mother's first attempts at being more American. After all, she had little choice; from the beginning we kids decided that we wanted to be like the "American" kids. I remember being invited to dinner at a girlfriend's house and being shocked at what was served. Where was the rice and beans? I came home that evening full of new ideas for my mother. "Mammi, you don't have to cook rice all the time, cook 'hotz dog' like over at Kathy's house," I remember telling her. It would not be until many years later that my mother allowed hot dogs in our home. Meat loaf, on the other hand, did make its way in one unexpecting day. The smell of the meat cooking hit me before I walked through the front door. The scent was very familiar, like the school cafeteria, yet it was nothing I had ever smelled from my mother's kitchen. There she stood, next to the small kitchen table we had gotten from the Salvation Army, a smile on her face, as she replied "es loaf meat."

Childhood for myself and my brothers was different. My parents, not always comfortable with their surroundings, would remind us not to become too much like the Americans. We just wanted to fit in, to be like the other kids, and this scared them. Yet I never recall hearing them express any regret over their move to the United States. Just like the "hot dogs," certain American customs were also never permitted in our household, such as sleeping at other children's homes or going to the movies alone, or especially eating sandwiches. According to my mother, sandwiches were not real food.

As different as my upbringing was—eating fried bananas, rice, and pigs feet for dinner, being allowed to speak only Spanish in our house, and always wondering if we were wrong to want to be like the other (American) kids—I had the best of all worlds. I have had the honor of knowing what it is to be different.

THANKSGIVING DINNER: TURKEY, MASHED POTATOES, GRAVY AND RICE AND BEANS

Recently, I returned to Puerto Rico. I went to offer my nursing expertise to my dad, now in his seventies and battling cancer. While there I discovered how American I had become and how comfortable that felt and how wonderful it was to be in Puerto Rico and to feel equally proud to be part of this world. It was on my third day in Puerto Rico that I came to this realization. My dad, hospitalized the day after I arrived and feeling stronger, requested that a telephone be placed in his room. The procedure for securing a telephone in a patient's room required a visit to the hospital's admissions department. I arrived in the admissions department, money in hand. I approached the counter and was taken aback when two individuals stepped in front of me and began their transaction with the admission's clerk. For a brief moment, I was in the United States and thinking, "didn't these people believe in lines and waiting your turn?" Then suddenly I remembered I was in Puerto Rico and here you did exactly as these two individuals standing in front of me had. I acknowledged and respected the difference and my dad got his phone.

I now understand that the one thing I so highly resented as I grew up, being different, is one of the reasons that I have become a more understanding and caring person.

REFERENCES/ADDITIONAL READINGS

Achebe, C. (1959). *Things Fall Apart.* New York: Fawcett Crest.
Bean, F. D., & Tienda, M. (1987). *The Hispanic Population of the United States.* New York: Russell Sage.
Rand, A. (1943). *The Fountainhead.* New York: Bobbs-Merrill.
Rosenfeld, P., & Culbertson, A. L. (1992). *Hispanics in the Military.* In Knouse, S. B., Rosenfeld, P., & Culbertson, A. L., *Hispanics in the Workplace* (pp. 211–230). Newbury Park, CA: Sage.

4

Immigrant Women

Janice T. Thomas

Courageous women from Haiti, setting forth in 1980 from their native land to face the dangers of a sea voyage, miraculously arrived safely, though soggy and sunburnt, to face the dangers of a new land, the United States. The "boat people" had left behind their young children, their aging parents, their mates, and other loved ones in order to escape repression and poverty. Like many immigrant women before them, they came with only the clothes on their backs, but with a strong sense of who they were and what they were capable of given a glimmer of opportunity.

For many, this glimmer faded as they were turned away from the land of opportunity. Most were denied political asylum by the United States Immigration and Naturalization Service (INS), incarcerated in detention centers both here and in Guantanamo, and some were even sent back. Some, however, escaped the net of the INS. Classified as "entrants," they were allowed to stay in the United States until further decisions could be made about their future status. Thirty of these women were interviewed several years after their arrival in South Florida, in order to chronicle their experiences living in a foreign place, and to gain more understanding about their cultural beliefs and practices, especially as they influenced health care (DeSantis, 1985, 1986; DeSantis, & Thomas, 1990). From these interviews, it is possible to gain insights about what life in this country was like for these pioneering women.

STARTING OVER

With no extended family or kin living nearby, the women had to find jobs for economic survival. They also felt a responsibility for providing for their families left behind in Haiti, who were living in deep poverty, some of them hiding in the barren hills in fear for their lives. With an average of five years of formal education, unable to speak English, afraid of deportation, possessing few job skills, how could they survive? They quickly found Haitian mates, who spoke to the women in their soft Creole patois, and eased the loneliness of living in such a strange, fast-paced country, with its fast-food emporiums, shiny, new autos, and its impatience with the status quo. Working in low-income jobs, such as domestic workers, field hands, restaurant workers, the new family was able to make its way to the bottom rung of the economic ladder in South Florida. Anxious to acclimate to their new homeland, the women ate their Big Macs and fries, stayed out of the way of the shiny, fast new cars, and were glad, as hard as things were, not to have to eat the stray dogs and cats that roamed about unmolested in the land of plenty. They also enrolled in English classes when they saw that very few of the inhabitants could speak Creole.

STUMBLING BLOCKS

With the economic situation marginal at best, these immigrant Haitian women had other stresses to overcome—initially, the social stigma accorded to Haitians in South Florida. Immigrants from third world countries were thought to be carriers of AIDS and tuberculosis. Haitians were accused of imposing additional burdens on the health care system, especially in the use of the large, public hospital serving the urban indigent population. Actually, most Haitians avoided public hospitals and clinics for fear of being deported. They had their own traditional healers and home remedies that seemed to work. There was no need to expose themselves to the dangers of the American health system, when all Haitians knew you weren't ill unless you felt bad. Before you knew it, you were whisked away to Krome Avenue Detention Center, there to languish until you were packed off to Haiti to face your fate.

Because Haitians were willing to assume menial tasks at low wages, they were accused of depriving other South Floridians of work. Often, these jobs had gone unfilled because of the low pay and social undesirability associated with them. Working for minimum wages or less was disadvantageous to those Americans who were eligible to receive welfare benefits if unemployed. In other instances, employers were reluctant to hire Haitians for fear of governmental fines for hiring illegal aliens.

Governmental policies were different for Cuban immigrants, who had been welcomed with open arms as they fled Castro's repression. This gave rise to cries that the Haitians were being unjustly discriminated against because they are black. Even the highest achieving Haitian family would feel this stigma in the United States. Stigmatized by the upswing in communicable diseases, facing racism and discrimination, and begrudged the most menial of jobs, these long-suffering women and their mates nevertheless persevered.

RAISING CHILDREN

Haitians consider children gifts from God. Almost all of the mothers interviewed had left small children behind in Haiti with relatives rather than exposing them to the uncertainties of travel by sea in rickety, overcrowded boats. To their sorrow, they were not allowed to send for these children once established in South Florida. New liaisons in this country for these adult women soon resulted in the birth of more children, more gifts from God. The mothers were then faced with the prospect of raising children in the new country, without the extended family and kin support that had been available in Haiti. Mothers had to recruit neighbors or friends for child care. Children were sometimes left alone so the mother could work. Mothers often had to rely on others to care for sick children, and to spend time with them while she was away.

These American-born children would grow up without ever knowing their Haitian sisters and brothers, or other relatives in Haiti. They would have only tenuous ties to their parents' homeland, and find it difficult to identify with the Haitian Diaspora. Some suffered from low self-esteem and some were at odds with their old-fashioned parents. Many heeded their parents' urging to apply themselves at school so that they could get ahead and bring esteem and honor to the family.

Children achieved early independence, but often lacked appropriate supervision. The mothers found the most difficult aspect of raising children in the United States was trying to provide appropriate discipline without family support. They traditionally utilized three methods of discipline—spanking the children; having them kneel for long hours behind a chair; and verbal reprimands which they described as "screaming." It was not uncommon for the mothers to slap, paddle, or hit their children with leather belts or wire whips. Haitian childrearing is based on unquestioned obedience to parents or other adults in the family. Since corporal punishment is frowned on by American culture, Haitian mothers found it impossible to censure their children in the time-honored ways of their culture. Many of the mothers said that it was difficult to raise children in this country due to early independence of the children, the prevalence of drugs and other temptations, the breakdown of discipline, and the lack of parental or family supervision during long working hours. These same factors have impacted childrearing for other groups in this country as well. Families must work hard to succeed in the land of opportunity, while children are often left to rear themselves.

THE FUTURE

As the political situation in Haiti stabilizes, the future holds promise for these hard-working women. Some of them have managed to blend into the American culture, advancing themselves and their children through education and work. Centers of Haitian pride have risen including an elementary school named for a Haitian hero, Toussaint L'Ouverture; Haitian markets; Haitian newspapers and radio stations. New friends and families have been added to complement those so far away in Haiti, some of whom may not have survived the political upheavals.

Yet ties to the homeland remain strong. Undoubtedly, some Florida Haitians will return to Haiti when they feel it is safe to do so. If they do, they will remember their experiences here, and be empowered by their accomplishments in spite of major obstacles to their success. The women of our story, who have survived in spite of it all, will contribute their great strengths to bring about changes for the betterment of Haiti and for the United States.

REFERENCES

DeSantis, L. (1985). Childrearing beliefs and practices of Cuban and Haitian parents: Implications for nurses. In M. A. Carter (Ed.), *Proceedings of the tenth annual transcultural nursing conference* (pp. 54–79). Salt Lake City, UT: Transcultural Nursing Society.

DeSantis, L. (1986). A comparison of cultural beliefs of Cuban and Haitian parents: Effects of acculturation on childrearing and parent-child health. In M. A. Carter (Ed.), *Proceedings of the first annual Virgin Islands nurses' association conference on contemporary nursing* (pp. 58-87). Memphis, TN: Virgin Island Nurse' Association.

DeSantis, L., & Thomas, J. (1990). The immigrant Haitian mother: Transcultural nursing perspective on preventive health care for children. *Journal of Transcultural Nursing, 2*(1), 2-15.

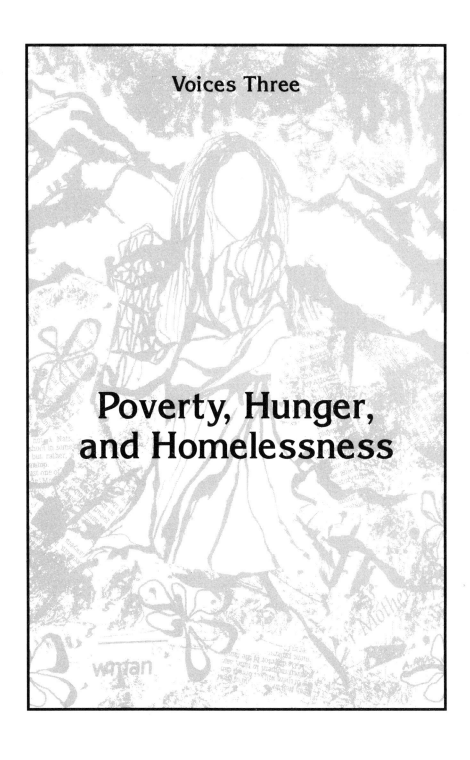

Voices Three

Poverty, Hunger, and Homelessness

5

World Starvation and Our Moral Bankruptcy

Simon Glynn

*A*pproximately 15 million people, mainly women, children, and babies, die from starvation or malnutrition-related illnesses every year. Put another way, the death toll is equivalent to 100 fully laden Jumbo Jets crashing every day without survivors, or one Hiroshima every 2 to 3 days, as 40,000 people a day, 1,600 an hour, or approximately one person every two seconds dies in this manner. Unfortunately, however, it usually takes each victim much, much, longer to die. Many children die slow, agonizing deaths, from dehydration following long bouts of vomiting and diarrhea, or from the effects of a starved stomach trying to ingest its own intestines, a death almost as harrowing to the mothers and fathers who have to watch, helpless, as their babies and children die.

A further 40% of the children under 5 in the developing world suffer from malnutrition while millions suffer from inadequate protein for proper brain development. It has been estimated that about 400 million people currently lack the proteins, vitamins, minerals, and calories necessary for a normally healthy life. Only one half of the children in the developing world have access to clean drinking water, and fewer have access to sanitary toilet facilities. Little wonder then that the infant mortality rate there is 7 to 10 times higher than that in the developed countries, and that the life expectancy of those who survive into adulthood is ⅓rd lower.

While at some earlier time in history it might have been possible for us to claim that we did not know the facts, or that we lacked the technological capacity to deal with the problem, the Presidential Commission on Hunger, the "Food and Nutrition Study" of The National Academy of Sciences, the Executive Director of UNICEF, and some 52 Nobel Laureates, have all stated that the know-how to end world hunger is currently available. Nor should this come as any great surprise. World grain production alone is already enough to give everyone on the planet well over 3,000 calories a day, while, with a world-wide military expenditure of $800 billion/year, enough is spent every minute on weaponry alone to feed 2,000 children for a year.

All that is lacking for us to eradicate world hunger is the political will to do so. But there is no tangible personal or national advantage to be gained from cutting the death rate in the third world. And unlike many other interests, the dying children of our world have no strong and influential lobby in the political capitals to represent them. Again, the political will continues to be absent; missing, at least in part, because of a failure of moral conscience, compounded by ignorance or misunderstanding of the facts. And the excuses for our failure are endless:

1. Charity begins at home, and anyway we can't feed our own poor.
2. We are not responsible for their problems, and there is no reason why we should help them solve them.
3. After all, we do not owe the world a living.
4. If we feed them today there will only be more of them for us to feed tomorrow.
5. They only have themselves to blame as they do not limit their families.
6. Anyway, the environment cannot support that number of people on the planet at the moment, so death will reduce the population to a sustainable level.
7. Their own governments won't help them, and in some cases won't even allow them to be fed, therefore there is nothing we should or can do.
8. Most of the aid will not get to them anyway but will end up in administrative costs, or the pockets of third world despots or bureaucrats, or be maladministered.

9. Why should *I* give? After all I am not nearly as well off as some of the . . . Foreman . . . Clerks . . . Teachers . . . Deans . . . Managers . . . Dentists . . . Lawyers . . . Doctors . . . Surgeons . . . Businesspeople I know, and many of them don't give anything.

Let us then examine some of these arguments.

1. Charity begins at home. It is a sobering thought that fully 55% of the world's population have a per capita income of between $60 and $440 per year. Thus the poor nutrition and adverse health effects suffered by *the majority* of those regarded as "poverty stricken" by U.S. standards, severe as they may be, are not likely to be so severe as for those regarded as "poverty stricken" by third world standards, which seems a good reason to concentrate on the "poverty stricken" of the third world first. Moreover, the cost of purchasing the resources (e.g., housing, or the materials and space to build a house, basic medical services, food) required to raise such people above the absolute poverty level is usually much greater in the industrialized nations than in the third world.

It is worth noting that, according to James Grant, Director of the United Nations Children's Fund UNICEF, about 7,000 third world children die *every day* because their parents do not have the knowledge, or the 10 cent package of saline solution, that would enable them to deal with dehydration; another 7,000 a day die because they don't have a dollar's worth of antibiotics; and approximately 8,000 die every day because they do not have enough low cost vaccines in them to prevent six common diseases. A further 1,000 children a day go blind because they don't have 20 cents worth of vitamin A. The marginal utility of resource in the third world is clearly very much higher than in the industrialized nations.

2. We are not responsible for their problems, and there is no reason why we should help them solve them. The first point to be made in reply to this argument is that even if the initial assumptions were correct, the conclusion would not necessarily follow, for if I am in a position to save the life of another at little cost to myself, it is at least arguable that I am under an obligation to do so, regardless of whether or not I am responsible for the threat to their lives. Moreover, it is by no means clear we are not, in fact, responsible for starvation in the third world.

For example, much of the soil erosion that has so adversely effected crop production in the third world is a direct consequence of adopting agricultural practices and technologies urged upon them by the industrialized countries and agribusiness. Deep plowing, for instance, breaks up soil structure, a problem exacerbated by the use of synthetic nitrates and other artificial fertilizers which increasingly replace composting as a

means of soil nutrition. This results in soil becoming increasingly partic-
ulate or "sandy," and prone to erosion by floods and wind.

Moreover, the activities of foreign lumber interests and the attempts of
agribusiness to urge industrialized agricultural practices upon traditional
farmers often leads to deforestation, the removal of trees that previously
acted as wind breaks, and to a dying back of thick forest undergrowth,
with the result that rains flow more quickly downhill, taking more soil as
they go, while the vegetation and leaves that had previously contributed
to soil stability are gone. Not only has this led to the loss of agricultural
land, but also to the silting of rivers, waterways, and irrigation systems,
with the consequence that in the rainy season further agricultural land is
lost to flooding, while in the dry season the land that does remain is insufficiently irrigated.

Further, increasing releases of carbon dioxide, emanating mainly from
the burning of fossil fuels by the industrialized nations, as well as from the
burning off of much of the smaller and lower quality timber, together with
the fact that there are now far fewer trees to reconvert this carbon dioxide
back into oxygen, has, it is argued, already begun to trigger the "green-
house" effect. This, together with ozone depletion due to the release of
chlorofluorocarbons and other pollutants by the industrialized nations,
may be producing global warming, resulting in climatic shifts that are
claimed to be responsible for much of the drought in Africa, for example.

Furthermore, while the adoption of "high tech" agricultural practices
has often led to increased food production, this has not always resulted in
a decrease in third world starvation. Take, for example, the introduction
of high-yield monocultures. While fields planted with a number of different strains of corn or rice may not have had such a high yield, this was
a small price to pay for a diversity that insured that some strains would
be likely to survive drought, pestilence, or other adverse conditions to
which other strains succumb. While the industrialized nations are able to
store surpluses produced in good years to compensate for years when
yields are poor, third world countries lack the storage and other facilities
of the industrialized nations. Consequently, surpluses produced in good
years often go to waste, and therefore can in no way compensate for poor
years, no matter how infrequent, when the well-bred high-tech strain happens to fall victim to adverse conditions.

Moreover, the susceptibility of monocultures has often led to an increasing prophylactic use of pesticides. This trend is further encouraged
by the tendency of agribusiness to replace crop rotation with single crop-
ping, which has led to an increase in natural pestilence, and by pests exposed to so much pesticide developing greater resistance. This leads to
increased costs for the farmer, a problem exacerbated by the fact that soil

supporting the same crop each year quickly runs short of vital nutrients, and thus requires additional use of, usually synthetic, fertilizers. The result has been that many small farmers have been forced into bankruptcy, which, in societies with no welfare or social security has meant that they and their families face starvation. Acquired by bigger farmers and agribusiness conglomerates, small farms are amalgamated, making economies of scale possible. Labor-intensive agriculture is thereby replaced by capital-intensive mechanization, the product of industrial societies with great capital wealth and comparatively high employment and labor costs.

The net result then is not only that more and more land passes into fewer and fewer hands, but that less and less labor is required, forcing yet more workers off the land to starve, while dependence on capital-intensive technologies means that, even though agricultural production may rise sharply, more and more of this is of nutritionally valueless cash crops, such as flowers, tea, coffee, tobacco, cocaine, marijuana, rubber, which, together with whatever nutritional foodstuffs are produced, are exported to the industrialized countries, in order to pay for the technology that makes such production possible. Consequently, Asia, Africa, and Latin America, where the vast majority of the hungry are concentrated, export $40 billion worth of food each year to the richer nations, 36 of the world's poorest 40 nations exporting food to the United States, which despite having very much more rich agricultural land per head of population, finds it cheaper to import from these countries, where labor costs are low, and to allow much U.S. agricultural land to go uncultivated,* and this despite the fact that over 30% of the world's population does not receive enough food to eat. For these reasons, it is not uncommon to find increased agricultural production in some third world countries accompanied by rising levels of starvation and malnutrition.

In sum then, it seems clear that many of the food problems facing the third world are very definitely *not* of their own making, but of ours.

3. We do not owe the world a living. This brings me to what, I anticipate, will be an even more controversial part of my analysis, and that is to the claim that we in the industrialized world do not owe the rest of the world a living.

It was upon the minerals, cotton, rubber, timber and other raw materials and labor, often extracted extremely unwillingly from foreign countries and their inhabitants, that early industrialization, and the subsequent affluence that still continues to flow from it, was based. And if we now

---

*The U.S. government pays $2 billion/yr in subsidies aimed at taking agricultural land out of production.

recognize slavery, and the exploitation, against their will, of other's land and labor, to be wrong, as we say we do, then it would seem to be wrong that we reserve to ourselves the benefits and prosperity that continue to flow from an industrial revolution fueled by such exploitation.

If the forebearers of those in and from the third world contributed, albeit against their wills, labor, land, and resources to the industrial revolution, it would seem *no less* reasonable that their descendants should share in the affluence continuing to flow therefrom, than that we should share by virtue of our forebearers contribution.

If alternatively one were to argue against such inheritable rights and privileges, on the basis of utility* as some do, then while one might thereby justify taking land from the American Indians, for example, on the grounds that their hunter-gatherer techniques were underutilizing the productive capacity of their land at the same time that many Europeans, who were willing and able to make the land more productive, were starving, then exactly the same argument could now be made to justify giving much of the land of the United States, and many other industrial countries, to starving peasant farmers in the third world.

Thus not only would redistribution of this land to peasant farmers bring it back into production, but it would result in the application of labor intensive agricultural methods, which for reasons we shall see in detail later often produce much higher yields per acre of cultivated land than does capital intensive agribusiness, a fact which would argue, on utilitarian grounds, for redistributing not only unutilized U.S. land to third world peasant farmers, but also much of the underutilized land presently farmed by agribusiness in the United States and elsewhere as well.

Moreover, while the 5% of the world's population who are U.S. citizens, own approximately ¼th of the rich agricultural land of the world, they in fact consume approximately 40% of the world's resources, or about 12 times as much per capita as the rest of the world on average.

Indeed, more generally, current investment and trade policies, the critics argue, insure the continuing flow of cheap goods and resources to be consumed in the industrial, or post-industrial, nations, from the third

---

*The argument to utility was formalized by "Utilitarians" Jeremy Bentham and John Stuart Mill, who supported social arrangements, actions, etc. which lead to the "sum total of human happiness" or well being, against those that did not. This, together with the "Law of Diminishing Marginal Utility," which argues that in most cases the *degree* to which any given resource etc. increases one's happiness or well being *decreases* the more of it one has, (e.g., that while $200 can, to a poor person, make all the difference between life and death, but to a rich person it makes no significant difference), tends to support a rather even distribution of resources in many cases.

world where they are produced. Yet third world wages remain low, transport and food costs high, and health care and education scant as they must if billions of dollars in profits are also to flow to the post-industrial nations to pay off the interest on the loans we have made to them so that they could afford to invest in the technology necessary to produce such goods and resources for us.

In sum, in view of earlier colonial and imperial practices relating to the acquisition or resources, labor and even lands, as well as of contemporary economic practices, it is at least plausibly arguable that we do indeed owe the world, or at least much of it, a living.

4. If we feed them today, they will become dependent upon us. It is, perhaps unfortunately, the dramatic that most often captures the attention of the media. Consequently we tend to equate the response to world malnutrition and poverty with airlifts of food to feed the starving. The Chinese, however, have the following saying; "Give a person a fish, and you feed them for a day; give them a fishing rod, and you feed him for life."

Thus aid projects currently underway in the third world include the drilling of deep wells and the construction of irrigation systems to fight drought, the provision of "intermediate," "appropriate," "alternative," or "convivial" agricultural technologies*—which enable greater, though perhaps not necessarily maximum, productivity, without tying the producers to vast capital debts—and some modest industrialization projects aimed, not simply at maximizing the returns on capital by the production of luxuries for mass export, but at the production of basic necessities, most of which are consumed domestically. In such a way, it has been found to be possible to help many in the third world to set up community workshops and small agricultural collectives, so that they may better help themselves.

5. In any event, there will only be more of them to feed tomorrow as they do not limit their families. Nevertheless some remain skeptical, for despite all attempts to help the poor so far, the number of people requiring aid continues to far outgrow the aid available.

This being the case however, givers of aid are in a position to choose between, or, if they find it morally acceptable, even to "educate" or otherwise attempt to influence the behavior of, the would-be recipients. Faced, for example, with some groups who will more than willingly practice

---

*Such terms, coined by Ernst Schumacher, Ivan Illich, and others refer to comparatively simple and inexpensive technologies—technologies that can in general be owned by the individuals or communities who operate them, rather than involving either outside ownership and control, or / and high capital debt—which are designed to maximize social utility or benefit rather than productivity or profit, and to minimize excessive resource use, pollution, or other adverse environmental impacts.

birth control, and others which will not, many relief agencies reason that their long-term goal, of reducing the number of malnourished and starving people in the world, is better served by directing their aid to the former groups. Furthermore, as experience in North America and Europe shows, birth rates go down anyway as living standards increase, and for a number of discernible reasons.

First, many in the third world have children in order to insure that they will be provided and cared for in their old age. An increase in the standard of living, which makes it possible to make provision, with pension and geriatric health care plans etc., for old age, removes one incentive for having large families.

Second, the drop in the infant mortality rate that accompanies a rise in the standard of living means that parents, who can be more confident that their children will survive into adulthood, will have fewer children. Thus a temporary surge in population growth, a consequence of the time that it takes the society as a whole to adapt its behavior in response to the increased survival rate of its young, is followed by a sharp decline, not only in the birth rate, but in family size.

Third, increases in the standard of living increase economic expectations, which sooner or later, almost inevitably outstrip the increases in the standard of living that produced them. This results in pressures to have smaller families so that the material expectations thus engendered can be more nearly fulfilled.

Fourth, the increasing specialization and formal labor arrangements symptomatic of industrializing societies mean that more children have to learn specialist skills, and that in any event entry into the labor market is regulated. Consequently children, who in a rural economy begin to "pull their weight" from the time they can walk, become an increasing economic burden, thus turning what was a considerable incentive into a considerable disincentive to having large families.

Fifth, the increase in education, on the model of the industrialized nations, along with the job opportunities that arise, mean that women will increasingly find possibilities other than child bearing and rearing competing with these traditional roles. This, together with the incentive to find employment outside the home in order to achieve economic aspirations, will result in a growing number of women either abandoning these traditional roles altogether, or, at least, restricting them.

Therefore, as we have seen, we may perhaps reasonably require, and in any event ultimately expect, countries receiving aid to limit their populations.

6. The environment cannot support the number of people on the planet at the moment, so death will reduce the population to a sustainable level.

This claim can be usefully broken down into three parts: the first concerning the amount of food that the world can produce, the second concerning the amount of energy and other resources consumed, and the third concerning the level of pollution.

Turning first to the question of food production: The Chinese currently support ¼th of the world's population on considerably less than ¼th of the world's rich agricultural land. The European Economic Community's "wine lake" and "butter mountain," produced by farmers in pursuit of subsidies, is kept out of the market in order to maintain food prices, while billions of dollars are paid to U.S. farmers to take land out of production entirely. Furthermore, much of what is produced are nutritionally valueless cash crops, or, is produced in order to maximize the profit per dollar invested rather than the net agricultural product; thus maximum production (or total output) is sacrificed to productivity (the *ratio* of output to input).* The result is that in those countries, such as the USA, where labor is relatively expensive, and land relatively cheap, the average acre of even that land where nutritionally valuable crops are cultivated by agribusiness produces about ⅕ the yield per acre as the average, labor intensive, English country garden for instance.

This problem is further exacerbated by the fact that, in pursuit of profits, many of the edible crops produced by agribusiness are then fed, at conversion ratios of approximately 8:1,† to cattle destined to become meat for the inhabitants of the wealthy nations. Therefore meat eaters who derives as little as ¼ of their dietary protein from meat indirectly consumes enough vegetables to provide the protein for two other people. Thus 70% of the world's grain is consumed by 15% of the world's population, the vast majority of it indirectly, while more humanly edible food, mostly grain, peanuts, cassava, soya, etc., is consumed by livestock in the United States of America and what formerly was the USSR.

Nor is only agricultural produce fed to livestock, but fish, too. Thus, while many in South America suffer from protein deficiency, the agribusiness is able to pay more and therefore buys the available fish to be fed to

---

* Thus like the motorist, who, recognizing that mileage (output) per gallon (input) begins to drop off as speeds exceed 50 mph, decides not to travel at the maximum 100 mph attainable, farmers, recognizing that the *ratio* of the cash value of their output to that of their input (or productivity), begins to drop off (due to diminishing marginal utility) well before they approach anything like the maximum yield (production) of which any given acre of land is capable, immediately switch investment of additional labor and capital to other, as yet uncultivated, land.

† It takes approximately 8 lbs. of edible vegetable protein to make 1 lb. of meat protein.

cattle or used as fertilizers. Up to 90% of world protein deficiency could be met by grain and fish fed to U.S. cattle alone. It is, I am afraid, a sad fact that many women in the third world die, or have to watch their children die, because they are unable to spend as much on food to sustain their lives as we spend on our pets' food.

We could indeed easily produce enough food to support the world's population many times over. This being so, let's now see whether the current consumption or resources and emission of environmental pollutants is sustainable.

With many of the earth's key resources in shorter and shorter supply, and 1 in 5 American and British deaths attributable to cancers, 80 to 90% of all cancers being environmentally caused, it would seem that a reduction in the human population of the planet is called for if we are to survive. However, with the consumption of such resources and production of pollution so much greater in the industrialized nations than in the third world—the average inhabitant of the United States, for example, consumes about 50 times as many resources, creating about 75 times as much pollution as most of the citizens in the third world. A reduction of 1 in the U.S. population would have the same impact on resource use and pollution as a reduction of 50 and 75, respectively, in these third world populations. Clearly, then, it is to the industrialized nations that we must look for the population reduction necessary to save the planet, while it should be equally clear that current economic strategies aimed at introducing resource, energy and capital intensive industrial technologies into the third world, are unsustainable, and must be replaced by "convivial," "appropriate," "intermediate," or "alternative," technologies if not only they, but we, are to survive and prosper.

7. *Their own governments won't help them, and in some cases won't even allow them to be fed, therefore there is nothing we should or can do.* While some third world governments seem to care little for the well-being of their populations, these seem to be in a distinct minority, and many more have certainly tried, albeit with varying degrees of commitment and success, to help their populations escape poverty and starvation. We should continue to provide resources to these latter countries, regardless of the behavior of a few governments.

8. *Most of the aid will not get to them anyway but will end up in administrative costs, or the pockets of third world despots and bureaucrats, or be maladministered.* Nor can any charity entirely escape administrative costs. It does, after all, cost money to collect money, to direct aid, and to deliver it to where it is needed in the form in which it will be most beneficial. Indeed those charities which spend a little money on doing their research, on insuring that charitable contributions go to truly needy cases,

or to projects that promise long-term success, are clearly to be preferred to those which spend good money after bad on projects that have little hope of long term success, or that could have functioned far more effectively and efficiently had there been more adequate planning in the early stages. Thus, while admittedly there are a few charities that seem to exist almost entirely for the benefit of their administrators, far from providing an argument against contributing to charity, such considerations simply provide reasons why we should investigate the charities which we may be thinking of giving to.

9. *Anyway, why should I give? After all I am not nearly as well off as some of the . . . Foreman . . . Clerks . . . Teachers . . . Deans . . . Managers . . . Dentists . . . Lawyers . . . Doctors . . . Surgeons I know, and many of them don't give anything.* Such an argument is clearly ludicrous as it seems: To suggest that no one should feel any obligation to give anything until *all* those who were better off have contributed, or to give any more than the least given by anyone better off. Indeed the converse, that while there are many in the world with much less who have given far more than us, we should feel ourselves under some obligation to give more.

The standard of living in the United States, and much of Western Europe, as well as Japan, much of the Middle East, and a few other countries, is so high that even the average industrial worker has an income undreamt of by all but the most wealthy in many third world countries, where the vast majority of the population have a per capita income below $200 a year. Therefore, most of us who are residents of these rich countries are in a position to save the lives of many in the third world at little cost relative to our own incomes.

CONCLUSION

I have argued that, (a) we have contributed, and still contribute to third world poverty, (b) much of our wealth derives directly or indirectly from the third world, (c) that help, when intelligently directed, can produce self-sufficiency and an increase in prosperity that, (d) will result in a drop in third world birth rates, and (e) is therefore compatible with the long-term survival of the planet and its population and is consequently sustainable, while (f) our wealth is such that we can provide such help at little cost to ourselves.

Consequently I submit that we can no longer credibly excuse the deaths of 40,000 people a day, mostly women and children, from poverty on our planet.

58 SIMON GLYNN

REFERENCES

While the arguments that I make here may be contentious, the information and statistics etc. with which I illustrate them, being widely confirmed by a number of sources, are fairly well agreed upon. I have not referenced each individually, but include here a highly selective, short bibliography, in which most of this information is available.

Ehrlich, Anne, & Paul. (1972). *Population, resources environment.* (2nd ed.). San Francisco: W. H. Freeman.
Epstein, Samual. (1978). *The politics of cancer.* San Francisco: The Sierra Club.
Schumacher, Ernst. (1975). *Small is beautiful.* New York: Harper & Row.
Singer, Peter. (1979). *Practical ethics.* Cambridge: Cambridge University Press. Chapter 8.
Human Development Report. (1993). United Nations Program. Oxford: Oxford University Press.
Hunger 1994: Transforming the politics of hunger. (1994). Silver Springs, MD: Bread for the World Institute.
World Development Report. (1993). New York: Oxford University Press/World Bank.

Many excellent pamphlets produced by Oxfam America, 26, West Street, Boston, MA 02111.

6

Lessons on Life as Women as Taught by Women Who Are Homeless

Glenda Kirkland

*T*he first shelter for homeless women I was in charge of was located in "the last block in town." Over the years, I have observed that homeless shelters usually are in the last block in town. This shelter was on the border of the cities of Newark and Irvington, New Jersey, a mostly abandoned square city block consisting of my shelter; dilapidated, three-story frame walk-up apartment buildings; vacant lots overgrown with weeds, cans, bottles, and soggy mattresses—household trash thrown from windows above. This landscape was dormant in the cold months, with very little moving on the streets or sidewalks. However, in the warmer months, life bounced around everywhere—stray cats, feral dogs, unattended-to-toddlers, portable music boxes balanced on strong teenage shoulders. Just across the street from the entrance to my shelter was a miniature "tunnel" entrance in the cement curb. This was the doorway to the underground lodgings of a sizable rat population. The shelter had no parking lot and those of us on staff who owned cars parked on the street. Fortunately, only on street cleaning mornings were we required to park on the opposite side of the street. I made sure I did not have any food or groceries in my car on those alternate-side-of-the-street parking days. My staff told me rats would chew up through the floor of an automobile to get food. This was one of the few precautions I took in the inner city.

My shelter was a four-story 16-unit apartment building with one- and two-bedroom apartments. It was cream-colored brick with a black roof. I eventually painted the large double front door a bright red hue. This is a color scheme for houses that I observed in the Yorkshire villages in the United Kingdom. My own house was also a cream-colored stucco with a black roof and a bright red door. I deliberately painted my house these Yorkshire colors upon my return to living in the United States after three years in the United Kingdom. I did not realize until sometime later that I had similarly also painted the front doors of the shelter red.

The building had been burned to a shell during the Newark race riots in 1967 and had been hollow for some years. In the late 1980s, city administrators were successful in obtaining a federal grant to rehabilitate the building to provide shelter for the homeless. The 16 apartments were completed in early 1991. The basement floor, half submerged in the front, totally above ground in the rear, contained a maintenance person's apartment, a laundry room, a small classroom-type room we named "the Seminar Room," and a small but delightful daycare room that led to a fully enclosed playground area, accessible only from the building. High around the play area was chainlink fence, topped with swirls of razor-sharp barbed wire. The right-front apartment was converted to an office for staff.

LIFE UNFOLDS

Becoming the director of this shelter seemed at the time to be purely an instance of being "in the right place at the right time." I came to see that this directorship was a series of very deliberate decisions motivated by what was then an unconscious drive to be at home in the world myself. I came to the church-based, non-profit organization indirectly. My first encounter was delivering hefty Thanksgiving boxes artfully decorated by the Sunday school children and filled with seasonal produce, canned goods, and a frozen turkey. (I came to learn that these thoughtfully created meals labeled "family of four," "family of eight," were immediately broken down when reaching the shelter, the nonperishable goods stored on the pantry shelves, the perishable produce cooked in the soup kitchen, and the turkeys not immediately used were frozen. None of our clients had cars to transport the heavy boxes, carfare to spare or the strength to haul the goods on city buses. Most of our nonresident clients did not have pans in which the turkeys would fit nor ovens to hold the pans. Few had the knowledge to properly thaw and cook the turkey. I delivered the boxes in my large, blue station wagon on a cold Sunday after church. With frozen fingers and red-tipped noses, my husband, nine-year-old daughter, and I went on to our exclusive golf club for lunch. I had never been to a blighted inner city area and the contrast between the soup kitchen building and the golf club burned in my mind.

I felt compelled to do more. I volunteered to do some fundraising and to write some grants. I was successful and energized with having an "activity" during the day that was mine, rather than my husband's and my daughter's. I had done only volunteer work for the previous nine years since my daughter was born. I had finished my MBA in 1975 and had many years of business experience to my credit by the time my daughter was born. I left work to devote myself to motherhood rather than live the hectic life of a "supermom." I felt fortunate at the time to be able to rely on my husband financially and not have to earn a living. After nine years, I was bored and had allowed my dependency on my husband to be more than for money. My concept of myself did not exist in my own mind apart from my husband. I did not know this at the time.

My brush with meaningful work outside the home motivated me to seek part-time employment, something that would not interfere with my responsibilities at home. But my main objective was that the work had to be interesting and meaningful, not merely for money. All my personal goals and efforts in this regard were met with hostility and disdain by my husband. His goal for me was to cut my hair shorter and learn to play golf, so I would "fit in."

In the late 1980s, Wall Street employment was turbulent to put it mildly. Suddenly my husband became more agreeable to my being able to earn my own "pin money." We still disagreed on the type of job I should seek, however. I called the agency where I had been a successful volunteer and applied for any available position. There was an opening for a part-time housing relocation manager, someone who would investigate landlords and apartments, verify documents and disburse rental assistance and security deposits. I took the job. After four months at work, I heard that the agency had been awarded an operating contract for the City of Newark's new homeless facility and would be recruiting a new director. I stepped into the meeting of the small group of trustees, and applied for the job. I was hired on the spot. My reaction after sheer joy was

deep terror! I had not gotten "permission" to take a full-time job no matter
how wonderful and I had so little time to find household/childcare help. I
knew quality dependable childcare was the only key to guilt-free work.

I left the agency's main offices in the safe North Ward of Newark and
went as a lone white woman to the havoc of the Central Ward and my new
full-time job—my first in over 10 years. My husband was displeased with
my defiance, my foolhardy decision to go where grown men are afraid to
go. With full-time help, I was free of the domestic responsibilities and answered only to myself. More than half my salary went to the housekeeper,
but I was still making more than working part-time.

A WHITE WOMAN LIVING IN TWO WORLDS

I soon became one of the more interesting people at cocktail parties. My
husband privately showed no interest in my new job or industry but publicly talked for me and answered questions about homeless issues that
were addressed to me. The more interesting I became to listen to in my
white, upper-middle-class suburban town, the less willing I was to engage
in dialogue of any sort about homelessness, poverty, teenage pregnancy,
drugs, or crime. No white person I knew at the time was the least bit interested in discussing issues of racial intolerance.

The first few months of the shelter's life was a hectic, 24-hour cutting
edge environment—inventing the wheel for long-term, comprehensive,
rehabilitative services to a tattered group of homeless women, 13 African-
American, 1 hispanic, 2 white. All had children and histories of chronic
homelessness. Most had serious addiction issues. Only one had finished
high school. Several had GED degrees. The goal of the program was to determine what services were necessary, then offer them for the length of
time necessary to "make it work."

Each family was assigned one of two case managers; I also worked directly with each mother. Each woman worked to develop a comprehensive plan for herself and her family. Education, socialization, job skills,
health needs—all were examined and addressed. The highest level of services was engaged to meet the needs of this "experimental" program.
Round-the-clock staff was available to observe and listen, advise and counsel. Aptitude testing, job-training, or educational placement and full-time,
free daycare were available to all participants in the program.

I was the only white staff member. I chose a staff mostly of recovering
addicts and formerly homeless individuals to work with the residents.
These individuals were initially handpicked mostly on instinct. They later
helped identify new staff additions. (I continue to staff my agency this

way.) I knew programmatic issues, how to deal with other agencies and bureaucrats, how to raise money; my staff knew the turf. They did not need to know what I knew; I learned all I know about homelessness from my staff and that first group of residents. I went from being invisible to someone whose insight was so valuable, her ability to make decisions so crucial, that I needed to carry a 24-hour beeper at all times.

The first societal behavior trait that I had to shed at the shelter was my dealing with people superficially, at arms-length. In my culture, this is a well-honed skill. Never discuss anything intimate, never talk about money or sex. Rather than masking an emotional response, it became necessary for me to express whatever response was elicited by the conversation or behavior of a resident or child. I was so well-trained not to display feelings that I had for the most part, ceased to feel anything. The stark truths of these women's lives and the intensity of the bond created when such truths are shared caused feelings that were too big to surmount or repress. From brief, reactionary moments of intense feelings brought about by a resident, my emotional state grew to a more immediate, "here and now" level of awareness all day and long after I arrived home.

LIFE'S MIRRORS

The sharing of life's experiences became a contrasting of life's experiences. The early summer had arrived at the shelter. By now, residents were well-known to me and for each one I felt deep caring and concern, if not love for some of my favorites. Their favorite activity was sitting on the front stoop of the building with all the children playing on the sidewalk. At six-thirty or seven, the residents would trickle down to the wide front stoop to watch the traffic. Before I left for home, I would join them. This became for me a most enjoyable way to spend time—the energy, the friendship, the laughter and cavorting—woman to woman was pristine joy to me.

One evening on the stoop, I was watching the apartment building residents who lived across the street. There were four or five adult women and twice that many children of all ages. Mostly the children picked on each other, harassed dogs with sticks, and invented elaborate tumbling routines on the mattresses scattered around the weedy lot. The women had carried a formica-top kitchen table with metal legs, several matching kitchen chairs, some more straight-back wooden chairs, glasses, pitchers of Kool-Aid, cards, tablets, pencils, and a large radio to the sidewalk. They played a very animated game of cards—hooting and screeching with each hand won. As the evening wore on, the men would come home, scoop up a straight-backed chair and straddle it or sit in it straight, leaning far back on the back legs. They would talk quietly to each other, occasionally take a child up on their laps or pat a dog. Observing this scene, I pictured my own wide and deep front yard in the suburbs. My house sat back on a small hill. There was never hint of human activity on my front lawn except for the landscaping service that came once a week. The same with all my neighbors. Seldom was human life observed even peeking through the heavy trees and rhododendrum concealing the backyards!

I was very amused imagining the neighbors' facial expressions had I hauled my kitchen table to my front yard and invited friends over for a game of cards. As the summer deepened, my daughter went away for camp and I stayed until building curfew most nights—on the stoop.

WHY HOMELESSNESS?

Homelessness does not have a single cause and often it is a syndrome. The easiest women to rehabilitate were drug addicts (not alcoholics—that was another issue). Addicts for the most part had learned to function as clever human beings, finessing their way in the world, manipulating systems and other people to obtain drugs. Long-term drug addiction, regardless of one's socioeconomic status at the onset, requires the finest honing of conning skills—"getting-over" in street talk. Addicts are usually attractive individuals, cunning, with efficient observation and analytical skills applied to their quest for drugs. Women sell their bodies and domestic skills at homemaking; men trade the convenience of living with these women for cooperation in getting the drugs for them. The trade-off is understood by all. The "sizing-up" can be nearly instantaneous. Thievery and acting pitiful are an art form for addicts. Self-indulgence becomes a religious experience.

Once a physical addiction is conquered, the long road of emotional recovery begins. The only successful format I ever observed was 12-Step Narcotics Anonymous. Fancy residential facilities or long-term therapeutic communities were artificial environments that had little lasting power for the addict. These clever skills, when properly directed and not under the influence of searching for drugs, support the former addict in the new real world of school or work. Most importantly, the ability to achieve at something has been experienced, especially for women.

Women from domestic violence situations were the most injured by their environment. Many could not understand the dichotomy of love and physical abuse and most experts at the deepest level could not explain it. Most women I saw still loved the abusing partner, wanted to patch a relationship back together and felt they were a causal reason for the abuse.

They displayed an almost nonexistent level of self-reliance—disbelief that it was possible for them to take care of themselves.

I experienced the lowest success rate with women crippled in the foster care system. These women, products of foster care situations from early years and most especially in their teenage years, came to the shelter as older teenagers with one or two children. Many had been pregnant as early as the ages of 13 or 14. The division of youth and family services would often place mother and child in separate foster care situations when the baby was born. No substantial bonding occurred in early infancy. A typical pattern was that the mother was emancipated (declared an adult for legal purposes and put on her own Aid For Dependent Children grant) with the birth of her second child.

The typical young mother is entitled to a grant of $448 per month in the City of Newark with additional food stamps. Studio apartments start at $450 per month. A single room without a bath is approximately $90/week at the YMCA. An adult with brilliant coping skills would have difficulty managing a household on this amount of money.

This young mother typically has not had the benefit of another adult teaching her the life skills necessary to cope on her own let alone raise two small children at once. Daycare has long waiting lists, even for those who can afford to pay. Jobs for the unskilled are virtually nonexistent. Few of these young girls had finished high school nor had the motivation, support, or wisdom to seek this diploma through an equivalency program. But the most debilitating factor remained the lack of parenting or guidance at the right time. These young women were the most difficult to achieve success with behavior modification. They were in the shelter the longest and made only slight gains upon exiting our program. The only successful technique was to "reparent" on an intense basis. This entailed offering constant support and direction starting at a preadolescent level and working through the maturity goals achieved in the teenage years: priority setting, decision making, delaying gratification, self-control, consideration of others. The children were placed in daycare for at least part of the day in order for the girl to focus on her own growth. Most of these young mothers treated their children as dolls rather than children. We worked with them largely through role modeling and mentoring to see different, more responsible patterns of parenting.

There were 15 women in the first year of our program. One was unable to function financially on her Army allotment and was given no additional funds by her husband who was on duty in the Gulf War. Two residents were prostitutes, both of whom had cancer. One of these women was found to be "selling" her 14-year-old daughter for drug money as she was too sick to sell herself. One woman was homeless due to domestic violence and one left her partner to protect her 5-year-old daughter from further incidences of incest. Two women in their late thirties were chronic alcoholics; four women were in recovery from drug addiction. (Only one has since relapsed.) The remaining four women were 25-years-old or younger, who had children as teenagers, and now had 2 or 3 children. Two of these four women were brought up in foster care. None of these four had attended school as far as the tenth grade. Two of the 15 women were married; the remainder had never legally married.

With the exception of the former drug addicts, all shared underdeveloped social and living skills, including household management and decision-making know-how. They all shared the sense of depending on others or "the system" for survival and connection to the world. The most striking causal factor in their homeless predicament was the overwhelming reality of child-care responsibilities—24 hours a day/365 days a year. The City of Newark at that time did not offer any extended day programs through the public school system nor programs for school holidays and vacations.

WHAT IT ALL MEANS

A home is not bricks and mortar and being homeless is not about losing an apartment. Being able to provide a home for one's self is possessing the skills to leave the house to look for a job, to be hired for a job and to achieve passable results on the job. First a woman needs a sense of being capable to pull off the above achievements—to have self-expectations of managing a roof over your head. Without entry level jobs and job readiness and skills training, employment does not become a reality. Without affordable daycare, jobs cannot be accepted.

The striking similarity between clients and myself was not in life skills, education, or job training. It was the self-assessment of being responsible for yourself. It was a self-esteem issue. I did not believe myself capable of keeping a roof over my own head or making my own decisions.

I did not believe myself differentiated enough from my husband to have any decisions of my own to make. I was not technically homeless, but I was invisible in someone else's house.

What a global experience it is for all women. We are invisible. We exist on the fringe of the world of men—even in our own home, we live on the last block in town.

7

Housing for the Single-Parent Family: A Blueprint for Women's Educational Support

Judith Mathews, Maureen Hreha, and Marilyn Burk

SINGLE-PARENT HOUSING: ONE FORMULA FOR WOMEN'S DEVELOPMENT

Each year qualified applicants to the Muhlenberg Regional Medical Center School of Nursing in Plainfield, New Jersey, include single parents. These individuals inquire about student housing for themselves and their children. They withdraw their applications when they find out that the

Grateful acknowledgment is made to the Robert Wood Johnson Foundation, Inc. and the BARD Foundation.

traditional dormitory residence halls available for the nursing students
have no accommodations or facilities for children. The lack of appropriate housing for families creates a barrier that prevents some qualified applicants from pursuing their degree.

Judith Mathews, Dean of the Schools of Nursing and Allied Health at
Muhlenberg, directed a study that would determine the feasibility of providing housing and other services for single parents. The study was a
component of Project TLC (Transcultural Leadership Continuum), an ongoing project funded by the Robert Wood Johnson Foundation involving
Muhlenberg as well as Union County College, Kean College, and Elizabeth
Regional Medical Center, all New Jersey based institutions.

Project TLC proposed to increase the retention of minority women in
nursing education by supporting the students' academic and economic
needs, enabling them, thereby, to return to their communities as independent professionals. These students will also increase minority representation in the administrative ranks of nursing as they progress in their
profession. The ultimate goal of Project TLC is to increase the representation of minority nurses in leadership roles within the profession. Attaining the nursing degree is the first step in that process.

Project TLC's Feasibility Study for single-parent nursing students included three goals:

- To determine the requirements for converting existing student
  residence space into housing for single-parent students and their
  families.
- To determine the need for such housing.
- To determine the needs for additional support services for the
  single-parent students and their children.

Accomplishing the first goal required identifying physical space and planning the renovation. Addressing the second and third goals required research into the nature of the single-parent student and the needs of that
student.

BASIC PEACE: A ROOF OVER OUR HEADS

The number of young, single mothers in the United States is increasing according to the Census Bureau of the Department of Commerce of the
United States. The Census Bureau counts "other families" as a category of
households. "Other families" is defined by the Census Bureau as households not headed by married couples. Single mothers head about seven
million of these families. The Census Bureau projects that by the year

2010, eight million households will be headed by single mothers. The number of these families headed by single mothers under the age of 25 will increase by 50% by the year 2010.

The 1990 census showed that households headed by single mothers are often low income households. About 45% of single mothers with children under eighteen live in poverty. (*Single parents*, July 1992). The number of families headed by single mothers is increasing and many of these are families in need.

These families are frequently minority families. In 1992, " . . . 67% of births to African-American women were out of wedlock, compared to 27% for Hispanic women, and 17% for white women . . . it is among Hispanic and white women that the greatest increases have registered" (Patterson, 1993). If Project TLC proposed to address the needs of minority students in nursing education, Project TLC had to address the single parent as well.

Does the single mom with her children require support services? Corporate America thinks so. Twenty-five percent of today's American families are headed by single parents (*Single parent support*, 1994). Employers who address the issues of diversity in the workforce often find that some of those issues include family demands. Employers are willing to invest in supporting workers affected by various family issues to enable that employee's productivity and well being. Demographics indicate that single parenting is now recognized as one of those family issues (Dow, 1993).

Single parents' needs are often addressed by employers who provide assistance, such as child care programs or flextime scheduling arrangements. Dow Chemical provides daycare programs, school age child care, flextime, and even lactation support programs at a number of its plants to assist single parents and dual career families (*Occupational*, 1992). Sony is another company that provides daycare facilities at some of its sites (Jorgensen, 1993). American companies are taking advantage of the diversity of the workforce and addressing employees' lifestyle concerns to enable increased success on the job. Companies want to " . . . harness the diversity of the U.S. workforce to increase productivity and profit share" (Dow, 1993).

Single-parent students have needs as students, as parents, and as individuals. Colleges that have begun on-campus residential programs already know this and address these needs.

Single-parent housing, child care, and other support services for nursing and other post-secondary students are already provided at schools such as Trinity College, Goddard College, Texas Women's University, and St. Catherine's in Minnesota. Douglas North of Goddard College wrote:

Everyone who works with single parents recognizes that among their primary needs are relevant education, skilled counseling, quality child care,

and a job that pays enough to make it financially advantageous to work.
(North, 1987)

Texas Woman's University program for single-parent students in need is a quality program in increasing demand. Nancy Murphy-Chadwick of Texas Woman's University describes her school's services which support not only the adult single woman student but the child of that student.

The on-campus family population has grown yearly with a 363% in-crease since 1983. [This is written in 1989.] . . . Single parents have a se-cure environment to make a home while attending classes. . . . The accessibility of quality child care and convenient, secure housing can re-lieve two of the major pressures students with young families face. . . .
(Murphy-Chadwick, 1989)

The College of Saint Catherine recognized a need for special housing and additional services for its population of students, several of whom were single mothers. St. Catherine's programs include several health-related degrees, including an associate's degree in nursing. St. Catherine's recog-nized the need for:

. . . odd hour daycare . . . necessary for students who must take early morning clinicals in hospitals in support of their school work. . . . Living . . . with other single parents and having access to regular and odd-hour child care would reduce scheduling hassles and enable a community of support to occur. . . . the support and people connections that provide a 'safety net' for . . . students. (Wroblewski, 1990)

A 1989 doctoral study from Ball State University compares the imped-ing and enabling factors for the traditional fresh-out-of-high-school stu-dent to reentry students in Ball State's nursing program. The older, reentry students list the cost of college and arranging for child care as im-peding factors, or barriers, to their enrollment in the nursing program. Two potential enabling factors listed by reentry students are encourage-ment from college personnel and change in responsibilities at home (Scott, 1989).

All of these programs recognize that housing and child care are basic requirements for the single parent in need who wants to enroll in post-secondary college and nursing programs. Additional support services allow that student to succeed, increasing not only enrollment, but reten-tion and successful completion of the programs.

As Muhlenberg Regional Medical Center addressed the issues of hous-ing for its single parent students, it also addressed the issues of programs to support those students. Based on information from these colleges, Muhlenberg Regional Medical Center's Feasibility Study Team developed plans for three counseling approaches which would address the single parent as student, person, and parent.

A BLUEPRINT: THE MUHLENBERG PLAN

Once Muhlenberg decided that the physical change was feasible, it developed its support services plan. Students admitted to the nursing program are fully qualified applicants as well as single parents in need. Support services also include housing, child care, counseling, and academic support. The program addresses the well-being of the children living at Muhlenberg. The program was called Project HOPE (Housing Opportunities for Parents in Education).

This program targets the enabling factors cited in the Ball State Study—child care and support from college personnel—as well as housing as the basic needs of these students and their families. In many cases, however, these single parent students have extraordinary needs.

Local New Jersey shelters who also provide housing for single parents were surveyed. They all affirm the necessity of providing support services, such as counseling. Several of their residents are from a world of poverty, abuse, or other crisis situations. Identifying the potentially successful student is not enough. The single-parent student may have a history of complex problems to overcome.

Project Hope respects the single parent as a person. A Personal Counselor is available for scheduled individual and group counseling sessions. The sessions focus on improvement in self-esteem, problem solving, interpersonal relations, and conflict resolution within the group. This counselor helps students adjust to dormitory living and enables each to function as an individual, student parent in a communal public setting.

The program also supports the single parents as parents and that begins with safe, dependable child care. The women have the services of the Muhlenberg Child Care Center which provides care from 6:30 A.M. to 6 P.M. for children from the ages of 3 weeks to 5 years of age Monday through Friday. Evening child care is included and scheduled for two week-day evenings twice a week within the dormitory setting. A cooperative program of babysitting was organized for week-end, odd-hour and sick child care, gradually assuming more of the child care responsibilities.

Project Hope facilitates additional parenting support by providing a Family Mentor. The Family Mentor is available formally and informally for the purpose of fostering the family unit and supporting the student as a parent. Formal sessions are presented in parenting, safety, child growth and development, decision making, goal setting, health and wellness, socialization, team building, and peer interaction. The Family Mentor also assists in an initial orientation period for the incoming families.

Finally, this project supports the single-parent nursing student in academic and clinical training matters with an Academic Counselor. This counselor focusing on the student as a student identifying and addressing any learning problems or disabilities. The Academic Counselor also builds study skills, test taking strategies, and time and project management skills.

CONTRACT FOR DEVELOPMENT: FAMILIES TOGETHER

The TLC project has family residential and academic policies in contract form that ask the women and their children to commit to academic performance and housing responsibilities.

Accepted women enter the program screened for motivation, sense of responsibility and aptitude for college academic work. This screening process is in addition to a preparatory six-week period before classes begin. It is essential that both the women as single parents and their children are familiar with their new living conditions and expectations. This orientation period gives the families time to get to know one another before the entire class meets as a whole.

Careful screening of single women/parent applicants combined with a full network of professional support for the women and their children enable these women to achieve their educational goals.

The program is not simply a gift. It demands from the student the ability to study and achieve academically as she copes with communal living and parenting.

The program asks that the woman return to her community as an educated nurse ready to serve as role model of achievement and independence.

REFERENCES

Dow programs address child care, dual-career couples, and other work-family issues. (1993, October 23). *Chemical & Engineering News* (p. 47).

Healing's bedside revolution: Health care reform could further expand role of nursing. (1993, December 31). *Washington Post* (p. A1).

Health-care reform should bode well for nurses. (1994, January 11). *Wall Street Journal* (p. A1).

Hennenberger, M. (1994, August 21). For nurses, new Uncertainties: Managed care means fewer openings, specialized needs. *New York Times* (p. 45).

Jahn, B. J. (1990). An investigation of changes in perception of career mobility with advanced formal education by registered and vocational nurses. East Texas State University Ph.D. Thesis.

Johnson, S. (1991, August 28). Helping single parents find success in college. *Wall Street Journal* (p. B8).

Jorgensen, B. (1993, September). Diversity: Managing a multicultural work force. *Electronic Business Buyer* (pp. 70-76).

Mathews, J. (1993, September). Dean of Schools of Nursing and Allied Health. Muhlenberg Regional Medical Center, Plainfield, NJ.

Murphy-Chadwick, N. et al. (1989). *Family housing and services.* Washington, DC: American Association of State Colleges and Universities. ERIC ED316148.

New Jersey Administrative Code. Chapt. 126, Sub. 1, 5, 6. Manual of Requirements for Family Day Care Registration. Provider edition. (1988, Nov. 7). Trenton, NJ: NJ Dept. of Human Services, Division of Youth and Family Services.

North, D. (1987). AFDC goes to college. *Public Welfare, 45*(4), (pp. 4-12).

Occupational outlook handbook, 1992-1993 Edition. (1992). Chicago: VGM Career Horizons.

Patterson, M. (1993, July 14). Single motherhood on the rise. *The Star Ledger* (pp. 1, 15).

Scott, J. (1989). Traditional and reentry nursing majors: Motivational factors, vocational personalities, barriers and enablers to participation. Muncie, IN: Ball State Indiana.

Single parents. (1992, July). *American Demographic Desk Reference* (pp. 14-15).

Single parents. (1993, December). *American Demographics* (pp. 36-37.1).

Single parent support. (1994, September). *Small Business Reports* (p. 20).

8

Women and Social Action

Jacqueline B. Mondros

*B*efore long, anyone who joins a social action organization will notice the preponderance of women in leadership positions. While women are just beginning to occupy the top positions in major corporations, academic institutions, and philanthropic organizations, historically many of the top leadership positions of community organizations have been filled by women. Since the beginning of this century, women have built organizations to express their own grievances and advance their own causes (e.g., the Suffragettes). They have assumed leadership in some of the country's strongest unions (e.g., the involvement of Mother Jones in organizing the United Mine Workers); in the early part of the century, the leadership of the International Ladies Garment Workers Union (ILGWU) was largely women. Women have also played important roles in organizations that worked on broad community issues. Jane Addams, Lilian Wald, and other "settlement house ladies" were instrumental in improving urban living conditions before World War I. Lucretia Mott, Sarah and Angelina Grimkey, and Abby Kelly were strong and visible leaders in the abolitionist movement. Their work in the American Anti-Slavery Association convinced them of the need for a women's organization that also examined the "slavery" of women. Ethnic organizations such as Haddassah and mutual aid societies among Chinese, Japanese, and Native American Tribal Councils all had active women leaders. Women of color have also played significant leadership roles: among others, Ida B. Wells Barrett in the Black Women's Clubs, Fanny Hammer in the Welfare Rights Organization, and Rosa Parks in the civil rights movement.

The involvement of women in social action organizations continues today. Not only have women formed organizations dedicated to what we may call "women's issues" (e.g., reproductive rights, pay equity), but they are often the leaders of some of the country's strongest community organizations (Faye Wattleton of Planned Parenthood, Jill Ireland of NOW, Mary Moreno of COPS, IAF, Gail Cincotta of NPA, Ann Deveney of Northwest Bronx Community Clergy Coalition). In my own research, out of 92 organizers and leaders of 43 national, statewide, and local groups, 47 were female (Mondros & Wilson, 1994).

Why are women so well represented among the leadership of these organizations? After all, are women not the gentle sex? Have we not been described as timid and docile, pliant and agreeable? Aren't women known to be hesitant to argue their rights and push forward their grievances?

Experienced organizers suggest that is not at all the case. To the contrary, women seem particularly well equipped for leadership roles in social action organizations and particularly effective leaders. There are many reasons for their success.

- *Mothers' Role.* Until the latest part of the twentieth century, women's major roles in western culture have been as wives and mothers. Women kept families together; kept them financially afloat; kept children clothed, fed, safe, healthy, and whenever possible, happy. In order to realize this nurturing role and successfully carry out these family responsibilities, a woman had to assess how helpful or harmful was her family's surrounding environment. When the environment posed obstacles to her family's welfare, her role responsibilities required that she intervene. The safety and amenities of the neighborhood, the social and academic environment of the schools, and the predictability of the employment arena were particularly important environmental systems. Thus, it is no surprise that women have a history of activism in neighborhood organizing, in parent organizations, and in unions. These systems pose the greatest threat to family welfare, and, as a natural extension of their nurturing role, women sought, joined, and built organizations that helped them defend their families (Acklesberg & Diamon, 1987; Gilkes, 1981).

• *Connections Among Women.* Women effectively develop intimate and enduring relationships among themselves. Women are successful at cultivating these relationships and using them to trade needed information, and to obtain both emotional support and resources (Gutierrez & Lewis, 1994). Women are more likely to share openly their problems and the difficulties faced by their families. There is little stigma against such commiseration; in fact, problem swapping and solving often characterizes women's relationships. Wherever women congregate—in parks and playgrounds, in laundromats and grocery stores, in the waiting rooms of clinics and welfare offices, on the stoops of urban America and in its churches, kitchens, and basements—they share their problems and trade information. In the literature of community organization, such problem swapping is formally known as the first phase of "issue identification" in which grievances are expressed and validated by others.

• *Spirituality and Church Participation.* In most western religious and ethnic groups, it is women who make the connection between family and religious observance (Gilkes, 1986; Anzaldua, 1987). Women have traditionally played important, albeit not always highly visible, roles in maintaining religious institutions. Women are more frequently than not regular church and synagogue attendees, often prodding more reluctant family members into attendance. They populate the choirs, do the teaching at religious schools, run the fund-raising benefits. Through such experience they often become sophisticated about organizational development, and savvy about how to recruit, engage, and sustain a cadre of committed volunteers. These skills are especially valuable in social action organizations for which the ability to recruit new members is often an issue of survival. Further, women are often spiritually oriented, and therefore influenced by Biblical notions of social justice and charity (Gutierrez & Lewis, 1994). Such notions are embodied in the messages of most social action groups and their change agendas often flow from values of decency, equality, and fairness. Consequently, women find that the ideas that animate these organizations strongly agree with their own belief systems.

• *Consensus-Building Skills.* Finally, the feminist literature has long noted that women tend to reject hierarchial and authoritarian ways of operating, in favor of consensus building, negotiating, and compromise. Women are more prone to seek commonalities and to motivate people on the basis of common interest and stake. Again, these are crucial skills in social action groups that often require internal agreement among various ethnic groups, social classes, generations, and people with different needs and interests. People who can "barter" different interests and seek compromise when diverse interests are operating are highly valued socio-emotional leaders in these groups.

Consequently, women have both the self-interest in forming and joining social action organizations and the skills that are very useful to them. It is therefore no great surprise that, for the most part, in many social action organizations, women occupy both the top and second level leadership positions.

There are still differences about which women are active in which organizations (Gutierrez & Lewis, 1994; Mondros & Wilson, 1994). In general, white professional and executive women are most often found in organizations that are focused on "women's issues," (i.e., reproductive rights, women's political caucuses, equality in the workplace), while most working class and women of color are found in local community organizations and ethnic associations which work on "family issues," (i.e., local schools, low-income housing, utility rates, and access to community health services). This bifurcation suggests that social class still makes a difference in the arenas that women assess need their intervention and protection. While white professional women pursue their own interests in their workplaces, lower income and minority women still act out their traditional role and seek to protect their families in their neighborhoods and schools.

This division is unfortunate, particularly when we understand how much women have in common, and how many strengths and skills women bring to organizations. Social action groups that develop change agendas on issues which cut across class lines, such as the need for childcare and child safety and pay equity in the workforce, will attract women of all different races, ethnic groups, religions, ages, and social classes, and will be fundamentally enriched and strengthened by their contributions.

REFERENCES

Acklesberg, M., & Diamon, I. (1987). Gender and political life: New directions in political science. In B. Hess & M. Feree (Eds.), *Analyzing gender: A handbook of social science*. Newbury Park, CA: Sage.

Anzaldua, G. (1987). *Borderlands/La Frontera: The new Meztiza*. San Francisco: Spinsters/Aunt Lute.

Gilkes, C. (1981). Holding back the ocean with a broom: Black women and community work. In L. F. Rodgers-Rose (Ed.), *The black woman* (pp. 217-233). Beverly Hills: Sage.

Gilkes, C. (1986). Building in many places: Multiple commitments and ideologies in Black women's community work. In A. Bookman & S. Morgan (Eds.), *Woman and the politics of empowerment*. Philadelphia: Temple University Press.

Gutierrez, L., & Lewis, E. (1994). Community organizing with women of color: A feminist approach. *Journal of Community Practice, 1*(2), 23-44.

Mondros, J., & Wilson, S. (1994). *Organizing for power and empowerment*. New York: Columbia University Press.

9

The Culture of Poverty and Backyard Efforts

Pedro José Greer, Jr. and Patricia L. Munhall

*T*his is how I first met Joe. I was new to Barry University in Florida and had been asked to start a Primary Care Nursing Center for the School of Nursing. We were to be interdisciplinary in delivery and wanted a committed physician to be part of our team for the five schools we were planning to serve. The schools were in economically disadvantaged areas and the children were without any health care and in severe need of health teaching.

One morning I was reading the *Miami Herald,* the favorite paper in these parts, and there was a story about a physician who went under the bridges to treat the homeless people. The article announced that he had been chosen as a recipient of a McArthur Award, one of the country's most prestigious awards. He had gone to the people without homes, into their "backyard" in his jeans, shook their hands, introduced himself, and listened. Under the bridges of I-95, his own respect for the cultural aspects of poverty took shape.

He now practices and teaches what he heard. And in Washington, as well as Miami, the policymakers listen. I called Joe Greer and asked for an appointment. We met and when I complimented him on his award, he replied, "my mother probably nominated me." He seemed uncomfortable with accolades. He is determined to be a physician, the kind some of us have begun to think do not exist. He wants individuals to feel good. Joe enters a room and the feeling of care he exudes immediately has a healing effect. He is young, jovial, and self-effacing. He said, "Sure I will help you with this project." That was the beginning. We have had and still have our physician for the Center. Most important to this book project though is that Dr. Greer has developed a Theory of Poverty, which he teaches to health care professionals.

When planning this book, I asked Joe to write a paper on poverty, because it is one of the themes interwoven in the book. Joe moves too fast to write, does too much "hands on" work to write, teaches poverty medicine to the medical students, consultants, and advocates for the homeless, so I cornered him for an interview. This paper is the result of that interview.

"What we do is fundamentally misdirected. We attempt to solve the problems of disenfranchised groups, like the homeless, from a middle-class perspective," he begins, sipping a diet coke. "We think that they think the way we do or worse that they believe the same things we do. They just can't seem to get what it is WE think THEY need, when in fact we must first hear their own expressed needs. I mean a pint of whiskey may be the only thing on their mind, or heroin, and we tell them the importance of good nutrition. We are way off center and then we lose them."

Part of Joe's theory of poverty has to do with our taking for granted that a group such as the homeless and a group such as those with homes could possibly share the same perceptions. Not only do they not share the same perceptions, he explains, but the life in poverty is a culture unto itself. The culture of poverty has its own social hierarchies and a very separate language. Though the words might be English or Spanish, the meaning is entirely different and so the meaning of being-in-the-world is entirely different.

Then, we as honest "do-gooders" reach out essentially to foreigners without a clue as to what their world is about. He goes on thoughtfully, "This group that we call the 'homeless' is, in addition to comprising another culture, an extremely heterogeneous one. They are homeless for very different reasons and a one-shot approach or program is doomed."

"We do all these quantitative studies on this population but we need qualitative studies to find out who these people are and what meaning their culture has for them." At this point, I comment to him that anyone who knows me will think I coached that line. He looks puzzled and I tell him a little bit about one of my own crusades, the need for phenomenological studies. He sees on my desk a book on phenomenology (I'm not making this up!) and asks, "what is that?" And I say "that is what you have been doing under the bridges and in all the clinics from a philosophical realm. It is about meaning." I think Joe has thought about all his work as being completely logical: that if you are going to effectively help people you must first understand their culture and the meaning.

Back under I-95 Joe listens and observes. He finds a microcosm of the larger society: social hierarchies, good guys, bad guys, and horrendous violence. There is theft of all kinds, people who sleep with weapons, women and children are raped, and the weaker who are most vulnerable beaten and kicked about.

He goes on, "The realities that exist in the dark recesses of the inner city homeless range from human kindness to crack dealers, to women who will prostitute themselves for crack, and cracked lives. The most vulnerable are the elderly, the children, and the women. Not protected from the elements or offered protection by society as a whole, each must learn the rules of the streets and how to fend for one's own survival. Since the majority of those that are homeless are men, the day labor jobs go to them. As such, the women must seek other avenues of economic viabilities. Being homeless offers little in life's comforts, but much in life's quick comforts and subsequent long-term suffering.

Women who turn to prostitution must then live with the consequences of violence, arrest, addiction, and AIDS, as well as other communicable diseases. In a yet unpublished study, looking at over 2,000 patients in our homeless clinic, Miami had the highest rates of HIV seropositivity of 16 different sites in the United States and, among Blacks and Hispanics, there were equal rates of HIV infection between men and women. Lack of education, familial support systems, societal support systems leaves the most vulnerable in society at risk for suffering fear, and slow and lonely deaths. Unfortunately, the women top the list and their advocates too often know little about the realities that exist. They advocate for unrealistic solutions that fit well into a middle class society but not with the realities that exist in the dungeons that lie under the overpasses of the inner city," he concludes reflectively.

I ask him about pregnancy of the homeless woman and he says that often it is the one and only way a young girl or woman can receive love.

From our middle class perspective, especially about responsibility, how can we understand the women's need for someone to love and to be loved in return in this cold, dismal existence?

As Dr. Pedro José Greer, Jr. is riding around one morning, he decides to stop. The word "stop" here is not used literally but as a metaphor. It is a "Stop" what we can. Cammillus House is the place, a place where the homeless can be fed daily, counseled, and most important understood. Joe is Medical Director of all the medical and health care services. He understands that our middle class perspective is "out-in-space" to these people and his work is to make sure they stay alive. He knows that these people do not have transportation, a simple concept, yet one that seems to defy most of the best intentioned clinics, and that people need to be brought to the services, or the services to them.

Camillus House itself is located within walking distance of the area's homeless population. In this Culture of Poverty theory, one must look at the reality of the culture. Poverty itself should announce, without explanation, the lack of resources. Individuals do not have carfare. Resources also include abilities. Many of the homeless do not have abilities. The culture includes or is inclusive of the lack of middle class abilities and simple knowledge. Not because there is a cycle of poverty but because there is a culture of poverty. So you do what you can, but from their perspective, and begin a re-education program. I think the idea of rehabilitation when applied to these people is demeaning. Would we rehabilitate people from another culture? What we might do, if they decided to live in "our" culture, is to help them enter the culture with the most effective tool—education.

However, educating an individual requires a degree of physical and mental health. The medical services at Camillus House, under Joe's direction, recognize that and he has implemented not only programs that care for the sick, but programs aimed at immediate threats, such as HIV/AIDS, pre-natal dangers, drug and alcohol abuse, violence and malnourishment. This is part of the Culture of Poverty approach. Go in and do what you can right now, immediately, with a nonjudgmental approach and a respect for a different culture. Re-education can follow and with successful cases individuals may be educated into this other culture.

Some are too far gone. Joe makes sure they live out their life in as much comfort as possible. He still cares for them as much as he would for a person with a "good" prognosis. This is contrary to many theories of caring for the poor or homeless. Treatment in many places is geared toward those that have a possibility of a positive outcome. Joe's theory includes the idea that some people cannot leave their culture and yet they deserve food and medical treatment. This is not a reward and treatment program. This is recognition of a different culture with different beliefs, attitudes, values, resources, and abilities that is not evaluated through a judgmental lens as to how they became a part of that culture. Rather, efforts are made to educate and indeed improve their lives, but a person is not "dropped" because he or she is not "educable."

Everyone—doctors, nurses, psychologists, Brother Paul and his staff, the people in the kitchen, the people hanging around outside Camillus House—helps. They are volunteers. Sometimes grants come in to support staff members, but for the most part, this represents a backyard effort: individuals, giving of themselves, understanding this culture and practicing within it. Joe remarks, "Small private organizations affiliated with religious organizations offer help to some in compassionate, caring, patient arenas, truly reaching out to the individual woman and her children. Unfortunately they are small and overwhelmed."

The major concept of this theory is that middle class prescriptions for successful living are called into question. They are not the barometers of success, nor are they presumed to be even important in the culture of poverty.

Backyards are all over this globe. A culture of poverty theory makes sense in the evaluation of our social problems. For as long as I can remember the question asked was "How do we break the cycle of poverty?"

Listening to Pedro José Greer's Theory of Poverty, in this very brief description, has once again demonstrated the aftermath of asking the wrong question or perceiving the situation through a misleading paradigm. I have listened to him and have experienced an insight that, for me, is very important. Instead of the perception of a cycle, the perception becomes one of culture, "How do we understand the Culture of Poverty?"

Once we understand the concept of culture as it applies to poverty, the backyard efforts which we need globally for any group will be as they should be. Our efforts will reflect respect for a culture, no matter how contrary to our own. Then and only then can we be responsive to the characteristics and values of that culture. But, again and again, we fail because of a basic lack of understanding of meaning . . .

10

In Another Backyard: A Primary Care Nursing Center Without Walls

Patricia L. Munhall

About two years ago, I became associate dean of the graduate program in nursing at Barry University. I had been an associate dean before and in my own subjective evaluation had performed well enough, considering the quagmire that exists in Academia, so I was not particularly worried about whether I could do this job or not. In fact, I would never apply for a job I didn't think I could do. I'm just not that young, or put another way, I'm too old, like teaching old dogs new tricks. So I went into my office that July, two years ago, and wondered how best to get started.

Then, after a while, I walked down the hall and into Judith Balcerski's office, dean of the school of nursing, curious as to her conception of how best to get started. And she said, "I would like you to start a Primary Care Nursing Center."

I thought that a wonderful idea, however, I certainly did need to learn a whole new area. Foiled at the start!

I returned to my office and considered the possibility. I knew in some small, vague way that these Primary Care Nursing Centers were a lot of trouble. Faculty didn't want to work in them without additional pay or credit allocation. Patients, depending on the area of the country, could not get to the Centers, as described in the preceding Culture of Poverty paper. In fact, patients only came if there was an emergency and they lived very, very close. Patients most often did not return, if seen, for follow-up care. Once they received a prescription or directions for care, they did not return. Twenty-four-hour coverage created havoc with peoples' lives and was continually debated as whether this was appropriate for a university. I had seen many a Center in my travels, empty of people but furnished with expensive equipment—Centers that, for one reason or another, did not work.

Let me back up here. About ten years ago, some colleges of nursing started Nursing Centers to deliver nursing care to individuals in the community and/or within the university community. There were many variations on the theme. Faculty, usually Nurse Practitioner faculty, could practice at these centers. Students learning nursing, whether as a practitioner or as a bachelor's level nursing student, also had a clinical setting to deliver care. On the community side it seemed like an excellent way to meet health care needs. Since then, there have been huge successes with this concept, yet many have closed because of the previously mentioned problems and because of cost. The ones that did well survived on generous grants and not on income generated by patients.

However, the intent is good and the need is there, especially in economically disadvantaged areas where health care is delivered mostly in the emergency room. We know that is not health care, but for the poor, that is where they interface with medicine and nursing. From there, they are once again forgotten, until the next emergency.

Remember, from the previous paper, when individuals are not of middle or upper economic status, they may have different perceptions about health care. This is a generalization that I know could apply to people from all economic groups, but often people who are economically disadvantaged do not seek out medical or nursing care even when there appears to be an emergency. Home remedies, letting something heal with a large scar, or developing a no-turning-back complication comprises some of the economically disadvantaged individuals' attitudes toward health care. There is a critical need to do something, especially with high-risk groups, and especially with children. I truly believe that the poor have a right to health care. I wish I could allocate my tax dollars, but since I can't do that directly, I began to think this could be a wonderful opportunity to "walk the talk" of care. We formed a committee and began planning.

Commitment to the project was varied. Interest vied with exhaustion. The comment, "oh, no, not another thing to do," was not uncommon either at first. I really understood though. Women entering the 21st century are so overwhelmed with role responsibilities and expectations that they are enormously stressed. Academia is filled with demands that few people realize. But this is not what this chapter is about. Just let it be said, for the record, that such response was quite appropriate.

We did make one decision though that, based on the history of other centers, was crucial: The center had a better chance of succeeding if it were non-traditional, a true "center without walls." We also chose to focus first on children.

When we speak of culture, the idea of enculturation and socialization is inherent, and we believed in the importance of health and safety education as part of that enculturation. Thus, we made initial contacts with schools in Miami's economically disadvantaged areas, gathered data to assess what was needed, not from our preconceived assumptions, but from the principals and teachers. After some time, the children began to tell us what they needed in indirect ways. And being on site, we could observe and hear the actions and words of the participants in the different schools. They told us often what they needed, sometimes in heartbreaking ways, too.

A Nursing Center Without Walls offers many advantages in the effective delivery of health care, evaluation, and education. Miami is one of this country's most ethnically diverse cities. Each of our schools is a mixture, but primarily a majority of one group, such as Haitians, African-Americans, Cubans, White, mixed—all wonderful children with potential. Individualizing the needs of each school according to their cultural majorities enabled us to perform our roles and respect the customs of the various ethnic groups. Beliefs, values, and attitudes vary widely from school to school and if we were to bring in our way, we would not be effective and certainly less than compassionate. While we are on the subject of compassion, we do not stereotype a culture, rather, we know the predominant culture provides a beginning point, and a better one than our usual middle class perspective.

I can be more specific about the "without walls" concept. One critical aspect of being onsite is that we avoid the transportation difficulties that our population experiences. Let me throw in a statistic here. I am very proud and appreciative of all the people who made this number possible. This 1994-1995 year, our faculty and students had 4,000, yes, 4,000 contact hours with students, parents, teachers, principals, and members of the community. How could this be, you might ask? Being onsite at a school gives us the opportunity to teach to groups, to have entire days devoted to health education, as well as "one-on-one" contact.

If we were located on our own campus, none of this would be possible. More important, if the compassion, empathy, and enthusiasm of the faculty and students to participate in this way was not present, neither would such hours be possible. But these faculty and students are emergent 21st century individuals. If every College of Nursing and Medicine, as well as the other important health care providers in this country, volunteered some time to such an endeavor, the health care and level of health in this country would be quite different. I know this because of the changes our faculty and students have made.

The economically disadvantaged is often the most forgotten group in this country. In fact, to some people, they are just annoying, seen as a tax burden, a societal burden, and best out of sight. However, this is a country of immigrants and almost all our ancestors suffered economic deprivation unless they had a "rich uncle." Yes, we go to the schools and do immunizations, health assessments, programs on drugs, violence, and sexually transmitted disease, among many more, and while we all believe this will make a difference, often I think it is the "attention" that will make the most difference. Or such attention will make the other aims and goals possible.

Many of these children receive very little extra attention. It is not necessarily their parents' doings or their single parent's doings. They live in neighborhoods where it is unsafe to go out. A taken-for-granted activity of yesterday, play outside after school, is no longer possible. The danger is that real. One principal told me how a child stepped over a dead body on the way to school that morning. We were able to talk with that child. Another principal told a faculty member of violence in a home, a very common problem, and we were able to see that child that day. It is the same with children who were physically abused, thrown out of their house, asked to try drugs, bitten by a dog on the way to school, hadn't had a meal in two days, were attacked and robbed the night before—the litany goes on. We are able to assist the teachers with these problems. We can see the child alone. We can give a child individualized attention and we can follow up by our consistent presence in the schools. The children are beginning to know who we are and that we can be trusted.

Wanting so much and receiving not enough, they cling. The teachers are overburdened. We are a Primary Care Nursing Center with different locations and our faculty and students are becoming intricate parts of the lives of these children and the entire community.

First, we were strangers—to the children, another adult to be cautious about. Now they are beginning to know us. Their associations to us seem positive. They want to know when we will be back. And we try to be at each school more than once a week with some planned activity to improve the quality of their life. And if we receive a call from a principal concerning a need, we respond accordingly.

Let me return to the initial response of "oh no, not one more thing to do." Perhaps we were all strangers to the idea—center without walls—and it did seem burdensome. But faculty self-selected, as volunteers, and when those children's eyes light up from our attention, our lives have achieved a deeper meaning. The university students are of all ages and backgrounds and they too self-selected and seemed to blossom in the true spirit of reaching out to others. They were and are emerging in their own humanity and the children are emerging with them.

As faculty, clinical experiences have taken on a new vitality. These circumstances wake up our sensibilities: that children live this way, that there may not be parents, that they cannot leave their home or apartment, that some are sick, that some are not diagnosed, that some are abused, that some lack love and attention and at early ages some have already given up—certainly different than the predictable hospital environment. Many students have said to me that it is in the schools that they really feel like they are making a difference. From my perspective, when the students are free to design programs for the children, their enthusiasm knows few bounds.

Some readers might want to know how this is organized. When we say a "Center Without Walls," we mean this: our central location for meetings is on campus. We organize activities usually on campus. We recruit for volunteers on campus. The address and phone number for the Center is on campus. In branching out, within yet another concept, "going to the people," we have five schools and have managed with funding to equip a room at each site. We have plans for "our" Center's room at each school (one school has actually been funded for a capital grant to build a building and become a full-service school). So walls exist at each site. This structure, which is quite acceptable to us, also does not limit others from participating in the Center. The organizational structure is comprised of a director, site director, clinical director, and each school has a school coordinator. We are interdisciplinary. We have faculty working on evaluation, budget, and now public relations. We are very young and growing.

We have many plans to do many things. Sometimes I think even catching elementary school age kids is not early enough to prevent damage or be as effective in the promotion of health and safety. And then what can we do with the larger society? Remember, these children inhabit violent, drug infested, gangland neighborhoods. So there is a downside; one that seems beyond our control. Our effort though is to walk with them and to demonstrate how to navigate what is sometimes the unspeakable. We encourage them to give voice to the demons that might haunt them. We certainly have learned that primary care nursing is much more than we had expected. We have learned not to proceed with an agenda but to listen to the needs of the children, teachers, parents, and the members of the community and together establish an agenda. Without walls, communication and energy flow without interruption. Without walls, we are in the same place. Without walls, there is continuity to our relationship to one another.

Within this Center, there is an overwhelming commitment and compassion from the members that serve it. And in all reality there is more work. A small stipend is paid faculty from grant money. Grant money or federal funding is always needed. Both are hard to come by. Without primary care for children we know the price later on will be much higher for society. There is a whole group of individuals who have made this Center possible, who engaged in the "going to" and then giving of their multifaceted talents, care and love. I would like to acknowledge just a few of the individuals who joined our Center: Judith Balcerski, Dean; Claudia Hauri, Sandra Gibson, Susan Folden, Jessie Colin, Gigi Moneda, Margaret Bagardi, Carolyn Brown, Kathleen Papes, Joan Davis, Linda Perkal, Sheila Hopkins, Evelyn Hayes, Ann Lamet, Karol Geimer, and numerous faculty and students at Barry University.

Grateful acknowledgment is made to the Hugoton Foundation and to The Dade County Office of AHEC (Area Health Education Center).

Voices Four

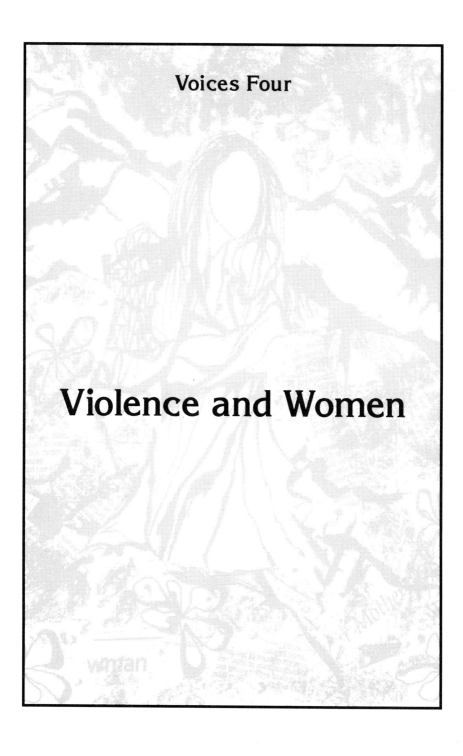

Violence and Women

11

Violence Against Women in Armed Conflicts: Genocide in Bosnia

Amela Sapcanin

The only thing that previously seemed so inconceivable to me was war. Unfortunately, I speak today from the perspective of a woman in the war. At the beginning of 1990 when I was expecting a child, I could not even imagine that my little daughter will not be able to virtually leave our house for two years, or go anywhere from 1992-1994. Since this is my first journey out of Sarajevo since the beginning of war and my first encounter with the outside world, it has become clear to me now how difficult it may be to grasp the Bosnian situation from your prospective . . .

> —Ms. Jasna Baksic Muftic,
> a Bosnian NGO's representative
> addressing the United Nations Development
> Program Panel Discussion that looked into the
> role of women in conflict situations;
> in New York, mid March 1995

*W*hen a year receives a certain attribute, as is the case with 1995—the international year of women—an opportunity arises that emphasis be put on certain topics. The year's attribute simultaneously puts issues into current prospective. In this year, the focus will emphasize a range of relevant issues for the current reality of women throughout the world. One such issue will be violence against women, and ensuring the appropriate mechanisms to eradicate it.

Before development and equity, there must be peace. The women in Bosnia and Herzegovina and, for that matter, in any part of the world afflicted by aggression, armed and nonarmed conflicts, have learned this all too well and in the most painful of terms. This year as the previous three years has been marked again by the continuous aggression against our country.

While the international community looks forward to the advancement of women in all spheres of their lives, or, while in some parts of the world, women have just begun to assert their status, Bosnian women's human rights, and most importantly their right to life, have been most brutally violated in the course of the aggression. In the besieged towns and villages, lacking basic food and medical provisions, with water, electricity, and gas cut off at will by the Serb aggressor forces, dodging Serb sniper bullets and shelled at while waiting in line for bread or water in the besieged "safe area" that have never really been made safe, and recently even more so proven unsafe, Bosnian women's priorities have radically changed.

Because of the inability or lack of will of the international community to deliver on its promises and live up to its commitments to protect civilians while simultaneously denying Bosnians their inherent right to defend themselves, Bosnia's women continue to be exposed to cold, hunger, and death and the fourth winter of war coming to their destroyed homes. In the occupied territories, they fear persecution, torture, expulsion, or death. Even when fleeing, they face imminent danger. Very often women refugees have to cross areas of armed conflict or are otherwise exposed to harassment and assaults, including rape, as pointed out in the report of the United Nations High Commissioner for Refugees. In a daily struggle just to survive, their lives continue to be dramatically limited and at constant danger.

Scars of this aggression are multiple and complex, bearing depth that will be felt by the generations to come. However, one of the most complex manifestations of this aggression is reflected in a particular form of crime against the female population of all ages: the mass and systematic rapes of non-Serb women.

94

Recognizing "that the major victims have been the Muslim women," according to the findings of the Economic Community's investigative mission lead by Dame Warburton, this can only be denounced as a form of genocide.

Ever since the first gruesome accounts by eye witnesses' and the media dating back to early 1992 that have reported of brutalities and atrocities carried out against innocent civilians in pursuit of the policy of "ethnic cleansing"—a euphemism for genocide, much has been said in great detail about the crime of rape and sexual abuse of women in armed conflicts. We have hoped that talking openly about this grave crime will help raise awareness of such unabated violence occurring before the world's eyes, in the heart of Europe, and that the aggressor would stop under the diplomatic pressure of the international community, or that the international community would take appropriate steps to put a halt to such despicable practices.

While the international community continues to respond to the war of aggression against the Republic of Bosnia and Herzegovina, by appeasement, for the fourth year, Bosnian civilians, including women of all ages, have been and still are subjected to unspeakable brutalities. In the Serb occupied territories in Northern Bosnia, such as Banja Luka, Bijeljina, Prijedor, and other areas, ethnic cleansing as characterized by harassment, beatings, rape, torture, and murder has not ceased. According to the various reports by the Commission of Experts, Special Rapporteur and numerous humanitarian and nongovernmental organizations that point out several typical patterns in which rape occurred as well as some common threads that run through the cases reported. A systematic rape policy existed in areas and this policy has been used as an instrument of war and executed in such a manner as to instill terror, shame, and humiliation on the entire nation. Testimonies of the survivors and witnesses confirm that in the campaign of violence neither 6-year-old girls nor elderly women were spared. There has not been a single norm of international law that has not been violated. Some of the crimes that have occurred are unprecedented and require international legal definition as well as mechanisms that condemn and prosecute their perpetrators. An example of this is forced pregnancy.

According to the data collected so far by the State Commission of the Republic of Bosnia and Herzegovina, there are an estimated 25,000 registered victims (though we fear the figure may be as high as some 60,000) of genocidal rape—rape as a political weapon of torture and as part of the policy of ethnic cleansing. Due to the nature of trauma, it has been difficult to ascertain this figure precisely. As pointed out in the Commission of Experts Report (S/1994/674, UN Documentation), "owing to the social stigma attached—even in times of peace—rape is among the least reported crimes . . . The victims may have little confidence in finding justice. The strong fear of reprisal during wartime adds to the silencing of victims. The perpetrators have a strong belief that they can get away with their crimes."

Recognizing the need to grasp the gravity of this crime, Ms. Jasna Baksic Muftic, a lawyer and a sociologist, pointed out in her article for "Zena 21," a Bosnian Women's publication, that:

> *the number of raped women is not a determining factor of the weight of this crime; insistence upon the figures leads to minimizing and turning considerations into statistics, thus, deviating from the essence of the crime. Woman is a target of the aggression, as a part of a unique, detailed plan according to which genocide against a non Serb population, that is, Bosniacs, has been the goal, not the onsequence, of aggression. However, in a similar fashion that the political interests of some have sought to convert the aggression into a conflict of warring parties, rape has also suffered from political manipulations. That can be detected in attempts to treat mass and planned rape as an incident—an excess—typical for war situations, or what is even more perfidious, drowning it into violence against women as women. In the case of Bosnia and Herzegovina, it is not only the women's being that is being aggressed against, but this attack is precisely directed against a particular nation—primarily Bosniacs—which in the light of other committed crimes increases its gravity . . .*

Women were victims of massive deportations and detentions in most of the 200 registered camps in the occupied territories of the Republic of Bosnia and Herzegovina, and, as a rule, those camps were the scene of large scale rapes and other abuses. Apart from being subjected to the brutality of rape, many women were killed after the rape had been committed. Many have disappeared and are registered as missing. One of the early reports of the Commission for War Crimes Investigation in Sarajevo has registered 200 executions of women and girls after they had been raped. The Commission has also registered numerous cases of suicide among women and girls after being raped.

These mass rapes have been premeditated and are results of carefully planned and organized actions, and under no circumstances are a mere byproduct of the war environment. Numerous testimonies of witnesses confirmed in the reports of the Special Rapporteur, indicate undoubtedly that the aggressor's forces had been given clear orders to rape women and very young girls before the eyes of their family members—husbands, children, siblings and cousins, in order to humiliate them in the most brutal fashion. In the report to the U.N. Secretary General of February 26, 1993, the Special Rapporteur, Tadeusz Mazowietski, while stating a variety of methods that have been used to achieve ethnic cleansing, a genocidal policy carried out by Pale Serb forces against non-Serbs, reported:

> *[R]ape is one of these methods, as has been stated from the outset. In this context, rape has been used not only as an attack on the individual victim, but is intended to humiliate, shame, degrade, and terrify the entire ethnic group. There are reliable reports of public rapes, for example, in front of a whole village, designed to terrorize the population and force ethnic groups to flee.*

The consequences of this genocidal rape are horrendous. Physically, the damage is severe. All the victims have suffered acute wounds inflicted by the perpetrators, and for many others the damage is irreparable, so much so that their future lives as mothers may no longer be possible.

But this systematic rape and torture is not only meant to hurt physically, but also psychologically. It aims at the honor of the whole Bosnian nation, as well as at the disintegration of our traditions and culture. Moreover, the victim faces unavoidable personal issues: how to relate in society again, how to take the role of mother, wife, sister, or daughter in the family after having undergone the trauma of rape, after they have been humiliated, and after their physical safety was at stake.

As noted by one of the legal organizations working on the issue of rape in the context of war crimes:

> *[A]ccountability for the crimes is the first step toward restoring the moral and political order of the society. Participating directly in that process helps restore the victim's sense of control over their own destinies while lifting their sense of shame and powerlessness. Thus, while silence—and even denial—may be necessary during the initial period of some victims trauma recovery, participation in rebuilding the moral foundation of their societies by establishing accountability for war-related atrocities may be critical to their and their country's longer term recovery.*

Toward this end, the long-awaited proceedings of the International War Crimes Tribunal established by SC resolution 827 (1993) is seen as a very significant step.

The U.N.'s Commission of Experts, the Special Rapporteur of the U.N. Commission on Human Rights, and various nongovernmental human rights and women's organizations have reported rape and other sexual violation offenses among the serious violations of international law in the current conflict in the former Yugoslavia. Rape is specifically named in the Tribunal's statute as one of the crimes within the competence of the Tribunal.

Various women's groups and other nongovernmental organizations working on the investigation of and collecting testimonies on the war-related crimes look to the International War Crimes Tribunal to take action to ensure that rape is investigated with the same thoroughness as other violations, that all the members of the Tribunal are trained and supervised in the proper investigation of these crimes, and that rape and other sexual assaults are characterized and prosecuted as a form of torture and among the most serious of crimes.

Thus, a number of recommendations have been put forward, including the need to facilitate the appropriate financing for the International War Crimes Tribunal so that it can carry out its functions without any impediments; the need for the appointment of qualified women to the staff of the Prosecutor's Office as well as the staff of the Tribunal; the strengthening of the protection of witnesses; the preparation for the stresses of trial and related measures and providing counseling services during the trial; and finally, the ensuring of appropriate rehabilitation and compensation for the victims.

These are all very critical measures that merit the utmost consideration. If implemented, they will be important steps toward the recovery of the victims.

The issue of violence against women has received due attention in my country. Despite the lack of resources and in conditions of continued aggression, attempts have been made toward offering financial, medical, and psychotherapeutic help. There have been centers organized in some areas, which are addressing this issue among other things. These include "The Counseling Department for Psychotherapeutic Help and Social Adaptation" in Sarajevo, aimed at helping all of the traumatized. There are 10 women's organizations in Sarajevo with varying programs and structures. The number of these organizations has risen to 47 in the territory of the Republic of Bosnia and Herzegovina as a whole. As a result of networking and mutual cooperation, and toward the goal of participating in decision making by actively working toward finding the solutions to unified and organized protection for women, children, and family, these 47 organizations have joined into a Federation, which is nonpartisan, voluntary, and nongovernmental association, bearing the symbolic name "Phoenix"—the mythological birth that rose from the ashes. The Federation has been successful in promoting dialogue by way of open seminars and panel discussions with topics that among others, deal with the plight of Bosnian women, families, and children.

At this national level, Bosnia and Herzegovina's women have taken the initiative to rehabilitate their integrity and have chosen to battle back from their victimization. They have articulated this suffering and the plight they have been subjected to, and thus taken an active role in offering responses and solutions for the current political, cultural, and economic situation.

They have exerted all of their efforts to transform themselves from being a political object into a political subject, taking stands, developing policies, and carrying out responsibilities. One example is a very lively publishing activity that encompasses literary, essayist, media, and scientific works by women writers. A new theme magazine that would deal with the issue of Bosnian woman and war is being initiated.

Based on our tragic experiences, we believe that this crime of rape should be checked by the highest level of international legal protection and that it should be denounced as a specific crime against humanity and as a crime of genocide. The Beijing Conference should take this step forward in denouncing such violence both on the national and international level. Thus, one of the tasks ahead will be to recognize, condemn, and specifically clarify that rape, which is a part of strategy and ideology to destroy a nation and is one of the goals of the aggression, is not a mere byproduct of war for which only individual responsibility will be called for, but is comparable to a crime against humanity or crime of genocide. We should seek to condemn not only the perpetrators of this crime, but the instigator—the ideologist behind it. Such clarification will bring at least moral satisfaction to the victims in Bosnia and offer to the women of the world who may be threatened again in this way, the adequate form of international criminal protection.

But the final stage of recovery for all who have suffered and been severely traumatized will come when a peace, a just peace, is achieved. When we wake up in the morning without the resounding sound of shells and sniper bullets, when the streets cease to be called "Sniper alleys," when we no longer fear for the lives of our families, friends, and ourselves.

The role of women in peace making and peace building is in the promotion of the values of peace, human rights, tolerance, political dialogue, and many others. It is because of this that the emphasis should be laid on the quality of peace. Is peace going to be a foundation for stability or a mere introduction to new conflicts? Peace has to be based upon at least a minimum justice. Therefore, the fascist ideology has to be defeated legally—by means of The International Criminal Tribunal, politically—by means of promotion of democracy for all citizens, respecting all cultural, ethnic, and national diversity; culturally; and militarily—by ensuring the capabilities of the victim to defend these values.

The principal role of women is not to remain victims. They have the real power to articulate their own suffering and to find solutions to it. Only then will they overcome their tragic pasts in favor of a brighter future.

12

Domestic Violence: A Loss of Selfhood

Evelyn Ortner

I am Evelyn Ortner, Founder and Executive Director of The Unity Group, Inc., advocates for battered women and their children. Prior to founding Unity, I had been an advisor and speechwriter for then Secretary of Health and Human Services, Margaret Heckler. My area of concentration was women's issues and domestic violence, in particular. Even then, through the Reagan period of the 1980s, Surgeon General Koop referred to Domestic Violence as the No. 1 health problem and leading cause of death and injury for women in the United States.

When I returned to my home in suburban New Jersey, I founded Unity, a non-profit all volunteer group (no one is on salary) which provides a multitude of services, all without charge, to meet the daily needs of our clients. We offer support group services, other monthly public service programs, and referrals to pro bono legal and medical services.

I first learned of the nightmare of abuse and its pervasive nature while in Washington. You need to know just how pervasive and perhaps these statistics will enlighten you.

- Every 15 seconds a woman is battered in the United States.
- Between 1959 and 1975, 58,000 American soldiers were killed in Vietnam. During that same period, 51,000 American women were murdered by their male partners.
- Each year, approximately 1,400 women die as a result of domestic violence.
- 95% of domestic violence victims are women.
- Industry loses $3 billion to $5 billion per year through absenteeism because of injuries caused by domestic violence.
- Two to four million women are beaten each year by their partners.
- Domestic violence is not limited to any geographic area, income level, or religious affiliation.
- Each year more than one million women seek medical assistance for injuries caused by battering.
- 15% to 25% of pregnant women are battered.
- Approximately 35% of women with injuries who use emergency room services are abused women.
- Battering is the cause of one of every four suicide attempts by women.
- There are three times more animal shelters in the United States than shelters for women.
- 87% of children witness the abuse of their mothers.
- Children in homes where domestic violence occurs are physically abused at a rate 1500% higher than the national average.
- Boys who witness the violence are more likely to batter their female partners as adults than others raised in nonviolent homes.

During the period I served in the federal government, I read countless books and articles on the subject of domestic violence including Dr. E. Shein's *Coercive Persuasion and Brainwashing, Conditioning and DDD (Debility, Dependency and Dread)* by I. E. Farber, Harry F. Harlow, and Louis Jolyon West; and Biderman's "Chart of Coercion." Having digested these materials, it became obvious that hostages of any variety (battered women are hostages) are kept imprisoned by the means described in this literature. As you read this, there are literally thousands of women who are being held hostage in their own homes.

Though there may not be bars on the windows and doors to keep them in, they are not necessary because there are invisible bars that keep them prisoners. These invisible bars control the minds of these victims and they are stronger than any iron bars could be.

Let me describe the function of the 3 Ds. They are, in order,

- Debilitation—This first D is induced by semi-starvation, fatigue, disease, isolation, chronic physical pain, loss of energy, all of which leads to an inability to resist minor abuse which then leads to inanition and a sense of total exhaustion.
- Dependency—This second D is produced by the prolonged deprivation of sleep, food, fresh air, social contact, factors necessary to maintain sanity and life itself. Occasional respites from the abuse teaches the victim that, should he want to, the abuser can stop the abuse. This leads the victim to harbor false hopes of change and keeps her there eternally hoping for release from her agony.
- Dread—This final, ultimate D is the fear of death or of permanent disability or deformity.

The 3 Ds keep a victim in her place in a constant state of panic hoping to please, never knowing what will incur the wrath of her abuser. Dr. Saul Shengold has termed this condition, "Soul Murder"—a victim's soul in bondage to someone else. Jefferson said, "I have sworn upon the altar of God eternal hostility against every form of tyranny over the mind of man." And what, if anything, has society done to practice what that great patriot preached so very long ago? Precious little.

A victim is told that she has provoked him and therefore must be punished, that if she did not provoke him, he would not be forced to hurt her, but she persisted, and therefore she must be punished. She, in fact, made him do it. One abuser actually told me that his victim now hits herself, also; he has trained her to do that. Dr. Biderman's "Chart of Coercion" encompasses DDD and depicts the descent into hell of emotional imprisonment.

These methods can reduce anyone to a slavelike condition. I have often drawn the comparison between Holocaust victims and domestic violence victims. The macro as opposed to the micro, but is it really the micro? After all, the Hitler Holocaust had a beginning and an end, while the victimization of women, like a mobius strip, seems unending. Anyone undergoing DDD is a dehumanized being who is unable to distinguish herself as a separate person and often is unable to distinguish right from wrong. These women are survivors in the same way that Holocaust survivors are. They do what they need to do in order to survive. One of my clients has referred to herself as a sacrificial lamb.

Table 12.1 Biderman's Chart of Coercion

General Method	Effects and Purposes
Isolation	Deprives victim of social support (for the) ability to resist.
	Develops an intense concern with self.
	Makes victim dependent upon interrogator.
Monopolization of perception	Fixes attention upon immediate predicament; fosters introspection.
	Eliminates stimuli competing with those controlled by captor.
	Frustrates all actions not consistent with compliance.
Induced debility and exhaustion	Weakens mental and physical ability to resist.
Threats	Cultivates anxiety and despair.
Occasional indulgences	Provides positive motivation for compliance.
Demonstrating "omnipotence"	Suggests futility of resistance.
Degradation	Makes cost of resistance appear more damaging to self esteem than capitulation.
	Reduces prisoner to "animal level" concerns.
Enforcing trivial demands	Develops habit of compliance.

Unfortunately, there are those ignorant among us who insist and persist in calling the battered woman a masochist—a shocking lie that the public must be disabused of.

I would like to introduce to you a few of my clients. The very first call I received was from a woman who had two daughters, one about 3 years old and the other about 18 months. Her husband, unbeknownst to her, was having sexual relations with their 3-year-old daughter. One night the husband took his two sleepy daughters out of the house, locked his wife in her room after beating her unconscious, and set the room afire. Fortunately, she regained consciousness, jumped out the window, and fled to a hospital. Those horrible events took place over six years ago. To this day, the older daughter has severe emotional problems. Her mother suffers from the physical after-effects of the fire and innumerable emotional problems. She is a strikingly beautiful woman and is still struggling with a court system to keep custody of her daughters.

Another equally beautiful young woman from a cultured upscale family met her abuser in 1982. He is an uneducated, perennially filthy drug user and dealer, unemployed and from a dysfunctional family. Being the con man that all abusers are, he convinced her of his loneliness and his needs. Within a month or so she was reduced to abject servitude. He said, "Call me Mr. Jones of Jonestown. I can do all this by drugs, starvation, and beatings." Currently she lives in poverty, has had major surgery, is losing her teeth, and is not permitted any connection with her family or friends. She is free only to work and support her abuser.

One client in her mid-fifties has been brutalized for years. Her story is unique in that her husband first told her she was too thin and insisted upon her gaining weight and forcing her to eat only high calorie foods. Once she was truly obese, he took her to the hospital and had her undergo intestinal bypass surgery to help her reduce her weight. As a result of that surgery, she suffers innumerable disabilities and currently weighs 180 pounds and is five feet tall.

Another client, beaten while pregnant, aborted at home and carried the foetus about, crying for help. Her husband, who had caused the tragedy, called her names, and refused to take her to the hospital.

These behaviors are not without repercussions. The trauma of victimization is a direct reaction to the aftermath of the crime. When victims do not receive the appropriate support and intervention, they suffer secondary injuries or, what I call, revictimization by the system. The victim feels numb, a kind of paralysis sets in, she is unable to make rational decisions, feels vulnerable, lonely, and confused. Her selfhood is gone. To question a victim's response or lack thereof is to inflict a secondary injury. Even those who escape suffer from post-traumatic stress disorder (PTSD). Some symptoms of PTSD involve sleeping and eating disorders, nightmares, flashbacks, extreme tension and anxiety, nonresponsiveness, and memory trouble.

Support from the medical professionals, the court system, law enforcement, and lawyers, to say nothing of friends and family, is essential. To blame the victim is a crime in itself. Failure to recognize the importance of the crime is to invalidate the victim who requires that very validation to recover.

The AMA has admitted that they are delinquent in recognizing and providing the necessary help that victims require. Doctors do not even ask how the injuries that they are treating have been inflicted. I think we can safely say that it is indeed a rare occasion when someone runs into a door or does a somersault in the tub. The reluctance to address the real issue increases the sense of isolation of the victim and discourages her efforts to leave the abuse. This refusal to recognize and validate the victim is a significant factor in the development of subsequent psychopathology.

Research shows that in 96% of the cases, there is no psychosocial history taken and no psychiatrist is consulted. In 92% of the cases, no social worker was consulted and in 98% of the cases, no referral was given. Dr. Malcolm G. Freeman of Emory University said, "Probably the greatest thing physicians can do to help victims of domestic violence is to be emotionally supportive." Prescribing tranquilizers and pain medicine is not a remedy. It is a bandaid solution and a poor one at that.

Triage nurses often are aware of the abuse, but refuse to get involved and instead refer the patient to police.

Anne Flitcraft, M.D., states that 45% of the women in alcohol treatment started out as battered women who drink or succumb to the drugs that doctors prescribe to make them feel better. The previously mentioned client who referred to herself as a sacrificial lamb has been calling doctors constantly, none of whom has recognized her problem. A prominent specialist to whom she went for ultrasound for three consecutive months decided she is in need of mental therapy. Furthermore, he says that she is suffering from Munchausen's syndrome, a feigning of ailments. And so, doctor, can you not decipher her clues, her silent call for help? By concluding that she is unstable, he is colluding with her abuser. The doctor is simply not listening.

Who are these women who become victims? They are all about us and can be anyone and everyone. Customarily, these are women who want to please, have low self-esteem, someone who defines herself in terms of others, but none of these factors is essential. All women are potential victims. As the saying goes, flattery will get you everywhere. By the time the victim is aware that conditions are abnormal, it is usually too late. Wooed by the silky tones of adoration, lulled by champagne and flowers, she descends step by hideous step down the path to hell.

Who are these abusers? They can be anyone and everyone, the mayor, the teacher, yes, even the clergyman.

A major characteristic of assailants in domestic violence cases is their capacity for self-deception and deception of others. They are masters in the art of finding ways to blame other people and external events for their inappropriate behavior. A lifelong pattern of avoiding consequences for their own behavior effectively limits a sense of personal responsibility for their actions as well as limiting their motivation for change. An abuser has an intense desire to control an individual. This individual becomes the repository of all of the abuser's inner conflict. In a kind of symbiotic dance, the abuser and his victim feed off of each other. The victim often thinks by being "good" she can eliminate the next beating. But as long as the abuser blames the victim for his own problems, the beatings will continue. The assaults are a product of the abuser's personality and bear little relationship to the victim's behavior. Unless the abuser takes responsibility for his own behavior, the violence will continue.

It is a misconception to believe that the abuser "loves." The attachment to the victim has nothing to do with love. It represents a pathological dependency on the victim. This factor is so extreme as to result in murder if the victim should leave or even speak of leaving. Often she is persuaded to stay by his pleadings of his absolute need of her. This bolsters her shattered sense of self. Often she is moved to remain as he fills her need to be needed. A "honeymoon" phase may ensue when no assaults take place, but that is short-lived and the tension and assaults are renewed. Society tends to blame the victim, and fix the responsibility on her to leave. We fail to hold the abuser responsible for criminal behavior. Claiming alcohol or drug addiction as an excuse for their behavior is outrageous. There is no excuse for abuse. Abusers abuse because they want to abuse.

Here is a list of the abuser's common characteristics:

- Jealousy of their partner.
- Control and isolation of their partner.
- Jekyll and Hyde personalities.
- Explosive tempers.
- Have legal problems, served time in jail.
- Projection (blame others for own behavior).
- Verbal and physical abuse.
- History of family violence.
- More violent when partner is pregnant.
- Denial (he never did anything wrong).
- Cycle of violence.

There are some early warning signs to be aware of and to run away from as fast as possible should you see them:

- Physical abuse during courtship.
- Violent family environments.
- Cruelty to animals.
- Inability to handle frustration.
- Poor self-image.

- Extreme possessiveness and jealousy.
- Police record for a violent crime.
- Overt and excessive concern (a cover for control).
- Chronically unemployed.
- Use of force in sex.
- Past relationships in which there were indications of abuse.
- Sees women as inferior to men.

Though society constantly berates the battered woman for not leaving and all manner of reasons are given for her staying in the abuse, the basic reason for her remaining is mind control and the aforementioned methods employed by all abusers, young and old, rich and poor, ignorant and educated. They are one and the same, hideous. Women are not born with this ailment, domestic violence, nor do they contract it like TB. It is visited upon them by vicious men.

And what can we do as a society to hold back this tide? We must train all of our professionals—including medical, legal, judicial, educators, the clergy, and so on—in the dynamics of domestic violence. We must do as they have done in some parts of the United States, and that is to practice vertical prosecution. What that does, in essence, is to employ personnel who are trained in domestic violence dynamics, from the district attorneys, prosecutors, judges, to the police officers. That unique group works only on domestic violence cases, and their success rates are outstanding. It is understood that domestic violence is a crime against the state and not a private matter. It will therefore be prosecuted to the full extent of the law. Victims need not press charges, nor appear in court, and charges are never dropped. In jurisdictions where vertical prosecution is practiced, battered women have a better chance of survival than in other parts of the country. Since that is the case, it must be implemented throughout the country.

Crisis intervention teams are another tool to save the lives of women and children. Here, trained volunteers from each municipality are on call on a rotating basis. Once they are notified by the police that a victim is waiting at the station, a volunteer goes there to offer practical information as well as solace to the victim. Such help and validation is essential.

One of the easiest methods to avoid future violence in our lives is to raise our children as equals, to let our daughters know that they do not have to marry into status, that they can and should be able to achieve on their own. And when Johnny destroys Mary's castle in the sandbox, he must be chastised publicly for that infraction. Mary needs to know that she need never accept that kind of abuse and Johnny needs to know that he was wrong and that everyone believes him to be wrong.

If that kind of misbehavior is not stopped in the sandbox, Johnny may grow up to be an abuser in some Mary's bedroom, and Mary, if not validated, will grow up thinking that abuse is okay. One might as well hang a placard around her neck which says, "Here I am. I'm a victim." Dr. Carol Gilligan, an expert on female adolescents, says that young girls sacrifice truth on the altar of niceness. Being nice is one thing, being subservient is quite something else.

We cannot allow our young people to grow up with the possibility of violence as a virtual fait accompli. We cannot sacrifice even a single female to this horror. We cannot afford it because our children are our future. Remember the teaching of the Talmud, "He who destroys a child, destroys the world, but he who saves a child, saves the world."

13

Cancer of Violence: Power Differentials and Family Values

Patricia L. Munhall

We've celebrated the twenty-fifth anniversary of Earth Day, even though our land was on fire, blood splattered in the air, human lives lost. Progress on the condition of the environment was noted and accolades given to those who are working diligently on conditions of the land, air, water, and trees.

We can worry about just so many things at any given time. As far as the environment is concerned, we need to expand our conceptualization of the environment and prioritize what is most important.

My worry is not so much the trees, soil, water, and air, as what it is that keeps people out of the natural environment, behind multilocked doors, off public transportation, out of parks, and living in a state of fear. My

---

This speech was delivered at the United Nations, New York in April 1995.

worry is about the "cancer of violence." And like cancer, violence comes when we are least aware, or when we thought we took proper precautions, and/or when we are trying to convince ourselves that "it" could not be happening to us. The suddenness, the unpredictable event, or the predictable event we were denying could happen—like cancer, violence, dark, scary, lurking in the micro and the macro environments.

This paper is on the cancer of violence as it affects women in particular. We are well aware that this cancer is pervasive in the world and is not gender determined. However, women pose specific considerations that call to us to respond rapidly and swiftly. We cannot bury our heads in the sand. Some may be survivors of violence, however, many women have not survived. The survivors bear scars, have nightmares, and carry a lack of trust.

This is not meant to scare you; most women and men are already scared. I hope to raise your consciousness to a critical women's health problem and environmental, societal, cultural bloodbath—in Burundi, in Rwanda, in Mozambique, in Nigeria, in Bangladesh, Cambodia, Afghanistan, and today in Bosnia. Since World War II, 23 million people have died in 150 wars. *One* unnecessary death or other act of violence is a tragedy and a travesty.

Today I am writing of other war zones, the "cancer of violence" and women. Women were killed and raped in those 150 wars. Their children and families were taken from them. And the same phenomenon happens to them in another war zone—often their own home, often their office, often their own neighborhood.

Every day, every hour, every minute, a woman in this country is violently assaulted. Every six minutes a woman is raped. Spouse abuse is more common than automobile accidents, muggings, and cancer deaths combined (U.S. Senate Judiciary Committee, 1992). When we re-cast this problem into a women's health problem, which it has not ordinarily been thought of, one now has a disease that affects 3 to 4 million women. Not only do *we have a major health problem,* but a major crime problem that receives little attention, unless it involves a celebrity. Yet, those who keep statistics on these kinds of crimes often discount them as domestic squabbles and trivial. Yet, one third of all female homicide victims are killed by their husbands or boyfriends (FBI, 1990).

I would like to share a story about a friend of mine. I'll call her Nancy. You have a similar friend or you may share some of her story. None of this is fictitious except her name. Nancy was abused as a child, not sexually that she can remember, but severely physically and psychologically. She grew up with little self-worth or feelings of safety. Though paradoxical, because her father never protected her, she married to feel safe. This man brutalized her, forcibly raped her (just recently declared a crime), hit her, and verbally demoralized her at every turn. "Battered women" was not a term known at that time, though I do remember her calling the police when she feared for her life. She was told they could not do anything until something actually happened.

Eventually she left him. She left him because she believed it was harming the children. Living at this time with a shattered ego, she could not leave to protect herself. Around this time, the term "dysfunctional family" came into vogue and divorce was commonplace. Nancy had a mental health problem from her childhood and was still pretty much doomed, which is part of the tragedy of domestic violence.

Nancy had lived in a fortress, feeling trapped, sensing suffocation, impending doom, but not entirely a victim. Still attempting to survive, she was caught up in the huge power differential that is the earmark of violence against women.

Nancy was able to leave, but was scarred. It was not long before she found herself in another abusive relationship. This is all too common; it is part of a cycle of demoralization and dehumanization that continues until someone helps the woman. This situation does not respond to rational explanations. The perceptions of an abused child or woman are so skewed that they become part of the damage. Once again abused, depressed, feeling worthless, she lived in a dungeon of debasement and powerlessness. Nancy had one night that I want to tell you about because she is fairly normal in every other aspect. But it tells you about violence and the powerful and unbelievable collusion of men to maintain power. Nancy eventually left this man. One night she was sitting at an outdoor cafe in Greenwich Village and he came up out of nowhere and hit her hard across the face, while shouting obscenities at her. A man came to her rescue. The old boyfriend went to her place, broke into it, and rampaged it, while the hero sat and consoled the visibly shaken Nancy, whose eye was beginning to swell. Her hero took her back to her place and she said "goodnight," but he said he would feel better if he saw her into her apartment. He then proceeded to rape her. He did not see this as rape, although she said "no." He thought in his powerful way that it would actually be good for her.

In these instances, the women are often blamed. People ask what is wrong with her? Few ask *what was wrong with these men?* A 1992 report by the Senate Judiciary Committee revealed that women aren't only being shoved and slapped but, "They are beaten with fists, burned with cigarettes, scalded, slammed against walls, dragged by the hair, hit with hammers, broomsticks and gun butts, pushed out of moving cars, run down by cars, sexually assaulted, strangled, stabbed and shot—*by men they know best.*"

What women are contending with is the recognized or the unrecognized, the conscious or the unconscious, use of violence as the maintenance of power—the power differential. It's old, but it's still with us and it seems to be coming back in insidious ways that we all must be on guard against. Men's superior strength and their control over economic resources still hold women hostage. Throughout the world, women who refuse their husbands sexual intercourse are raped or worse, killed. And we talk of women's sexual autonomy and reproductive freedom. According to the World Health Organization, more than 84 million women alive today have undergone sexual surgery in Africa alone (Rushwan, 1990).

What about this power differential? In the legislature of this country a bill called The Violence Against Women Act went into committee in 1990 and came out of committee in May 1993. What does that tell us? Anita Hill relates her story and the all white male Senate Judiciary Committee sits stonefaced quietly reinforcing our understandings about who controls the rules for social discourse. How precarious is the future for the woman who dares to speak aloud. Anita Hill gave public language to repeated experiences of sexual harassment in the work place. For this she is called self-serving, a destructive woman, a vindictive woman.

Power has always been an intricate part of women's oppression. This we know. Collusion among men has reinforced the power of power. The use of words spoken by women to the holders of power are conveniently suppressed or marginalized. But that is the power men possess and use. And they know it and they are not going to give it up until there are enough resources to resocialize them and develop a male consensus against the suppression or marginalization of women. A major consciousness raising is essential here as well as severe prosecution for these crimes.

We are walking on land mines. They are on the streets of our cities and the floors of our homes. They are most often planted by men . . . in our minds. Some men are outraged at violence toward women. They would never, and this is said as though it is a virtue, "raise a hand against a woman." Is this not still part of their context, of their power? Paradoxically, women also need the powerful to protect them. Women need men to feel safe. Each time a woman is assaulted this becomes reinforced for the unassaulted woman. The land mines: do not go out at night; do not go out without me to protect you; ask my permission and I will ascertain if you will be safe. And on it goes. The powerful then protects the weaker, at least the one perceived to be physically weaker. Men actually believe this at home, certainly in the office, and in society.

That is the *power differential.* Now I must refer to something very closely related to that. Something that we as women and good men want to watch very closely and analyze—the return to *family values.*

Let me tell you about a patient I have who today still suffers greatly. Lisa was sexually abused as a child by her father. She was also physically abused and, of course, her perceptions of the world are so altered that the sequences of her adult life have brought her close to death on several occasions. This is not uncommon for adults with this history. Lisa believes she deserved this. She was the oldest of four children and in a way took her mother's place. Her mother was an alcoholic and Lisa had to assume responsibility for her siblings. She cooked, cleaned, and took care of the household. The role reversal that we now know about is very apparent in these kinds of homes. By outside appearances this was an "intact" family. Lisa had nowhere to go and her survival depended on this. After all, she really was a child.

In my clinical practice and in my personal life, I have encountered enough fallout from the so-called traditional family that the thought of returning to this condition (family values) that existed before the sixties is frightening. The most frightening aspect of such a return is its hypocrisy— the secrets that were the most intricate part of the maintenance of the appearance of the "family." Of all the myriad of secrets to keep, the most important to appearance was incest or child abuse. The abuse, because of the threat of power differentials and/or lies, had to be kept secret. Once kept secret, because of a no-way-out scenario, the secret allows the repetition and the secret to continue. Other family secrets are parental alcoholism and, what we would call today, the battered women.

Returning to family values is to return to keeping secrets and to allowing abuse to continue. Also, I suspect that a return to family values is a return to the patriarchal family.

Society has not become violent because of a loss of family values. We now know more about family violence because we opened the Pandora's box of family secrets. This is incredibly important. We abandoned the idea of loyalty for mental health. What a step backward into mental illness and women's oppression and other scary possibilities under this rubric of family values. This is not political posturing or an ideological statement. When professionals began to look beneath the appearance to what was concealed, healthy actions could be taken. Today a child is encouraged to come forth if someone is doing something that does not feel right. Women are encouraged to seek help and, when they are ready, go to a shelter and save their lives and do better for their family in the long run. If a parent has a drug problem, a child is encouraged to seek help for herself in this situation. Where does a child learn violence, prejudice, or hate? These are not family values and neither is patriarchy. Incest is not a family value. Drunkenness is not a family value. *Father Knows Best* is a work of fiction—so might be family values. If there is love and respect, no one will argue. But we must be ever vigilant about loyalty and the toll it takes on women and children. We opened up the family. Let us keep it opened for the protection of the least powerful.

All I have shared with you is aimed toward empowering women and understanding the meaning of violence in our lives. War zones are where the powerful demoralize and dehumanize the less powerful. Women have enormous strength, but they must have places to say the unsaid, and women must feel safe. We cannot and we have not gone backwards. We must continue to move forward. Our consciousness is sometimes raised through tragic experience. Women must raise the consciousness of men. Another woman's rape is my rape and a man's mother's rape or his wife's rape by another man or his daughter's rape. Men need to know that they are intimately related by blood to women. Power is power. Do they want someone to use that power on the women of their blood, on the women whom they care for and about? Let us keep the family of humans open to values that are about survival and the quality of existence.

Dialogues have started. Bills have been passed. It will take a lot more— I would hope not with more bloodshed in the home, in our cities, in the country, in the world, but I am not naive. The power differential must shift. We must be very vigilant to its various appearances and attempts to maintain it. We must critically analyze this concept of family values. And we must allocate greater funding for a war against violence. In fact, a war against violence is an oxymoron. We must allocate greater funding to find ways to channel violent energy toward working for peace. How many times must it be said? How many women must be degraded? How many children must die? To answer this question we must continue our work. We must be heard around the world.

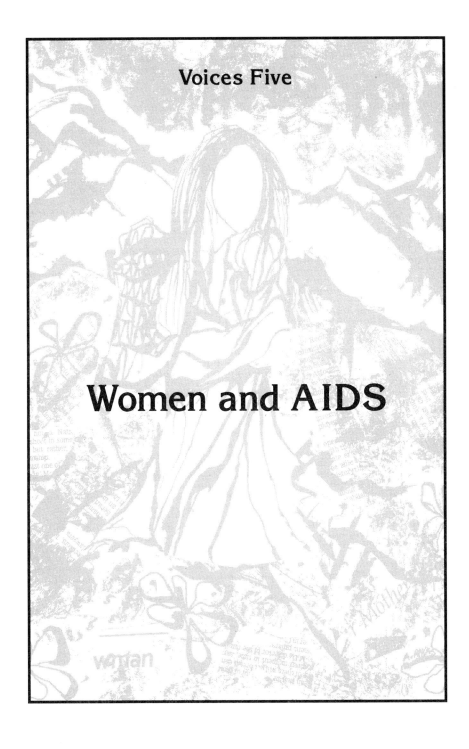

Voices Five

Women and AIDS

14

Beliefs and Attitudes about AIDS: Tatuape Adolescent Clinic, Sao Paulo, Brazil

Veronica Magar

*I*n Sao Paulo, the highest number of reported AIDS cases are among adolescents. Between 1983 and 1992, 1,532 females and 7,241 males between the ages of 20 and 29 were reported to have AIDS. Adolescent females are the emerging new high-risk group. In 1985, the ratio of males to females with AIDS was 38:1. In 1992, the ratio increased to 4:1 (Paiva, 1992). The largest number of cases are in the 20 to 24 and the 25 to 29 age range. To a large extent, these cases have been exposed during their teen years. Of the group reported to have AIDS, as many as 37% of the adolescent females contracted AIDS from heterosexual contact and over half (52%) from intravenous drug use (Centro de Vigilancia Epidemiologica,

SES-SP). Teens from this area face the added risk of poverty, violence, and gender discrimination.

I conducted a descriptive survey at the Tatuape teen clinic located on the periphery of Sao Paulo to determine adolescent girls' attitudes, risk perception, beliefs and reported behavior related to HIV/AIDS. I selected Tatuape clinic because it is a public sector clinic that integrates family planning, prenatal, STD, and child-health services in a holistic framework. The clinic's multidisciplinary team includes gynecologists, pediatricians, a urologist, social workers, a literature professor, and a psychologist. The team explored and created innovative and effective kinds of interventions within the clinic setting.

Tatuape Adolescent Clinic

Descriptive survey
  • Attitudes
  • Risk perception
  • Beliefs
  • Behavior
Integrated services
  • Family planning
  • STD/RTI
  • Pediatrics
Multidisciplinary staff
  • Gynecologists
  • Pediatricians
  • Urologist
  • Social workers
  • Literature professor
  • Psychologist

Clients are monitored with close follow-up. It is not unusual to see first-time clients as young as 13 years old. They are generally seen for a first pregnancy and subsequently followed over the course of 10 years for family planning, prenatal care, RTIs, and for well-child care for their children who are attended by the pediatrician. Clients describe the clinic as the only place they can go for help and have often said that the supportive atmosphere and the continuity of care draws them back.

METHODS AND RESULTS

The sample group includes 42 sexually active adolescent females between the ages of 12 and 20, attending the clinic between July 15, 1993 and August 15, 1993. This sample represents the clinic population only.

After conducting informal qualitative interviews, we administered in-depth, face-to-face interviews with open- and close-ended questions. We met with clients for 25- minute private interviews in an area outside the clinic waiting area before they saw the physician.

The average age of attenders in the sample was 17, and their average age of first sexual contact was 15. The average family income was less than US$200 per month and over a third of the adolescents worked and contributed to the family income. Most live in small communal quarters with other family members. The majority (68%) live with their mothers who are single parents.

In response to interview questions almost all (90%) of them said that they had someone in whom they could confide: 38% said that this person was their mother, 24% said husband or boyfriend, 26% said friend. According to the social workers, many have repeated their mother's adolescent history. Their mothers, who had been pregnant teens themselves, also faced the ridicule and discrimination these girls were facing from their fathers, brothers, and the community. Subsequently, many of these mothers became the sole social and economic support to their pregnant adolescent daughters just as their mothers had been to them.

Almost half the girls (42%) had never been pregnant, about a third (35%) were either pregnant or had a history of at least one full-term pregnancy, and the rest (23%) had an abortion. Excluding pregnant teens, almost half (47%) stated that they are currently using a contraceptive method, and only 3 of these said they used condoms as their method of birth control. Of ever-pregnant teens, only about one-quarter (26%) used a birth control method before becoming pregnant. Taken together, almost one-quarter of the clients use or used a condom to prevent pregnancy. Although 40% claimed that they currently use condoms, only one-quarter reported using a condom during their last sexual encounter. Condom use was found to be unpopular among the teens. The primary reason for not using condoms included, "my partner doesn't like to wear condoms" (20%); "I do not like condoms" (35%); "I trust my partner" (17%).

The adolescent girls attending Tatuape are well-informed about AIDS transmission and prevention. When asked what using condoms prevents, three fourths (74%) selected only and all the right answers (AIDS, STD, pregnancy), and the rest selected varieties of the correct answers. Like many teens worldwide, Brazilians have a high level of knowledge about AIDS that is not reflected in their behavior.

DISCUSSION

There are three cultural distinctions to keep in mind in terms of AIDS within the Brazilian context when addressing the reproductive health needs of adolescents:

Gender Character Conflict

Girls must remain virgins until they marry.

Brazil's colonial history of patriarchy and gender-biased beliefs maintains the feminine/passive and the masculine/active which has been well documented in Vera Paiva's research with Brazilian adolescents within the schools. Today, a woman is required to assertively confront her male counterpart in negotiating condom use for her own self-preservation. I believe that this conflict must be resolved in the broader framework of a woman's life rather than merely in the isolated and susceptible moments before sex. Condom negotiations, counseling, and support should be expanded to include all gender-related negotiations in a woman's life. AIDS educators should not be concerned only with a fleeting moment. If a woman is not empowered, she will not have a 5 to 10 minute transformation while she insists her partner wear a condom. It requires a commitment from those providing services to facilitate this empowerment.

An attitude reflected in the interviews demonstrated that to be male is to be aggressive without having to control personal sexual drives. It generally appears that men are excused from being "fair" or "honest" about their sexual lives, particularly if they are not married. Paiva's research with adolescent boys indicates that for boys to consider their partner's needs, by using a condom, is "artificial" and counter to "maleness." In response to the statement, "it is possible to believe what my partner tells me about his sexual past," over half (57%) disagreed.

On the other hand, many girls identified with the social pressure to be naive and acquiescent while having absolute control of personal sexual drives. Although things are changing in urban areas, maintaining virginity is the cultural ideal. One half of the teens believed that, in her neighborhood, a woman with a condom in her purse is considered "loose" or "easy." On several occasions, I was told that a condom identifies a woman as being sexually active with an eager interest in having sex. A single woman must always resist sex, but when she is married, she must always be ready and willing. Consequently, both in and outside of marriage many women have little sexual negotiating capability. Of our sample, 43% believe that it is too difficult to convince a partner to use a condom.

Permissible and Prohibited Sexuality

I don't use condoms because he is a good guy.

Most of our findings were consistent with other research. However, we found interesting results that should be considered when discussing AIDS with teens at Tatuape clinic. Paiva has documented that Brazilian adolescents generally believe that certain groups behave in ways that make them at high risk for HIV infection and that AIDS evokes a fear of contamination by "unhealthy," "inauspicious" people. This cultivates denial of personal vulnerability while also placing blame on "promiscuous practices" of people with AIDS. In our sample, a third of the group agreed with the statement, "Only homosexuals, bisexuals, and prostitutes get AIDS." When asked whether one can have AIDS and appear healthy, 83% agreed. However, when the question was placed in their own context, 60% claimed that a *limpinho* (clean) partner would be free of STD/HIV. In exploring meanings behind "clean," we discovered that a *limpinho* partner is "well groomed," "comes from a decent family," and is well behaved. By choosing such a partner, girls remain detached from the notion of their vulnerability to AIDS.

The "Ideal": Marriage and Motherhood

I want this baby so I can love him and he will love me.

Marriage and children are highly valued. Many stated that they wanted to be married or have children and face much pressure to get married. These girls must balance the social pressure to seduce their future husband and the maintenance of virginity in order to be marriageable. Motherhood is also essential in the construction of a woman's identity. In the field of family planning, we know that adolescent girls become pregnant for many reasons besides lack of knowledge and access to contraception. Often, having a child provides an illusionary "perfect love." A child symbolizes a teen mother's initiation into adulthood and womanhood. These subconscious intentions to become pregnant are in direct conflict with condom use to prevent HIV infection. Of those that were pregnant, not even a third used some kind of birth control prior to becoming pregnant.

In terms of risk perception, almost all of the girls stated that they were preoccupied with the possibility of getting AIDS and all felt that they could keep themselves from getting AIDS. Paradoxically, however, the majority claimed that their partner could not infect them with an STD. The majority do not use condoms; instead, they said they choose partners carefully.

CONCLUSION AND RECOMMENDATIONS

With the increasing threat of AIDS, adolescents may be expressing an "unrealistic optimism" generally common in Brazilian culture and especially among adolescents. While these girls fear getting AIDS, they also believe that they are protected through their choice of partners, loyalty to their partners or through their desire to maintain their virginity. These beliefs which often result in high-risk behavior are an outcome of their denial of actually engaging in sexual activity. Almost two thirds (60%) believed that a *limpinho* partner could not transmit STD/HIV. While most of the girls do not believe they can trust their partner to tell the truth about their sexual past, most do not believe that their partners can transmit an STD to them.

Because of the multidisciplinary nature of Tatuape clinic and the attention paid to holistic care, an AIDS prevention intervention can be easily adopted. A successful program must go beyond AIDS and HIV infection to direct messages effectively. I have concentrated on two important recommendations:

1. Placing AIDS prevention in a broader health context.

Parker describes Brazilian erotic ideology in the context of carnival and body exhibition. This takes place in a beach culture where passion, sex, and seduction are a central concern. Seduction, rather than medicalization of sex and condoms, is a key ingredient to success of a program in Brazil. In a clinic setting, issues such as AIDS must be addressed by also dealing with fertility awareness, sexuality, and contraception.

Condom negotiations must be addressed through self-esteem issues by looking at all aspects of a girls' life rather than merely the moment she must ask her partner to wear a condom. This also means that information about AIDS must be provided together with information about reproduction, contraception, and the body's erotic features.

2. Community-based education—a tradition in Brazil.

There has been documented success with using community-based education among adolescents, such as Paulo Freire's method of raising consciousness and Riviere's psychodrama techniques (Paiva). Tatuape has successfully incorporated these techniques related to pregnancy. In group interactive work, such as this, young women rise out of seclusion, become empowered and find solidarity as a way to overcome feelings of inadequacy. These are fundamental components to successful behavior change and maintenance.

3. Turning occasional condom use to conventional use.

In order to normalize condom use, health professionals should demonstrate the ways that condoms can be fun and experimental as well as serious.

Paiva has successfully used strategies that include making art, stories, songs, and games with condoms. These activities help make condoms touchable, ordinary, and even playful.

By examining attitudes and beliefs in terms of Brazilian sexual culture, outcomes regarding their perceived risks and self efficacy are useful in designing an educational strategy for this population.

REFERENCES

Centro de Vigilancia Epidemiologia (1993). Secretaria de Estado da Saude. *AIDS.* Sao Paulo: Estado de Sao Paulo.

Paiva, V. (unpublished paper). Sexuality, AIDS and gender norms among Brazilian teenagers. Sao Paulo: Universidade de Sao Paulo.

Williams, R. et al. (1992). HIV and adolescents: An international perspective. *Journal of Adolescence, 15:* 335-342. Estado de Sao Paulo.

15

Women Who Have HIV/AIDS Infection and Tuberculosis

Patricia R. Messmer and Jackie Moore

*T*he former U.S. Surgeon General, a Hispanic woman, Antonio Novello, M.D. (1995) expressed her concern about the impact of AIDS on women and minority groups. Novello further expounded that the number of infections recorded among racial and ethnic minority women is a national tragedy. There is a disproportionate increase in the number of cases of AIDS among women; in particular among African-American and Hispanic women who make up only 17% of the female population in the United States. In 1994, of the 79,674 persons aged 13 or older reported with AIDS, 14,081 (18%) occurred among women—nearly threefold greater than the proportion (534[7%] of 8153) reported in 1985; in addition, the proportion of cases among women has increased steadily since 1985. The median age of women reported with AIDS was 35 years, and women aged 15–44 years accounted for 84% of cases. More than three fourths (77%) of cases in women occurred among African-Americans and Hispanics, and rates for women in these groups were 16 and 7 times higher, respectively, than those for white women (MMWR, 1995).

124

The number of American women of childbearing age who are infected with HIV continues to climb, primarily because this is a sexually transmitted disease. Women also become infected through intravenous (IV) drug abuse as well as sexual contact with infected males who are IV drugabusers. As a result, AIDS cases attributed to heterosexual transmission are increasing faster than any other identified exposure risk. Heterosexual transmission now accounts for more than one-third (37%) of all cases among women (CDC, 1993). Over the next decades, heterosexual transmission will become the primary means of spreading HIV infection in most industrialized countries. Novello (1995) predicts that if these trends continue, the number of AIDS cases worldwide among women will begin to equal that of men by the year 2000.

Both in the United States and Europe, HIV-related tuberculosis has been closely associated with IV drug abuse (Casobona, 1990; Braun, 1990; Selwyn, 1995). This observation in part reflects high endemic levels of latent Mycobacterium tuberculosis infection in populations in which drug users are likely to be concentrated, although behavioral or other factors may also be involved. IV drug use was identified as a risk factor for tuberculosis before the AIDS epidemic; this risk factor did not appear to be explained simply by demographic or socioeconomic factors associated with drug use (Reichman, 1979). A more recent report described an association between tuberculosis and crack use, possibly due to environmental factors facilitating transmission of this respiratory spread disease, (tuberculosis) in poorly ventilated crack houses or other settings in which cocaine is smoked (CDC, 1993). This may be a particularly important risk factor for the subgroup of HIV-infected, drug-using women who are heavy crack users, engaging in sex-for-drug exchanges in crack houses and thus being at risk for tuberculosis through this environmental exposure. In addition, this group is equally at risk for sexually transmitted diseases (Chiasson, 1992; Chirgwin, 1991).

The early clinical manifestations of HIV infection are different in women than in men. In many women, the initial manifestations center around the genital area. The most common gender-related manifestations of HIV infection are vulvovaginal candidiasis, pelvic inflammatory disease, and cervical dysplasia (DeHovitz, 1995). In many cases, an earlier diagnosis is made in women due to their receiving annual gynecological examinations or prenatal examinations because of pregnancy, which usually includes STD screening (i.e., Hepatitis B, gonorrhea, syphilis, genital herpes, chlamydia, and HIV). In urban areas, reactivated tuberculosis can often appear in an immuno-compromised, HIV-infected patient. Therefore skin testing for tuberculosis should be routine at the earliest clinical visit for women at high-risk, (i.e., drug abusers, prostitutes, and recent immigrants from endemic areas). The Mantoux test (5 units of purified protein derivative) is the preferred test and an induration of 5 mm. or more is considered positive in HIV-infected patients (Selwyn, 1995). However, as the CD4 cell count declines, skin test anergy is common and patients with latent or active risk for tuberculosis should receive prophylactic isoniazid therapy (Selwyn, 1992). HIV-infected patients with tuberculosis typically present with pulmonary disease, although extrapulmonary manifestations are not uncommon, such as lymphatic, renal, etc. (Currier, 1995). Appropriate therapy should be determined by the frequency and pattern of drug-resistant strains present in contacts or the community.

According to the 1993 statistics in Dade County, Florida, 72 of the 246 reported cases of tuberculosis in HIV-infected people, were women, with a large number of those among African-American and Hispanic women. Preliminary data analysis for 1994 statistics, indicate a further increase among these minority groups of women. The following two cases admitted to our facility are characteristic of these epidemiological facts. The following case histories and course of disease for two minority HIV+/AIDS infected women who acquired tuberculosis are provided.

The first case was AC, a 38-year-old African-American female, who stated that she acquired her disease from her HIV-infected husband who had a history of IV drug abuse. AC denied all other risk factors. Although AC indicated that they practiced protected sex since her husband was diagnosed HIV+, AC also became infected. AC has a 15-year-old daughter in good health. AC was employed as a night nurse in a large teaching medical center community clinic facility for chronically ill children.

AC was first diagnosed HIV+ in December, 1990, after her second episode of shingles was evaluated at an eye institute. AC was started on Zidovudine in February, 1991, since her CD4 count was 290 mm³. AC had a febrile reaction to Bactrim in the past, so Dapsone was her prophylaxis for pneumocystis. AC was advised of chronic "patchy infiltrates" apparent in her chest x-ray and was bronchoscoped in March, 1991, yielding a diagnosis of lymphoid interstitial pneumonitis. AC's PPD was negative in February, 1991, but she was anergic. AC was also advised that her liver function studies had been abnormal.

In February, 1993, AC was admitted to our facility with a diagnosis of presumptive pneumocystis pneumonia with mild to moderate severity, and placed on respiratory isolation. This diagnosis subsequently was determined to be pulmonary mycobacterium tuberculosis for which AC was treated with a four drug therapy consisting of Isoiazaid (INH), Rifampin, Pyridoximide, and Ethanbutol. AC's other medications included Zidovudine, Dapsone, Retrovair, Pyrazinamide, Multivitamins with iron and Vitamin C. AC was discharged a month later and followed as an outpatient. There was a steady decline in T4 count and Zalcitibine was added to her regimen in March, 1993. AC's liver function enzymes were followed closely.

In June, 1993, AC was admitted through the Emergency Department in our facility with a two-week history of progressive shortness of breath and left-sided pleuritic chest pain without any other respiratory problems. The week prior, AC had experienced an intermittent fever of 102 degrees and was seen by her Infectious Disease physician who found her to have an O_2 of 83% on ambient air. The physician instructed her to use Albuterol and Beclomethasone inhaler. At that time, AC refused admission to the medical center because she felt capable to manage both at home and work and did not wish to take time away from her job or family.

One week later, however, her worsening respiratory problems and fever necessitated AC to be admitted to our facility. On admission, AC was alert and oriented in all spheres and exhibited no focal deficits with vital signs: B/P-^{100}/72, pulse-12, respirations-30, and temperature-101.4. ABG showed a ph of 7.42, PCO_2 of 31.5, PO_2 of 46, and O_2 saturation of 88%. The chest x-ray showed interval worsening of bilateral interstitial infiltrates when compared with previous examination one week earlier. AC's last CD4 count was 57 mm^3. AC was diagnosed with pneumoncystis carini pneumonia and started on Solu-Medrol 20 mg. IV q 6 hr and was given supplemental O_2 five liters via nasal cannula which maintained an O_2 saturation of 90%. AC was started on Pentamide IV 200 mg. daily and sputums were collected for lab analysis. AC was discharged one week later with IV Pentamide via a heparin loc, Solu-Medrol, Dapsone, AZT, INH, Rifampin, and Pyridoxine. AC improved rapidly and was followed closely at home by the private physician. AC returned to work approximately two weeks later.

Although the nurses caring for AC provided the standard supportive care, they seemed to identify more personally with AC because she was a nurse, and a very gentle caring professional. AC was an excellent patient who displayed a courageous and accepting attitude toward her illness and understood the importance of participating in her nursing and medical care. AC was anxious to return to caring for her daughter and resume her position in the community clinic. AC was one of the first patients admitted to the newly opened Special Immunology Unit. The nurses assigned to her care were in the transitional stage of receiving specialized education about all aspects of HIV/AIDS infections. Although the nurses were knowledgeable about HIV/AIDS, most of the nurses had not cared for a tuberculosis patient and had not received an updated educational program focused on tuberculosis as it related to the AIDS patient. Tuberculosis was thought to be declining prior to the AIDS epidemic and many nurses were apathetic about the consequences. Thus, AC served as a reminder to the nurses of the risks associated with the resurgence of tuberculosis which was very real and lethal, posing an occupational hazard to all nurses.

In a follow-up interview, AC stated that she had returned to work, but was serving in an administrative capacity on a part-time basis, working three days a week on the day shift. The change in her employment had reduced her stress level, and the change helped her maintain her physical well-being. AC related that she had experienced a bout of depression early in her illness at income tax time due to financial problems. AC felt this had a negative effect on her recovery during her first hospitalization in February, 1993. AC re-evaluated her life situation and changed her outlook on life to a more positive attitude and decided "to turn everything over to God." This positive attitude was evident during her second hospitalization in June, 1993, and made a tremendous difference in her early recovery. Since the second hospitalization in June, AC had another bout with pneumonia that lasted 3 days but was treated by the private physician. AC has a very optimistic attitude about her illness and prognosis. AC was very complimentary of the nursing and medical care she received during her two hospitalizations on the Special Immunology unit. AC strongly advocates that patients must participate in their medical and nursing care and try to do whatever they can for themselves to improve their "quality of life."

The second case involved MM, a 29-year-old Hispanic white female with an eight-year medical history of HIV positive status. MM, who lived in Puerto Rico, complained on admission that she had been suffering with high fevers, shortness of breath, chills, and cough for three weeks. MM had come on vacation to Miami a week prior to visit her mother and other relatives. MM also reported associated vomiting, nausea, and diarrhea for the past 8 to 10 days. MM had a productive cough and was unable to keep any form of liquid down. MM also complained of fatigue and malaise. MM's husband had AIDS and had died six months earlier. MM's husband also had been treated for tuberculosis. In addition, MM admitted to cocaine use but denied any needle sharing. MM had two children age 12 and 14 living at home in Puerto Rico.

On admission to our facility, MM's vital signs were: B/P-105/62, pulse-114, respirations-24, temperature-105 degrees and she was placed on Respiratory Isolation. ABG showed a ph of 7.49, PCO_2 of 28, PO_2 of 92, and Bicarbonate was 21. MM was tested in 1992 for PPD and found to be positive for which she was treated prophylactically with INH for six months. MM had a very complex and lengthy hospital stay. MM was diagnosed with tuberculosis and treated with Rifampin, Isoniazid, and Pyrazinamide. While hospitalized, MM developed a high-grade fever due to Candida sepsis and was treated with Amphotericin B. Simultaneously MM developed renal failure, with an elevated BUN and creative, secondary to pre-renal insufficiency. At that time the Amphotericin was discontinued and treatment changed to Fluconazole. MM's developed pancreatitis as evidenced by elevated levels of amylase and lipase. MM was placed on "nothing by mouth" but was very noncompliant, frequently sneaking *food against the nurses' and physicians' advise. MM would tell the nurses that the physicians allowed her to snack on apples which was not the case. MM was then placed on parenteral nutrition and she improved, at a steady pace. MM then became compliant and cooperative. MM developed anemia with very low hemoglobin and hematocrit and required blood transfusions. As MM's condition deteriorated, MM chose to be placed on "Do Not Resuscitate" (DNR) status. The doctors and nurses discussed this issue at great length with MM and her mother. The nurses found it extremely challenging to provide nursing care for MM because of her very uncooperative and noncompliant behavior, often refusing medications and treatments and at times complaining about her care.*

After a month, MM eventually became hemodynamically and cardiovascular stable. Thus, MM and her mother requested that she be transferred back to her home in Puerto Rico for further care so that she could be close to her two children. MM expressed the desire to die in her homeland near her children. On the day of transfer, MM was very weak and in poor condition and her prognosis was very poor. MM was transported by air ambulance with the following medicines: Fluconazole, Topical zinc oxide, INH, Rifampin, Vitamin B-6, Monistat vaginal suppositories, Benadryl, Zofran, and Vancomycin. Although parenteral nutrition was discontinued during transport, it was restarted at the receiving facility. The status after discharge is unknown; however, it is presumed that MM died in Puerto Rico.

These two cases demonstrate the challenges faced by nurses caring for women with AIDS diagnosed with tuberculosis. In the cases presented, one patient exhibited a positive attitude toward her diagnosis and prognosis, while the other patient displayed negative and noncompliant behaviors. Both received the same quality of care and support.

As Novello (1995) expressed so eloquently:

Women—even when they are sick—are asked to take care of their families. I believe the time has come to ask: who will take care of them? Although we may not know all the answers, a vital step is an increasing awareness among those who serve women regarding the complex circumstances faced by women at risk, or living with HIV/AIDS. None of us can ignore the impact of AIDS on women. Each of us must do more to fight the spread of this epidemic among women and care for those who are ill (xiv).

It does not help the situation to further burden the load of a woman diagnosed with AIDS to be told that she has the additional diagnosis of tuberculosis and the fact that this infection may be passed on to her loved ones through a casual kiss.

REFERENCES

Braun, M., Byers, R., Heyward, W., et al. (1990). Acquired immunodeficiency syndrome and extrapulmonary tuberculosis in the United States. *Archives Internal Medicine 159*, 1913-1916.

Casobona, J., Bosch, A., Salas, T., Sanchez, E., & Segura, A. (1990). The effect of tuberculosis as a new AIDS definition criteria in epidemiological surveillance data from South European areas. *Journal Acquired Immune Deficiency Syndrome 3*, 272-277.

Centers for Disease Control and Prevention. (1993). Update: Acquired immunodeficiency syndrome—United States, 1992 *MMWR42*, 547-557.

Chiasson, M., Stoneburner, R., Hildebrand, D., Ewing, W., Telzak, E., & Jaffed, H. (1991). Heterosexual transmission of HIV-1 associated with the use of smokable freebase cocaine (crack) *AIDS 5*, 1121-1126.

Chirgwin, K., DeHovitz, J., Dillion, S., & McCormack, W. (1991). HIV infection, genital ulcer disease and crack cocaine use among patients attending a clinic for sexually transmitted diseases. *American Journal of Public Health 81*, 1567-1579.

Currier, J. (1995). Medical management of HIV disease in women. In H. Minkoff, J. DeHovitz, & A. Duerr (Eds.), *HIV infection in women* (pp. 57-71). New York: Raven Press.

DeHovitz, J. (1995). Natural history of HIV infection in women. In H. Minkoff, J. DeHovitz, & A. Duerr (Eds.), *HIV infection in women* (pp. 57-71). New York: Raven Press.

MMWR. (1995). Update AIDS among women—United States, 1994 *MMWR45* (5), 81-82.

Novello, A. (1995). Women and AIDS. In H. Minkoff, J. DeHovitz, & A. Duerr (Eds.), *HIV infection in women* (pp. xi-xiv). New York: Raven Press.

Reichman, L., Felton, C., & Edsall, J. (1979). Drug dependence: A possible new risk factor for tuberculosis disease. *Archives Internal Medicine 139*, 337-339.

Selwyn, P., O'Connor, P., & Schottenfield, R. (1995). Female drug users with HIV infection. In H. Minkoff, J. DeHovitz, & A. Duerr (Eds.), *HIV infection in women* (pp. 241-262). New York: Raven Press.

16

Women Living with HIV/AIDS: The Third Wave

David Anthony Forrester

I do get tired and wonder
When my change is going to come.
But if the Lord says so
And the creek don't rise I know
I'll get better, better.

—*Maya Angelou*
Now Sheba Sings the Song,
(1994)

Women meet many complex challenges in their search and struggle for peace, equality, and personal development. It is within their situated contexts that women must strive to meet their personal challenges and obtain their future fulfillment. There is no greater challenge than living day-to-day within the context of a terminal illness. In fact, there can be no greater threat to the "personhood" of women than a stigmatized illness that destines them for eventual death. And yet, every day women meet this challenge with grace and dignity. They prevail—they must.

BACKGROUND AND SIGNIFICANCE

The human immunodeficiency virus (HIV) and the acquired immune deficiency syndrome (AIDS) it causes clearly pose some of the most compelling challenges imaginable. Some are unique to HIV/AIDS; some are common to other serious illnesses as well. For women, the issues raised by HIV/AIDS are amplified by the urgency associated with this rapidly evolving global pandemic and the complex psychological, political, legal, and social problems it engenders. For this and future generations of women, the ultimate challenge of HIV/AIDS will be to provide sensitive, compassionate care while balancing individual rights and liberties against issues of public health (Forrester, 1994).

In the United States, following gay men and intravenous drug users, women represent the third and most far reaching epidemiological wave of the evolving global HIV/AIDS pandemic. AIDS is spreading almost six times as quickly among women as it is among men, and disease transmission is fastest among black and Hispanic women. Worldwide, 50% of all new HIV infections are among women. New AIDS diagnoses are increasing at an annual rate of 17% among American women, compared to 3% for the nation's population as a whole (*The Advocate*, 1995).

DESIGN AND SAMPLE

This study is an exploration of some issues of importance to women with HIV/AIDS. Its existential/phenomenological design entailed investigator-conducted, confidential, unstructured, audiotape interviews of a racially diverse sample of 12 urban women either alone or in groups for no more than one hour's duration. These women were contacted through the investigator's nursing practice and community service activities. Physical and psychological safety, informed consent, and confidentiality were guaranteed.

These 12 urban women, living in the mid-Atlantic United States, were HIV-infected and had been diagnosed with AIDS for at least one year. Their ages ranged from 20 to 59 years with a median age of 28.9. Their ethnicity was black (8; 67%), Hispanic (3; 25%), and white (1; 8%). Their exposure categories were intravenous drug use combined with heterosexual contact

(8; 67%), intravenous drug use only (2; 17%), heterosexual contact only (1; 8%), and other/unknown (1; 8%). Ten (83%) of these women had dependent children living in their home.

FINDINGS

There is in every true woman's heart a spark of heavenly fire, which lies dormant in the broad daylight of prosperity, but which kindles up and beams and blazes in the dark hour of adversity.
                                                                    —*Washington Irving*
                                        "The Wife," The Sketch Book of Geoffrey Crayon
                                                                    (1819-1820)

The following are some of the salient themes and issues identified by the women participating in this investigation. They are accompanied by interview exerpts. For these women, issues of concern were an outgrowth of the psychologic and social stresses of living with HIV/AIDS.

Psychologic Stresses

Perhaps the major *psychologic stress* expressed by these women living with HIV/AIDS is their knowledge that they have an incurable illness that holds the potential for rapid decline and death. Their expressions of fear, anxiety, loss and grief, guilt, dependence, depression, and powerlessness and vulnerability were compounded by the uncertainty of the course of their disease.

Fear was universal among these 12 women with AIDS. Generally, expressions of fear centered around disease progression and diminished capacity. Specific expressions of fear were associated with fear of contagion, disfigurement, and death.

The progressive effects of HIV/AIDS, including symptoms, debilitation, and disability, figured prominently in almost all of these women's expressions of fear. One woman said, "I'm tired all the time—even on my 'good days.' I'm so afraid that I won't be able to get out anymore—afraid I won't be able to take care of my kids." Another woman said, "Every day that passes brings new worries. I'm afraid of every infection . . . I'm afraid every time that this may be the one that kills me."

A number of the women in the study expressed fear of contagion, and usually related to contracting opportunistic infections from others. For example, "I'm afraid everywhere I go that someone will sneeze or cough on me and that I'll get sick again. I don't go out a lot of times because of this." Occasionally their fears had to do with infecting others, even if they believed these fears were irrational. For example, "I've had other friends with AIDS and I haven't been afraid of them. But now that I have it [AIDS], I think sometimes that I'm afraid I'll give it to somebody else . . . I worry about my kids. I worry about using the same shower as them . . . using the same soap . . . letting them drink after me. I know I shouldn't worry about this, but I can't help it."

Fear of disfigurement for themselves and others was also mentioned. "I'm afraid every time I look in the mirror about what I might see. Every change is worse. My clothes don't fit . . . I don't look like me anymore," said one woman. And, "Other people I see [in the clinic] are changing too. I see it almost every time I go. So many people I don't even know begin to look like living skeletons. Sometimes it goes for a long time and then I don't see them . . . they just evaporate."

Whether overtly or covertly, fear of death was expressed by several of these women. One woman said, "When I first found out I was HIV-positive, I thought . . . Oh my God, I'm going to die!" Another woman reported, "Sometimes I feel like I'm already dead. Things move so fast—with or without me. I'm scared!"

Anxiety was expressed by almost all of these women. "I'm always nervous . . . nervous about everything, my health, the bills, the kids . . . everything. I'm never alone that I'm not worrying about something to do with AIDS."

Ambivalence was a feature of the psychologic stress expressed by a number of these women. One woman said, "It's hell if I do and hell if I don't . . . I don't know what's better, being sick—getting the treatments and taking my medicine, or being well [symptom free] and worrying about what's next." Another said, "Sometimes I'm actually glad I have it [AIDS]—at least I know. But then I think—no, nobody wants this . . . I hate it."

Loss and grief, including denial, anger, bargaining, resolution, and mortality awareness and value of life were common features of these women's experiences with HIV/AIDS. This grief was for perceived losses already experienced and anticipated losses. There seemed to be dimensions of both anticipatory and post mortem grief. For example, one woman said, "It seems so long ago that I was normal—healthy . . . I miss just being normal. I'd give anything if I could go back to just being normal." And, "I've had so many people [friends] die. I haven't been able to think about them so much now . . . I used to think about them a lot—before I got sick. Now I think about my kids. I don't want to lose them. I don't want to be taken away from them."

One woman described her shock and disbelief and subsequent denial upon learning of her HIV-positive status by saying, "How could this happen? There must have been some mistake!" Later, upon learning of her AIDS diagnosis, "I just couldn't believe my ears . . . I was numb—still am. I still just can't believe it!"

Frank anger was expressed by several of these women. It was sometimes expressed as time-limited and undirected anger leading to social isolation such as, "I went for a while there when I was mad at everyone and everything. I've never been so mad—and I didn't really know why. I just knew I was mad and that everybody should stay away from me. And they pretty much did [stay away]." Some of these women also expressed anger as being vague and ever present. For example, "I walk around tied up in knots about half the time. I want to hit something . . . hurt someone, but I don't know what or who."

At least one woman expressed anger and feelings of inner turmoil that were self-directed, "I hate my body for betraying me. I hate myself sometimes for giving in . . . for being weak." Yet another woman reported feelings of anger toward others, "I really hate other people sometimes just for being healthy. I'm jealous of them for that and I get mad at them."

Bargaining was a feature of at least one woman's experience of living with HIV/AIDS. She said, "I used to pray for Jesus to give me the strength to get off drugs . . . [I used to] think that if I could only get straight, maybe he would let me keep my life like it used to be. Now, I pray every day that he'll let me live. I try to make little deals with him every day if I can stay well, get better and live longer."

Resolution regarding their diagnosis and the probable eventuality of death was mentioned by several of these women living with AIDS. One woman said, "Once other people knew about my sickness, it was easier for me to accept it. It was like telling my secret [and] getting this huge weight off my shoulders. I was relieved and now I live with it [AIDS] better." Another woman said, "I know I'm going to die. I don't know really when or how, but I know I'm going to die of AIDS. Of course it bothers me, but not like it did at first. I've just come to accept it . . . I'm not giving up though. I'm still fighting it."

Increased mortality awareness and value of life were also of concern to several of the women in the study. "I'm just glad to be alive. I looked out my window last night at the moon through the trees and I was overwhelmed by the beauty and how lucky I am to be here to see it. Even though it hasn't been a hard winter . . . not like last winter—I still want to see spring. Life is so beautiful; it just means so much more to me now."

A number of these women living with HIV/AIDS expressed feelings of guilt. Some were experiencing guilt over behaviors which, as they perceived them, had placed them at risk of contracting HIV. For example, one woman with a history of intravenous drug use said, "I try to remember to be mad at the virus, but it doesn't always work. I keep thinking that it's my fault I have AIDS. If I had been able to get straight maybe this wouldn't be happening." Another woman expressed guilt over transmission of HIV to her children, "Now my babies have it. I don't know what to do for them. I feel like it's my fault; I don't know what to do."

Dependence, especially regarding care givers, health professionals, and the health care delivery system as a whole, was also mentioned. Comments often had to do with their perception that the "system" was in some way failing them. "Sometimes I don't think they [health professionals] know how much we [people with AIDS] are depending on them. I feel like I'm at their mercy for everything. I try not to let them know [that I feel this way] because I'm afraid they might use it against me . . . I know this is paranoid. I don't think they can really do very much for me anyway . . . I'm always hearing why this or that can't happen. Sometimes I want to shake them so they'll know that I'm counting on them. I have to count on them a lot."

Depression, episodic or continuous, was described by every woman interviewed. Expressions of depression included the entire continuum ranging from a sense of discouragement, to sadness, to impulsive thoughts and behavior such as suicidal ideation. One woman said, "I try to 'have good days' like you hear about—but I can't. I can't get away from having AIDS—it doesn't go away. There are no 'good days' because you can't forget you have AIDS. I'm so depressed; it's been that way for a long time." Another woman reported, "Once I finally got tested and found out I really had AIDS, I couldn't stand it . . . I just wanted to kill myself. If it hadn't been for my kids, I think I would have."

Powerlessness and vulnerability were expressed by these women in virtually every aspect of their lives. Feelings of helplessness, hopelessness and loss of control were frequent. These not only had to do with their health but their day to day lives. "It feels like I'm always the last to know what's going on in my life . . . When I see the doctor, sometimes I'm almost home before I think, 'I don't really know what she's doing to take care of me.' I mean, I'm out of the room and talking to the nurse before I'm told what the plan is. Most of the time, I just do what they tell me. I think a lot of other people [with AIDS] do better at telling the doctors and nurses what to do instead of [it being] the other way around like it is with me. I think they may do better . . . you know, get more and stay better."

Social Stresses

The major social stresses expressed by these women with HIV/AIDS included disclosure, stigmatization, prejudice, discrimination, alienation, and rejection and abandonment. These social stresses seemed to be subjectively experienced as fear, anger, and guilt as previously described, as well as human reduction and suspicion as described below.

A number of the women in the study expressed social concern regarding their disclosure of having HIV/AIDS in the community. Their concerns had to do with both self-disclosure and fear of others' disclosure of their illness within their family, friends, health care providers, and their larger social community. Their expressions of these concerns included a full spectrum, ranging from personal relief of finally being able to openly discuss their situations with others, to frank fear of the real or imagined repercussions of others' knowledge of their diagnosis. "When I first found out about my HIV, I didn't want anyone to know . . . and then, more and more, I just had to tell them—I couldn't keep it in anymore."

Several of these women felt that due to the physical changes they had experienced, they simply had no option as to whether or not they disclosed their illness to others. "My mother saw how much weight I lost and she would look at me funny . . . and ask me why. I didn't have any choice; I didn't have the energy not to tell her I had HIV."

Public identification as a person with HIV/AIDS also invites stigmatization. A number of the participants in the study were concerned about the social stigma associated with their illness. Comments such as, "I didn't think of myself as 'disabled' until I heard the social worker refer to my 'disability.' I don't like being thought of as disabled. I know that, technically—legally, I am [disabled]; but I still don't like it." And, "I don't always think of myself as a person with AIDS. Usually it's other people who think of me as an 'AIDS patient.' And always, they want to know how I got it. Some people ask about it in a round about way, but it always comes up . . . and soon. Sometimes I tell them I'm a gay man just to see what they'll say. It's surprising how many people pause. Some even say OK."

All of the women participating indicated that they felt that they had born the burden of HIV/AIDS prejudice of others. One woman reported, "I even feel it [HIV/AIDS prejudice] here [in the AIDS support group]. It's like it's the IV drug users versus the 'innocent' hemophiliacs or the straight sex partners versus the gay men. We even do this to ourselves and each other . . . If the 'IVDUs' take too much from the clothing bank or get ahead in the dinner line, we're looked down on." Another woman said, "Everyone I know with AIDS has lost something more than their health. They've lost friends, families, their homes, their jobs . . ."

Almost all of these women said that they had experienced some form of HIV/AIDS discrimination. This discrimination was not always directed at these women alone. For example, one participant said, "When my little girl's friends found out that her mother has AIDS, they were mean to her. You know how they [children] can be. Even her friends were ridiculed by the other children just for staying friends with my daughter. My little girl even thinks the teachers at her school reinforce this negative attitude. They may not say anything bad directly to my little girl, but I don't always think they try to help her either."

Social alienation in some form or other was a frequent complaint. "I've noticed in the hospital and in the clinic that the nurses and doctors don't really want to touch me. They don't ever ask how I feel about anything." And, "Sometimes people I know, who know [about my diagnosis] are overly happy to see me—sort of too friendly but stand-offish at the same time. It's really weird, like they're trying too hard to be nice to somebody they really wish would go away." One woman put it this way, "I don't relate to people the way I used to. I'm not sure if it's me or them . . . probably it's both."

In at least two extreme instances, the prejudice, discrimination, and alienation experienced by women in this study resulted in actual rejection and abandonment by family, friends, and/or co-workers. At a time when these women most needed social support, comfort, compassion, and closeness, they felt alone and isolated. One 20-year-old woman, who was now sleeping on a friend's couch, said, "When my family found out [that I have AIDS], they just shut me out. They just didn't want anything to do with me anymore. I don't know if it will ever get better." Another woman said, "The only people who will really have anything to do with me now are here [in the AIDS support group]."

All of these women expressed some sense of human reduction. Typically their sense of diminished self had to do with feelings of devaluation, and perceived weakness or worthlessness. They blamed themselves as well as others for their feelings of being diminished. "Sometimes I want to hide under the covers and play like this isn't happening to me. I feel dirty . . . damaged—like I'm less than human." Another woman said, "A lot of times I think it's other people that make me feel bad about myself . . . like I'm not a real person . . . like I'm a third class citizen." These women's feelings of devaluation, whether arising from the self or others, frequently were related to expressions of anger and feelings of inner turmoil.

Suspicion was expressed by some of the women in the study. For example, "I don't think they [health providers] tell me everything. Oh, I don't mean they lie to me—I just don't always think they tell me the whole truth about how I'm really doing." One woman was suspicious that her family members weren't being completely honest with her, "They [my mother and children] sometimes stop talking when I come around. They just stop—like they're keeping secrets from me. Sometimes I ask what they're talking about; sometimes I don't."

HYPOTHESES

Empirical hypotheses can now be generated to detect, explore and test potential relationships between these women's expressions of their psychologic and social stresses related to HIV/AIDS and their own personal/social contingencies and situated contexts. Contingencies of interest to women with HIV/AIDS include, but are certainly not limited to, their: gender, race/ethnicity, health, politics, relationships, culture, religion, education, social conditions, and economic status. Situated contexts of note for women with HIV/AIDS include, among other considerations: space, time, physical and emotional self, and rationality.

The following are examples of some of the broad contexts within which empirically testable hypotheses can now be posited:

1. The potential relationships between women's expressions of psychologic and social stresses regarding HIV/AIDS should be identified and described. For example, the relationships between expressions of grief, depression, suicidal ideation (psychologic stresses) and expressions of alienation, discrimination, frustration (social stresses) are likely to be of value to women experiencing HIV/AIDS.

2. Once these relationships have been identified and described, they can then be studied in relation to certain landmark crisis points (situated contexts) in the course of disease progression in women with HIV/AIDS. For example, the shock, disbelief and denial of the grieving process as they relate to the initial crisis of HIV/AIDS diagnosis would be relevant to the women who participated in this study. Subsequent crisis points of treatment, discontinuance of treatment, recurrence and relapse of disease, pain and dementia would all be worthy of investigation within the situated contexts of time and emotional self.

3. These women's expressions of fear and anxiety regarding their children was compelling. Virtually all of these women, who were living with HIV/AIDS and who had children, asked, "What's going to happen to my children?" Fear for their children and the social stigma their children potentially must bear may contribute to feelings of

"powerlessness" and "invisibility." Moreover, the sense of frustration experienced by women living with HIV/AIDS who perceive that they are unable to fulfill their maternal roles may lead to deep feelings of loss, grief and despair. These relationships are in need of further scientific exploration.

CONCLUSION AND RECOMMENDATIONS

Woman is woman's natural ally.
—*Euripides,* Alope
(5th c. B.C.)

Women represent the third and perhaps most far reaching epidemiological wave in the global HIV/AIDS pandemic. The resonating themes regarding these women's search and struggle for peace, equality, and development have been made more evident through this investigation. These women, living with HIV/AIDS, share with all women the same fundamental needs for hope, safety and security within their environment. Unique to these women's experiences, however, are the contingencies and situated contexts within which they attempt to meet their personal challenges for present and future self-fulfillment.

These women's desire to maintain their sense of "personhood" and "normalcy" in their daily lives may make them reluctant to share expressions of their psychological stresses (including fear, anxiety, loss and grief, guilt, dependence, depression, and powerlessness and vulnerability) and social stresses (including disclosure, stigmatization, prejudice, discrimination, alienation, rejection and abandonment, human reduction, and suspicion). For example, for these women living with HIV/AIDS, the first and perhaps most difficult psychological and social issues had to do with their children and their childbearing potential. Fear and grief for the physical and psychological health of their children combined with the social stigma they and their children bear may keep women silent and, therefore, invisible in their struggle.

A global HIV/AIDS research, care and educational agenda must be established which acknowledges women's perspectives, experiences and contexts. Gaps in knowledge regarding women's situations who are living with HIV/AIDS should be made a top priority. The totality of the context within which these women live their daily lives needs to be identified, described, and integrated into an agenda which has three main objectives: (1) to prevent further HIV infection among women; (2) to provide humane care for women already living with HIV/AIDS; and (3) to engage women in national and international efforts to fight HIV/AIDS and its associated stigma.

REFERENCES

Forrester, D. A. (1994). The evolving HIV/AIDS pandemic: A study in stigmatization and its ethical challenges for nursing. In J. C. McCloskey & H. K. Grace (Eds.), *Current issues in nursing,* 4th ed. (pp. 725-730). Philadelphia: C. V. Mosby.

The Advocate. (1995, March 21). A changing face, p. 10.

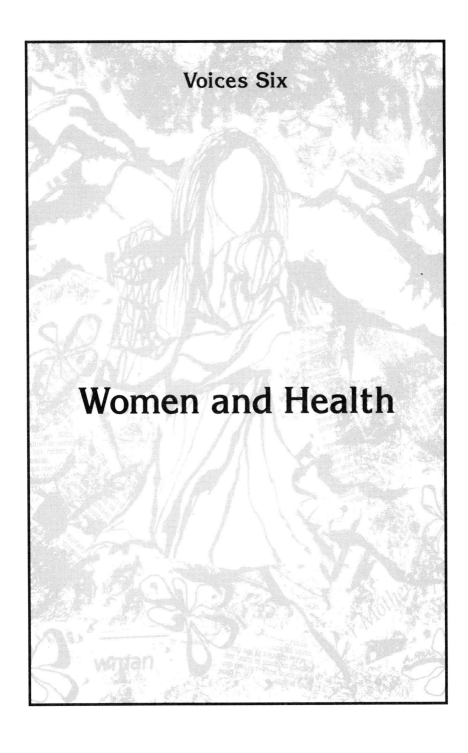

Voices Six

Women and Health

17

Assessing Well Women's Health: A Holistic Multidimensional Focus

Ellis Quinn Youngkin and Marcia Szmania Davis

*A*s women enter the next century, they face an ever-increasing life span, choice of opportunities and risks, and array of challenges and stressors. The assessment of a woman's health must be holistic. Indeed, all factors impinging on health and well-being must be considered to prevent significant omissions in detecting problems and offering care. Full opportunities for development and equality can only be promoted by this approach: "Wellness isn't a destination but a process" (Northrup, 1988). Women

Adapted with permission from Ellis Quinn Youngkin and Marcia Szmania Davis, WOMEN'S HEALTH: A Primary Care Clinical Guide, Appleton & Lange, Norwalk, CT, © 1994.

must become more attuned to their bodies and its cues, and the health care provider must use the assessment period as an opportunity for anticipatory teaching and counseling based on these cues.

CAUSES OF MORBIDITY AND MORTALITY IN AMERICAN WOMEN

In assessing any woman's health, the primary causes of women's mortality and morbidity, as well as related risk factors, should be considered. Understanding these influences enhances the assessment process and raises awareness of problem areas so that health-promoting and illness-preventing actions may be initiated.

Causes of death in American women differ significantly depending on age and race (U.S. Census Bureau, 1992). Young Women, 15 to 24, die most often from accidents and violence, with deaths from human immunodeficiency virus (HIV) rising rapidly. Cancer deaths (including HIV), heart diseases, and suicide begin to increase in young to mid-adulthood women, ages 25 to 44. Accidents and violence remain important causes, especially in African-American women.

Midlife to older adult women, ages 45 to 64, most frequently die from heart diseases, cancer, cerebrovascular diseases (CVD), chronic obstructive pulmonary disease (COPD), chronic liver diseases/cirrhosis, and diabetes mellitus. Accidents, violence, and suicide lessen slightly, but still remain significant causes. Suicide, highest among white women in all age groups as compared to other races, peaks between 45 and 64.

Women, 65 and over, have a dramatic increase in mortality from heart diseases, CVD, COPD, pneumonia, and diabetes. Accidents become a more serious cause again, and suicides lessen. Falls occur much more often among elderly women than men; 75% of deaths from accidental injury are from falls (Wyman, 1991).

White women have higher causes of death from COPD, motor vehicle accidents, and suicide (National Center, 1989). Deaths from homicides and legal interventions, HIV, heart diseases, CVD, and cancer (other than breast) are dramatically higher in African-American women. Asian and Pacific Islander women die most often from cancer (Horton, 1992).

Although the risk of dying from pregnancy and childbirth-related causes is very low in the United States (320 maternal deaths reported in 1989 and 3.8 million live births), nonwhite women are at a greater risk of death (threefold), and African-American women have the greatest risk (18.4 per 1000 live births as compared to 5.6 for white women) (Horton, 1992). Pregnancy-induced hypertension, hemorrhage, embolism, and ectopic pregnancy are the major causes of maternal death.

Lung cancer peaks at age 75 to 84; digestive system, breast, genital, blood-related, urologic, and oral cancers rise steadily from age 45 to peak in the 85 and older age group. (Census) The death rate for HIV quadrupled between 1985 and 1988 (Chu, Buehler, & Berkelman, 1990), and HIV-related deaths became one of the five leading causes of death for women age 15 to 44 in this country by 1991. Transmission from injection of drugs caused 46% of the AIDS deaths in women in 1990 (Horton, 1992). African-Americans had the highest incidence of AIDS deaths in women, followed by white, Hispanic, and others. Lung cancer became the leading cancer killer for white women in 1988 as women's rates of smoking reached all time highs. Smoking contributes to 25% of all the deaths from cancer in women.

All major causes of heart disease rise continuously from middle age through old age, with ischemic heart disease being the dramatic killer. Cardiovascular disease kills 500,000 U.S. women each year, yet until 1991, little research related to health issues for women, such as heart disease, had been done (Healy, 1992). Thirty-six percent of all deaths in women are due to heart disease (Horton, 1992). This major disease category must be considered in the assessment of every woman. NIH is now studying the relationships between diet, hormonal replacement therapy, exercise, and smoking and the major causes of death and disability in women.

For all acute conditions causing morbidity, except injuries, American women have a higher incidence than men. Infective and parasitic diseases, such as diarrhea, are more common in late adolescence through mid-adulthood, lessening after age 45. Upper respiratory diseases are more common in women under 45; lower respiratory diseases are more common in older women. Digestive tract diseases increase with age; irritable bowel syndrome is frequently seen.

The incidence of injuries, greatest in adolescence and young adulthood, decreases in middle adulthood, then increases again in older women. Heart diseases, hypertension, diabetes mellitus, and arthritis increase steadily in both sexes as they age with higher incidences in women. Other chronic conditions are more common in women than in men, such as constipation, abdominal hernia, urinary infections, migraine, sinusitis, asthma, hemorrhoids, and varicose veins. Osteoporosis along with heart disease and cancer are the three leading causes of disability in women after age 45 (Healy, 1992).

LEADING RISK FACTORS FOR WOMEN

An overall assessment of a woman's risk factors includes assessment of unsafe lifestyle behaviors, exposure to environmental hazards, negative

influences on emotional health, inadequate material resources, hereditary, cultural and ethnic influences, and current or past medical problems. Whether unhealthy behaviors or factors can be changed must be
evaluated.

Cigarette smoking is associated with lung disease/cancer, heart diseases, lowered estrogen levels, early menopause, cervical cancer, rapid
skin aging/wrinkling, and second-hand smoke risk to/from others (Stewart, Guest, Stewart, & Hatcher, 1987). Assessment includes what is
smoked, the number of cigarettes smoked per day for how many years, ill
effects, and others in the household who smoke and/or are affected. New
data indicts second-hand smoke in the development of respiratory disease.

Alcohol use is associated with cirrhosis, stroke, hypertension, accidents, an increased risk of cancer, use of other addicting drugs, and
psychosocial behavioral changes and their sequelae. Deaths related to alcohol use in women are primarily from cancer, cardiovascular disease, digestive disorders, and unintentional and intentional injuries. The use of
nicotine, caffeine, cocaine, marijuana, tranquilizers, and other substances is associated with health dangers for each. Damage to psychosocial relationships may be significant. Assessment includes the type of
substance, amount, years of use, unsafe associated behaviors, and effects.

Overuse of any medication may occur when clients fail to read or may
not be told warnings associated with excessive use of legal drugs. Examples include gastric mucosal irritation with nonsteroidal anti-inflammatory
agents (Bates, Bayer, Lang, & Ravinkar, 1986); and neurologic abnormali-
ties with excessive vitamin B6 ingestion (Schaumburg, Kapaln, Windebark,
et al., 1990).

Sedentary lifestyle and lack of exercise and personal fitness, associated
with cardiovascular, respiratory, gastrointestinal, and musculoskeletal
problems, require assessment. Exercise increases endorphins and improves the emotional health outlook. Americans tend to be very sedentary.

Nutritional excesses and deficits are associated with cancer, cardiovascular disease, diabetes, eating disorders, obesity, malnutrition, and deficiency diseases. Coronary artery disease in women is highly associated
with obesity (Manson, Colditz, Stampfer, et al., 1990). Binging, purging,
and anorexia are significantly more common in women (Plehn, 1990).
Clearly, nutritional assessment is essential.

Unsafe driving, inattention to precautions, and lapses in driving safety
are associated with a high level of morbidity and mortality for women up
to age 64, especially young women. Substance abuse, nonuse of protective devices (seatbelts), and reckless driving need to be assessed (Stewart
et al., 1987).

Violence is associated with homicide, suicide, sexual assault, physical
abuse/battering, and emotional trauma. Women are the most likely vic-

tims (Horton, 1992). Assessment should include asking about dangerous, conflictual relationships and living conditions (violent families/neighborhoods). Rape is the second leading violent crime. It is estimated that most rapes are unreported (Heinrich, 1987). Women who are young, single, students, African-American, and unemployed are at greater risk (Horton, 1992). Spouse abuse is anticipated in 66% of all marriages (Blair, 1986). African-American women are at a fourfold greater risk of homicide, often from partners, than white women. Elder abuse is a serious problem for older women with estimates ranging from 1% to 4% of the elderly (Horton, 1992).

Exposure to HIV, hepatitis, and sexually transmitted diseases may cause life-threatening, incurable, or disabling conditions. Assessment should include the frequency of sexual relations, the number of partners ever and currently, risk status of partners, forms of sexual expression, and use of barrier and chemical contraception.

Lack of health-directed behaviors, or poor personal care, is associated with a substandard health status and a lack of detection and prevention behaviors. Personal assessment should include breast self-exam, regular dental and eye exams, general screening physical exams, including pelvic examinations with pap smear and indicated cultures, vulvar self-examination, immunization status, and use of contraception and/or STD protection, and rectal examination with tests if indicated.

Inadequate, excessive, or unusual sleep is less a problem for women than for men (Ware, 1993). Assessment should evaluate breathing difficulties, snoring, smoking, neuroses, alcohol use, medication use, estrogen deficiency, time zone/shift changes, sleepwalking, stress and depression, heavy exercise near bedtime, and environmental conditions for sleep. Severe sleep apnea is related to possible cardiac arrest (Block, Nolan, & Dempsey, 1981).

Unsafe home environment encompasses falls, exposure to chemical/toxic/radon hazards, fire, excessive heat or cold, unsanitary living conditions, unsafe drinking water, lack of running water, rodent/insect infestation, and infections in crowded living conditions. Tuberculosis, which proliferates in crowded conditions, is on the rise again from the development of resistant strains of the causative organism and the deficient immune states of individuals with HIV infections.

Numerous occupational situations are associated with life-threatening, damaging, or debilitating conditions, such as asbestosis, lead poisoning, pesticide exposure, and radiation exposure. Assessment must include the individual's type of work, work hazards and conditions, and effects (Block et al., 1981).

Negative influences on emotional health vary widely from family crises to unrealistic values of thinness. Stress is associated with a wide array of physical and emotional problems. American women are increasingly stressed with multiple roles and pressures related to work, home, family, and other relationships. Crises in families are associated with increased physical and emotional risks for both the individual and the family. Assessment includes individual and family health, values, health care beliefs, cultural influences, stressors, and coping abilities. Poor or no support system is associated with feelings of loneliness, helplessness, hopelessness, and powerlessness. Social networks are known to decrease risks related to health associated with occupational stress, cancer, and pregnancy (Auslander, 1988). Assessment should include recent changes in life (such as marriage, divorce, birth, a move, a new job), distance from friends, relatives, cultural group, health resources, and access to support systems, such as church. Depression is associated with suicide, a leading cause of death in women. In the United States, depression is significantly related to social, psychological, and physical loss. Assessment includes typical signs and symptoms, such as eating/sleeping difficulties, unusual sadness, and suicidal thoughts.

The American ideal of youth, beauty, and slimness is associated with unhealthy, excessive concerns and behaviors relating to appearance. These concerns may also indicate an inability to accept the aging process. Assessment includes the client's appearance, age, weight, height, history of unusual or overuse of plastic/reparative surgery, diet and exercise history, and verbal or nonverbal cues, such as great concern with being overweight when in reality she is underweight. No recreational or relaxation activities is associated with stress, overwork, and anxiety, and possibly, depression. Assessment includes economic, social, physical, psychological conditions/barriers.

Being poor today is very much a problem of women and children, often called the "nouveau poor." Most adult welfare recipients are women (McElmurry, 1986). The fastest growing segment of homeless people is women and children. Poor people often delay seeking health care when ill, use fewer measures to prevent or decrease illness, have less information about health that is correct, and have fewer choices for access to health care. As women age, a greater chance for poverty exists. Assessment includes estimated income level, quality of nutrition and living conditions, untreated illnesses (acute and chronic), dental condition, disability, excessive sleep and sedentary living, depression and stresses associated with lifestyle, and inadequate self-concept and ability to change life. Choices for women are often limited due to family and child care needs.

Heredity, culture, and ethnic influences impact health. Familial diseases may be detected by assessing the family history of diseases such as diabetes, cardiovascular disease, and cancer. Significant health problems can be prevented or minimized by careful attention to family history. Some diseases are more common in certain races, such as osteoporosis in light- or yellow-skinned women, sickle cell disease in African-Americans; and G-6-PD deficiency in people of Mediterranean descent. Ethnic-cultural-religious influences may contribute to unhealthy practices. For example, eating uncooked meat, refusal to seek health care, lack of health-directed behaviors, and no understanding and/or education necessary for good health may be part of the client's ethnic, cultural, or religious beliefs.

Of particular concern are the risks of past and present medical problems, and the potential or real effects of current/past illness on new disease conditions. For example, recent research indicates a past history of smoking, even if the client no longer smokes, increases the risk of multiple myeloma by three-fold. Multiple drug interactions may cause increased risks and confusing presentations. This problem is often in the elderly, and is essential to assess.

THE HEALTH HISTORY

In taking the health history, good interview and interpersonal skills are required to gather accurate, useful data (Morton, 1993; Bates, 1991; Seidel et al., 1991; Fuller & Schaller-Ayers, 1990; & Eloipoulos, 1990). Any interaction with the client is considered a therapeutic intervention. Allow expression of issues/concerns; treat her with dignity and respect; be nonjudgmental, accepting, supportive, sensitive, and concerned; and be an appropriate role model.

Be clear and attuned to the client's level of understanding, culture, and background. Avoid medical jargon. Consider the client's age, education, response to the interview, and ethical-cultural-religious taboos. Clarify by restating confusing information. Use an interpreter, if necessary.

Open-ended questions used early in the interview promote broad information-gathering, are useful for mental status and general survey assessment, and provide an overview of the client's problems. Ask about her concerns; avoid interrupting her so that valuable data is not lost. Use pointed, directive questions to obtain specific data. Avoid leading questions, like "You've never had a STD, have you?" Phrase sensitive questions in a nonjudgmental manner: "How many partners do I need to notify about the risk of AIDS?" Note expressions, body movements, inability to make eye contact, reluctance to give information or avoidance of answering questions, and signs of anxiety. Such cues may indicate fears or concerns.

Physical and psychological factors affect the interaction. Provide a quiet, private place for the interview, if possible. Use measures to discourage others from intruding, such as a sign on the door. Allow the client to remain dressed during the interview. Provide eye-level, comfortable seating. Never obtain the history with the client in a prone position. Keep the interview focused to stay within a reasonable time limit. More than one session may be needed.

Components of the health history include:

- *Demographic-biographic data.*
- *Chief complaint (CC) or reason for visit.*
- *History of present illness or current health status.*
- *Past medical history or past health status.*
- *Family history.*
- *Psychosocial and personal history.*
- *Review of systems.*

Details of the interview techniques are covered in the reference materials.

SPECIAL ASSESSMENT GUIDES

- *Family assessment.* This appraisal involves assessing who lives in the home, relationships, cultural origins, religious preferences, health practices, education/occupation/role of each member, communication among members, home/money/material management, goals of the family, relaxation/recreational family activities, and strengths/weaknesses/conflicts/problems/past resolution methods (Morton, 1993; Berkley & Hanson, 1991). Use of an assessment tool is recommended. A shortened version (5 items) of the Family Environment Scale (FES) is reported to be useful for practice. The "Family APGAR" is another quick screening tool for identifying areas of difficulty with adaptability, partnership, growth, affection, and resolve in family (Sawin & Harrigan, 1994). The genogram is a family tree of a family's relationships, structure, health and other important data over a three generation period (Berkley & Hanson, 1991). Use effectiveness needs more research, but the visual picture provided may be helpful in identifying tendencies of conditions within families and, thus, risk factors for individual clients.
- *Nutritional assessment.* A 24-hour diet recall of food/drink intake for balance and adequacy of nutrients and fluids is indicated. For

nonpregnant, nonlactating women, governmental dietary guidelines suggest a daily intake of the following, with lower numbers for less active and/or older women (U.S. Department of Agriculture, 1992):

Bread/Cereal Rice/Pasta, 6-9 servings; Meats/Poultry Fish/Dried Beans/Eggs, 2-3 servings, up to total of 6 or less ozs; Milk/Dairy Products, 2-3 servings, such as 1 c. milk, $1\frac{1}{2}$ ounces cheese; Vegetables, 3-4 servings of dark green leafy, yellow, beans/peas, starches; Fruit, 2-3 servings.

Sugar and salt should be used in moderation; 30% or less of calories should come from fat with 10% or less of fat from saturated fats; no more than one alcohol drink (one ounce of liquor or equivalent) for a woman per day is advised. Six to eight glasses of water are needed daily. Added calcium is required for adolescent, pregnant, and older women.

Assess meals eaten, if she skips meals, uses vitamin and mineral supplements, wears dentures, eats snacks (how often and type), drinks caffeinated/carbonated beverages (type and amount), eats more beef than fish and poultry, takes in excessive fat and salt/sugar/substitutes, eats alone, eats too quickly, chews adequately, uses alcohol/tobacco/other substances or medications that could alter intake, has food intolerances, eats charcoaled or fried foods, has someone else who cooks for her, has wide weight fluctuations, abuses food when stressed, diets constantly, and knows what is included in a balanced diet. Correlate diet patterns to other history, physical, and diagnostic findings, such as high fat intake with obesity and abnormal lipid levels.

A "rule of thumb" for ideal weight calculation for women is that the woman should weigh 100 pounds for the first five (5) feet; add 5 pounds per inch for each additional inch (Star, Shannon, Samnors, et al., 1992). If her body frame is large, add another 5 pounds; if small, subtract 5 pounds.

• *Stress and risk assessment.* Assess the amount of healthy stress in the woman's life, and the amount of distress or stress overload (Pender, 1987). Examine factors increasing stress, such as financial problems, changing family or significant other relationships, employment problems/concerns (such as lack of control/input into job situation), personal information (age, race, hereditary factors, lifestyle, living conditions, habits), impacting life events, and coping strategies. Stress and ineffective coping are associated with hypertension, coronary artery disease, domestic violence, gastrointestinal disease, and substance abuse.

Use of an assessment tool, such as the Holmes and Rahe Life-Change Index which measures degree of change in one's life to predict the chance of illness, or Speilberger's State-Trait Anxiety Inventory, which measures the amount of anxiety a person feels at the time of testing, may be helpful in evaluating stress or anxiety (Pender, 1987). Be sure to correlate signs of excessive stress (mood swings, disposition changes, physical signs/symptoms) with other assessment findings (sleep, rest, appearance, nutrition, recreation, self-concept, social supports, use of medications/substances, unusual behaviors).

- *Fitness assessment.* Assess the types of activities at work, at home, or at play, for aerobic quality, stretching/flexibility activities, strength components, and intensity sufficiency to meet therapeutic cardiovascular levels without safety compromise. Look at the duration of the exercise session, frequency per week, and motivational aspects of exercise for the client (Dunn, 1987). Evaluate fitness within a framework of lifestyle, diet, weight, stress, and substance use for realistic assessment.

  Teach values of beginning slowly for short periods of time, then gradually building up with emphasis on increasing tone, strengthening, stress reduction, flexibility, and coordination enhancement, relaxation promotion, injury prevention, and improved self-concept. For the healthy woman with no contraindications, advise building up to 20 to 40 minutes of aerobic activity, with a warm-up for 5 to 10 minutes before the more vigorous activity, stretching after warming up, and a slow cool-down for 5 to 10 minutes after exercising, monitoring heart rate, and keeping it up for the rest of her life. The intensity of exercise is aimed at safely improving cardiovascular function. Referral to an exercise therapist may be necessary for a full assessment and program management.

- *Occupational assessment.* Assess for type of work, amount, duration, and type of physical labor involved, rest breaks, environmental risks, and stress overload related to job. Examples of problem areas include prolonged standing or sitting, heavy lifting, noise excess, heat/cold excess, exposure to toxins, chemicals, radiation; excessive hours on job, boredom, low pay, low recognition, demanding, and no or low control over work.

  Be especially concerned with the pregnant woman. Determine chemical, anesthetic gases, infections, and radiation exposure (Keleher, 1991). Consider the interrelationships of multiple variables, such as second-hand smoke, stress, nutrition, lack of sleep, and exposure to hazardous materials.

The physical examination and diagnostic studies, other integral components of the assessment process, provide valuable data.

CONCLUSIONS

To consider any facet of a woman's health out of context from her total life's picture, is to consider only a fraction of the whole. This is a disservice to her. Thus, for health care to be holistic and caring, the provider must examine all data within the framework of the woman's whole being. Then, it may be possible for the woman and the provider, as partners, to initiate health care that not only prevents illness and maintains the current health status, but fosters greater health and wellness.

REFERENCES

Bates, B. (1991). *A guide to physical examination and history taking.* (5th ed.). Philadelphia: Lippincott.

Berkley, K., & Hanson, S. (1991). *Pocket guide to family assessment and intervention.* St. Louis: Mosby Year Book.

Blair, K. A. (1986). The battered woman: Is she a silent victim? *Nurse Practitioner, 11:*38, 40, 42-44, 47.

Dunn, M. M. (1987). Guidelines for an effective personal fitness prescription. *Nurse Practitioner, 12:*9-10, 12, 14-16, 18, 23, 26.

Fuller, J., & Schaller-Ayers, J. (1990). *Health assessment: A nursing approach.* Lippincott: Lippincott.

Healy, B. P. (1992). The women's health initiative. *The Female Patient, 17:*36-38.

Horton, J. A. (1992). *The women's health data book: A profile of women's health in the United States.* The Jacob's Institute of Women's Health, Washington, DC.

Keleher, K. C. (1991). Occupational health: How work environments can affect reproductive capacity and outcome. *Nurse Practitioner, 16:*23-37.

Lichtman, R., & Papera, S. (1990). *Gynecology: Well-woman care.* Norwalk: Appleton & Lange.

McElmurry, B. L. (1986). Health appraisal of low-income women. In Kjervik and Martinson, *Women in health and illness.* Philadelphia: W. B. Saunders Co.

Manson, J. E., Colditz, G. A., Stampfer, M. J. et al. (1990). A prospective study of obesity and risk of coronary heart disease in women. *The New England Journal of Medicine, 322:*882-889.

Morton, P. G. (1992). *Health Assessment* (2nd ed.). Springhouse: Springhouse Corp.

National Center for Health Statistics. (1989). Age-adjusted death rates for selected causes of death, according to sex and race: United States, selected years 1950–1987. *United States, health and prevention profile* (DHHS Publication No. PHS 90-1232). Hyattsville, MD: Author.

Sawin, K., & Harrigan, M. (1994). Measures of Family Assessment, *Scholarly Inquiry for Nursing.*

Seidel, H. M., Ball, J. W., Dains, J. E., & Benedict, G. W., (1991). *Mosby's guide to physical examination.* (2nd ed.). St. Louis: Mosby Year Book.

U.S. Bureau of the Census. (1992). *Statistical abstract of the United States, 1992* (112th ed.). Washington, DC: U.S. Government Printing Office.

Youngkin, E. Q., & Davis, M. S. (1994). *Women's Health: A Primary Care Clinical Guide,* Norwalk: Appleton & Lange.

18

Girlchild

Sandra Gibson

*G*irlchild is a term of endearment used by some minorities to refer to adolescent females and the special place they hold in the hearts of their families. Their birth means a special child to be protected and taught about the world in a different way than boys and held close. They are extra special for the mother because girl children are reared to lead and nurture. Their lives sing songs of surviving in a world filled with contradictions and inequities.

TEENS THROUGH THE YEARS

Before discussing the psychosocial development of the adolescent female, we need to take a look at how we have viewed adolescence through the decades as our society has changed. From Plato's time in 347 BC, society has thought of the transition from childhood to adulthood as a journey filled with turmoil and stress caused by intense impulses thought to be constantly out of control (Violato, 1990). However, prior to the twentieth century, children were thought to be the parent's personal property. Children were controlled through stern discipline and spiritualism. It wasn't until the late eighteenth and nineteenth century that the child's development was broken down into stages. Rousseau (1712–1778) considered adolescence a "second birth."

Through the twentieth century, many of the stereotypes adults held of young people coincided with the major themes of any particular decade which are reflected in the following statements (Violato & Wiley, 1990):

- 1920s: The country was going through a tremendous expansion filled with prosperity and parties and teens were viewed as fun-loving, carefree, and self-indulgent.
- 1930s: During the bleak "dirty thirties," young people were viewed as socially conscious. The end of World War II threw teens in the war effort.
- 1940s: Post World War II teens were considered to be serious, committed, patriotic, and heroic.
- 1950s: James Dean era teens were thought to be rebellious without a reason, emotionally turbulent, and likely to strike out at any moment without reason.
- 1960s: The publishing of *The Vanishing Adolescent* by Friedenberg (1959) and *The Making of a Counterculture* by Roszak (1969) along with the media helped to portray the image of teens as visionaries. They were thought to be engaged in a struggle against the "establishment" (the adult world) as a force of evil.
- 1970s: The Me Generation teens were thought to endorse and exploit the establishment.
- 1980s: Teens were seen as troubled by the possibility of nuclear war, world famine, and the break-up of the family.
- 1990s: Seen as the "Impulse Culture," teens are often described as angry and lacking support systems.

We have been varied in our view of young people through the years. Note, however, that most of these views have centered around adult world events and not on the teen's individual responses to life's demands.

The transition into adolescence is not necessarily a homogeneous process. Although about 80% percent of adolescents cope well with the developmental process despite the blended periods of stress and calm (Neinstein, 1991).

The four major tasks of adolescence are:

1. Independence
2. Body image

3. Peer group affiliation
4. Identity development

For the most part adolescence is divided into three phases:

1. Early adolescence: approximately 12-14 years
2. Middle adolescence: approximately 15-17 years
3. Late adolescence: approximately 18-21 years

PHASE ONE: "LET THE DANCE BEGIN"

This phase is heralded by the onset of rapid physical changes, such as height spurts, breast buds, burgeoning muscles, new body curves, menarche, spermarche, and a variety of hormonal changes that stimulate the early adolescent's curiosity about how his or her changing body works (Gibbs, 1993; Strassburger & Brown, 1991). Adolescents have a lot of questions about the physical changes they are going through and usually turn to peers for answers. At this point, the teen clocks in a lot of time in front of the mirror examining their new found exterior. They are very concerned about how they compare with their peers who become the "all and all," especially those of the same sex.

Identity development is one of the primary tasks of adolescence and early teens start to pull away from parents in search of their individuality (Rice, 1993). It can be a sad time for moms and dads who suddenly feel that their otherwise brilliant, sweet child has turned into a moody alien who wants to move in the opposite direction (away from them). All this behavior is a part of the quest for identity. They test authority, values, politics, religion, and sex. It's not unusual for them to experiment with themselves by masturbating, trying out cigarettes, marijuana, or alcohol. They are very impulsive at this point and love the shock value of telling dirty jokes.

PHASE TWO: "BUCKLE YOUR SEATBELTS— THE MIDDLE YEARS"

The parents of middle adolescents are characterized by a knowing look in their eyes or bags under their eyes from all the sleepless, worrying days and nights. Middle teens have pledged complete loyalty to their peers down to their pierced noses and navels. Conformity in clothes and values is the norm, although they'll never admit it. You usually see them in crowds at the mall or at games, any games. Team sports are very important especially where the opposite sex is involved.

Most of the physical changes are over and they're polishing up the exterior with the latest in fashion and make-up. The strength of their physical selves promotes feelings of omnipotence and immortality which usually brings about different levels of rebellion, high risk behavior, and conflict with parents. Parents are intermittently viewed as the enemy, especially when it comes to religion, dating, school, family chores, and work outside the home (Rice, 1993).

The good news is that although teens generally give their parents a hard time, they really do depend on their parents' opinion (Rice, 1993). As they struggle to refine their identity, they begin to realize their limitations and search for realistic vocational aspirations (Neinstein, 1991).

PHASE THREE: "IN THE HOME STRETCH"

If parents can "hang in there" till the adolescent is seventeen or eighteen, they'll see a wonderful transformation. Puberty is complete and there is less concern with peers. You now have an individual who is more comfortable with his or her identity and has a totally different attitude toward relationships. Most late teens start to become more interested in one-to-one relationships with the opposite sex that involve sharing and understanding.

The poor impulse control they displayed earlier improves. They start to refine their ability to delay gratification. Also, it's impressive how they start to compromise and set limits. The vocational goals they set at this point are more practical and they may begin seeking financial independence (Neinstein, 1991). Parents will be glad to hear that although they separate from the family fold, they gladly come back to actually ask and appreciate advice.

IS THERE A SEXUAL AND CULTURAL TWIST?

Girls don't fit into the same mold, they never have. Every woman is significantly different from every man from conception to the end of the life course (Zilbach, 1993). Freud's classical theory postulated that the first three years of psychic life was the same for both sexes (Kleeman, 1976). However, a later concept of "primary identity" talked about a female's irreversible sense of female self between 18 months and three years (Tyson & Tyson, 1990).

Diversity from a developmental prospective may help us see how tradition and heritage fit into the challenges faced by adolescent girls.

Sarigiani, Camarena, and Peterson (1993) cited three major challenges facing adolescent minority girls: (1) adjusting to transformations of the physical body, (2) adapting to changing expectations for self and social roles, and (3) negotiating new standards and consequences of sexuality (p. 141).

Transformations

In America, puberty is not a time of formal celebrations as in many other cultures. American culture introduces menarche and associated secondary sex changes with privacy, anxiety, and awkwardness (Brooks-Gunn & Rieter, 1990).

Other cultures, like the Navaho Indians, have a history of celebrating four days when girls attain womanhood. Although this tradition and others are exercised in a variety of different ways, it still frames the experience of puberty in a different way (Richard & Peterson, 1987).

The pubertal experience also shows some variation across racial groups. There are a number of authors who suggest that black girls are more likely to develop secondary sex characteristics sooner than white girls (Rice, 1993). Although, this phenomena relates more to racial characteristics than culture, it still plays a part in the minority adolescent's quest for acceptance. Brooks-Gunn and Rieter (1990) explain that teens feel very stressed and self-conscious when they look different from their peers and the lack of confidence that results make adjusting difficult. A study by Phinney, Jensen, Olson, and Cundick (1990) found that early maturing teens engaged in dating and intercourse much earlier than their peers.

Although most teens in the majority culture compare themselves to the general American standards of beauty—thin, blond, and blue eyes—minority females have another viewpoint. Phinney and Rotheram (1987) verified this observation in a study they completed with African American girls. Japanese American girls may feel self-conscious about their racial characteristics, and in extreme cases resort to artificial means of creating a western-looking double eyelid (Nagata, 1989).

On the far side of the pendulum, there seem to be a small minority that are at risk for eating disorders (especially anorexia nervosa and bulimia) due to culturally conflicting standards for appearance (Hsu, 1987). The susceptibility for eating disorders in minority groups appears to depend on the close proximity of social/cultural references, and the degree to which they feel overwhelmed by negative stereotypes toward women of color (Silber, 1986).

Changing Roles

Included in the phase of adolescence is a brand new set of expectations, norms, and social roles. In most ethnic groups, these expectations center around a strong theme of "family." Hispanics view the family as the primary social unit and a critical source of social support (Brusch-Rossnagel & Zayas, 1991). African American and Native American families typically have strong ties with extended family members such as grandparents, uncles, and cousins (Davis & Voegtle, 1994).

Along with the close family ties come a variety of expectations. For example, the Mexican American female is prepared for marriage and motherhood in adolescence by close monitoring of her extra familial contacts (Ramirez, 1989). Native Americans, African Americans, and Asians emphasize the responsibility for extended family and friends (Davis & Voegtle, 1994).

The strong family theme is thought to give certain minority groups protection from depression and suicide due to their satisfaction with family life (Ramirez, 1989). For example, the Hispanic culture holds the reputation of having low suicide rates due to an emphasis to protect and honor the family (Brusch-Rossnagel & Zayas, 1991).

On the other hand, the unraveling of family ties can have a devastating effect on minority women. Smith (1989) found that the extended family role in African American families, that seems to be diminishing, has isolated many women from important sources of support as they take on adult roles. Similarly, Margolin (1991) reported that relationships between today's teens and their mothers are strained due to confusion about adolescent roles. She contends that the adolescent girls are angry and frustrated because the adults around them seem to lack the skills and sometimes the interest to give them direction. It has also been reported that minority girls that immigrate to America have far more stress than boys in the adjustment process (Zambrana & Silva-Palacius, 1989).

Your Sexual Self

Although the expectations for girls concerning sexuality come from family, peers, school, and community, the minority groups within the United States have been characterized as restrictive (Sarigiani et al., 1993). Consequently, the often conflicting messages obtained from these sources seem to leave the adolescent with a dilemma. Gibbs (1993) reports that many teens are in a state of confusion and distress regarding their sexual decisions. She quotes several teens requesting a discussion about the emotional issues of sexuality, that is intimacy, feelings, and opinions.

Overall it does not appear that minority families routinely engage in discussions regarding the physical or emotional changes surrounding sexuality. Asian families often view a discussion of sexuality as taboo (Nagata, 1989). Also, traditional Filipino American families emphasize chastity with their daughters and are very protective of their reputation, hence, they receive little direct sex education from parents or elders (Santos, 1983).

In traditional Mexican American families, knowledge regarding sexuality is viewed as inappropriate for girls. Girls are expected to remain virginal prior to marriage and any evidence of sexual behavior is considered to be a form of disrespect (Scott, Shiffman, Orr, Owen, & Fawcett, 1988). African American families maintain to their daughters that sex is best reserved for marriage with parenthood being highly valued (Scott et al., 1988). Premarital sexuality issues are emphasized as having a variety of consequences with the outcome having a great deal to do with socioeconomic status (Harrison, 1990).

The negative outcomes associated with the minority female as she adjusts to her changing sexual self are impressive. The amount of drug and alcohol use in Native American, Hispanic, and African American adolescents is at an alarming rate with associated problems of violence and depression (Freeman, 1990). In addition, the issue of teen pregnancy is overwhelming the African American community, especially the poor (Furstenberg, 1991).

CONCLUSION

An adolescent girlchild in this world holds a special place not envied by most. The role of acculturation (the acceptance of one's culture and others) holds special significance for minority girls in relation to their adjustment in their family and community. One theme that seems to be central to this issue is the need for the parent, especially the mother, to remain a very visible and active force in her daughter's life.

Strategies to strengthen communication between mothers and daughters is still an intervention worth pursuing. The violence and aggression we are starting to see in girls may be a symptom of frustration and anger regarding the alienation they feel. We need to make our daughters feel not only loved but valued and supported.

REFERENCES

Brooks-Gunn, J., & Rieter, E. O. (1990). The role of the pubertal process. In S. S. Feldman & G. R. Elliott (Eds.), *At the threshold: The developing adolescent.* Cambridge, MA: Harvard University Press.

Brusch-Rossnagel, N. A., & Zayas, L. H. (1991). Hispanic adolescents. In R. M. Lerner, A. C. Peterson, & J. Brooks-Gunn, (Eds.), *Encyclopedia of adolescence: Vol. I.* New York: Garland.

Davis, B. J., & Voegtle, K. H. (1994). *Culturally competent health care for adolescents.* Chicago: Department of Adolescent Health, American Medical Association.

Freeman, E. M. (1990). Social competence as a framework for addressing ethnicity and teenage alcohol problems. In A. R. Stiffman & L. E. Davis (Eds.). (1990). *Ethnic issues in adolescent mental health.* (pp. 247-266). Newbury Park, CA: Sage Publications.

Gibbs, N. (1993, May 24). How should we teach our children about sex? *Time,* 60-66.

Harrison, A. (1990). High risk sexual behavior among black adolescents. In A. R. Stiffman & E. Davis (Eds.), *Ethnic issues in adolescent mental health* (pp. 175-188). Newbury Park, CA: Sage.

Hsu, L. K. G. (1987). Are the eating disorders becoming more common among blacks? *International Journal of Eating Disorders, 6,* 113-124.

Kleeman, J. (1976). Freud's views on early female sexuality in the light of direct child observation. *Journal of American Psychoanalytical Association, 24,* 3-27.

Margolin, E. (1991, September) *Adolescent females: Where have they been?: Where are they going?* Paper presented at the women's studies annual conference, Bowling Green, KY.

Nagata, D. K. (1989). Japanese children and adolescents. In J. T. Gibbs & L. N. Huang (Eds.). *Children of color: Psychological interventions with minority youth.* San Francisco: Jossey-Bass.

Neinstein, L. (1991). *Adolescent health care: A practical guide.* (2nd ed.). Baltimore: Urban & Schwarzenberg.

Phinney, V. G., Jensen, L. C., Olsen, J. A., & Cundick, B. (1990). The relationship between early development and psychosexual behaviors in adolescent females. *Adolescence, 25,* 321-331.

Phinney, V. G., & Rotheram, M. J. (1987). *Children's ethnic socialization: Pluralism and development.* Newbury Park, CA: Sage.

Ramirez, O. (1989). Mexican American children and adolescents. In J. T. Gibbs & L. N. Huang (Eds.), *Children of color: Psychological interventions with minority youth.* San Francisco: Jossey-Bass.

Rice, P. F. (1993). *Human development: A life-span approach.* New York: MacMillan Publishing Company.

Richards, M., & Peterson, A. C. (1987). Biological theoretical models of adolescent development. In V. B. Van Hasselt & M. Hersen (Eds.), *The handbook of adolescent psychology.* Elmsford, NY: Pergamon.

Santos, R. A. (1983). The social and emotional development of Filipino American children. In G. J. Powell, J. Yamamoto, A. Romero, & A. Morales (Eds.), *The psychosocial development of minority group children.* New York: Brunner/Mazel.

Sarigiani, P. A., Camarena, P. M., & Peterson, A. C., (1993). Cultural factors in adolescent girls development: The role of minority group status. In M. Sugar (Ed.), *Female adolescent development* (pp. 138-156). New York: Brunner/Mazel.

Scott, C. S., Shifman, L., Orr, L., Owen, R. G., & Fawcett, N. (1988). Hispanic and Black American adolescents beliefs relating to sexuality and contraception. *Adolescence, 23,* 667-688.

Silber, T. J. (1986). Anorexia nervosa in blacks and hispanics. *International Journal of Eating Disorders, 5,* 121-128.

Smith, E. S. (1989). Afro-American and the extended family: A review. *Western Journal of Black Studies, 13,* 179-183.

Strassburger, V. C., & Brown, R. T. (1991). *Adolescent medicine: A practical guide.* Boston: Little, Brown, & Company.

Tyson, P., & Tyson, T. (1990). *The psychoanalytic theory of development: An integration.* New Haven, CT: Yale University Press.

Violato, C., & Wiley, A. J. (1990). Images of adolescent development: Clinical implications. *Adolescence, 45,* 253-264.

Zambrana, R. E., & Silva-Palacious, V. (1989). Gender differences in stress among Mexican American immigrant adolescents in Los Angeles, CA. *Journal of Adolescent Research, 4,* 426-442.

Zilbach, J. J. (1993). Female adolescence: Toward a separate line of development. In M. Sugar (Ed.), *Female adolescent development.* New York: Brunner/Mazel.

19

Eating Disorders Today

Fatemeh B. Firoz

Eating disorders are a "group of dysfunctional behaviors of nutrition." These unhealthy eating behaviors are characterized by crash diets, fasting, restrained eating, binge eating, purging, compulsive overeating, and craving nonfood items (such as clay or chalk). Distortion of body image and frequent exercise are common accompanying behaviors. All of these behaviors focus mainly on eating, getting rid of, or avoiding food. Eating disorders are psychological disorders that don't appear only in a person's physical appearance.

Many times it is difficult to determine who is suffering from a disorder and who is not. Since food and weight seem so important in our society, it is unusual to find a teenage girl or any female who is not or has not been concerned with her weight at one point or the other.

The pressure to be slim in order to look good and feel happy is continually reinforced through the media and publications. It is a constant struggle for some people to deal with the issue of their weight and appearance. Yager's (1992) survey showed that "about three quarters of women whose weights are fully in the normal range feel too fat and wish to lose weight" (p. 679). When an average young woman looks in the mirror, she sees a fat person. As Myers and Biocca (1992) explain, a young woman's perception of her body (body image) is a part of her self-schema and mental construction of herself. In a society where the ideal body is becoming thinner, it is not unusual to find women who are overestimating the size of their bodies (Birtchnell et al., 1987).

In general, an eating disorder exists when thinking about your body is endangering your health and preventing you from moving on in life. Most of us know how it feels to wish to look a bit trimmer or want to look fit for a special occasion. However if wishes, wants, and rewards become the basis of all decisions, then there are serious indications that a problem exists. In most cases of eating disorder, dysfunction is seen in social life, school achievement, and occupational life. Emotional instability and mood swings due to poor ability to regulate self-esteem are not uncommon.

Eating problems usually begin with the common wish to lose weight and maintain an image you have of your body. Many people go through a period of intense dieting, obsession with weight, or overeating that does not affect or interfere with their daily life. The most common eating disorders include anorexia nervosa, bulimia nervosa, pica, rumination disorder of infancy, feeding disorder of infancy or early childhood, and eating disorders not otherwise specified. A brief discussion of these disorders follows.

COMMON CAUSES AND DEVELOPMENT OF THE EATING DISORDERS

Although the exact cause of eating disorders is often unknown, practitioners must consider the role and effect of medical, chemical, genetical, personality, social, and cultural aspects.

Scientists have long known that clusters of nerve cells located in the brain's hypothalamus control basic eating behavior (Mosby, 1994). Researchers now believe that a predisposition to weight gain may be determined in infancy (Estroff-Marano, 1993). It is also possible that some eating disorders have genetic origins. In a recent study of the genetic aspects of eating disorders using a group of identical and non-identical twins, Kendler et al. (1991) studied bulimic patients and found that there is a 55% chance of inheriting this disorder. Holderness et al. (1994) investigated the relationships between substance abusers and familial eating disorders. There is a stronger positive relationship between eating disorders and substance abuse in bulimics than in anorectics. Among anorectics, the rate of occurrence is more common among sisters and mothers of those with the disorder than among the general population. A higher rate of Major Depression and Bipolar Disorder among first degree biologic relatives of sufferers has been reported (DSMIII-R). Frequently the parents of bulimics are obese and/or there is indication of obesity in adolescence as one of the major predisposing factors leading to the development of bulimia in adults.

Personality traits also play a major role in the development of eating disorders. For example, an anorectic personality is often associated with low self-esteem and with an external locus of control (life events that are not under one's control). They are particularly timid and avoidant, obsessional, or sensitive and moody (Yager, 1992). In addition, current evidence suggests that anorexia and bulimia are more likely to develop in women with panic disorders, alcoholism, and depression (Kendler et al., 1991).

Other causal relations might be fear of becoming an adult among adolescents. In an attempt to avoid the unfamiliar and uncertain events, the teens keep themselves looking like children: Small, thin, and androgynous. Another theory claims that those who are suffering from anorexia and/or bulimia are really suffering from a feeling of being without control of their lives. According to this theory, victims feel consciously or unconsciously that they may not have any control over the families they were born into, or a variety of other situations, but one thing they can control is their weight (Dowling, 1991).

Societal and cultural pressures can also relate to eating disorders. A recent survey conducted by Luppino (1992) indicated that children would choose to be crippled rather than be fat. A successful person in the world today has to contend with the cultural ideal of thinness. Brenner and Cunningham (1992) believe that the cultural expectation of unrealistic thinness continues to diminish a person's self-esteem. Often women express concern and anger over frequent teasing by their boyfriends.

The most highly paid and well-known faces are not immune to suffering from anorexia, bulimia, and/or compulsive exercising. Supermodels Kim Alexis, Beverly Johnson, and Carol Alt are some of those who have admitted experiencing eating problems at one point or the other (Sporkin, 1993).

In addition, many believe that advertising plays a key role in creating the emaciated standard of beauty that girls are taught from childhood to seek. Advertisements used for diet products use "Before" and "After" pictures of the people endorsing their products. Usually endorsers engage in describing their lives before the weight loss negatively such as being ashamed and embarrassed of their looks. Then the endorser tells of her new, happy life in which she looks and feels great leaving the impression and creating the stereotype that heavy and obese people are not happy or attractive. According to Armstrong and Mallory (1992), sales of diet-related products and services in the United States reached $33 billion in 1992. Stephens et al. (1994) demonstrated that advertising and marketing to promote thinness appears to foster and nourish an array of psychological and behavioral problems in young American women.

Cool (1992) demonstrated his result by showing that 30% of female participants chose an ideal shape that was 20% underweight. From this and other similar research, it is evident that an American female of average weight will often see herself as overweight and experience a high level of body dissatisfaction. Stephens et al. (1994) found that 15% of his participants used forced vomiting and laxatives as a dieting method to control their weight.

The distortion of body image may occur because of the psychological pressure that results from the contrast between the advertising created "ideal body" and one's objective body shape. As the ideal gets further and further away from the real body, we exaggerate the true difference, seeing ourselves as being heavier than we in fact are. This is the essence of body image distortion, and the media is believed to have a direct role in the promotion of it. Bell (1991) argued in his study that body image changes in response to social cues that are situational. Furthermore, his results showed that as the gap between the ideal and the average woman decreases, the apparent need for women to diet lessens, and therefore eating disorders may become less prevalent.

It is certain that marketing is not the sole factor for the growing problem of eating disorders. However, it has been shown that media and advertisements do influence the way women see themselves. They compare their own bodies to the ideal body and behave in response to this comparison.

EATING DISORDERS AND AFFECTED POPULATION

It was once thought that eating disorders were exclusive to white, middle/upper class, and over-achieving young women. Research is beginning to show that eating disorders affect women and men of all races and economic status (Reid, 1989). Gender, poverty, and race are among major risk factors that often contribute to the high prevalence of eating disorders. Eating disorders affect all races, classes, and genders. They are often triggered by a trauma (Kato, 1994). However, anorexia nervosa and bulimia occur at a higher rate among young, white, affluent females. There have been reports of more middle age bulimic patients than anorectic cases (DSMIII-R).

Cain (1994) reported in his study that compulsive exercisers are another group of population who are affected by eating disorders. These people preoccupy themselves with the perfect body—an image popularized by the fashion and diet industries. In order to achieve this image, they engage in intensive exercising to the point of obsession and compulsion which is often associated with eating problems.

Another population or group who have been affected by the eating disorders are young adolescents who fear fatness and who restrain eating. Arbetter (1994) estimated that eating disorders affect two million girls ages 12 to 18 and about 0.5 million boys in the same age level. In a similar study, Luppino reported that 80% of American 11-year-old girls feel overweight and currently are on diets.

As is clear through the studies, eating disorders are prevalent and widespread. Much of the public, as well as specialized population segments, are part of this potentially fatal cycle of weight-gain, weight-loss, and weight-gain pattern. Up to 20% of those who suffer from an eating disorder will die as the result of their illness (Siegel, 1988).

As mentioned previously, more than one factor contributes to the onset of eating disorders. Every case has unique and individual contributing factor(s) and should be studied carefully.

It is unfortunate that American women have been assaulted for more than 25 years with visual media reminders that being happy and successful means being thin. In addition, the vast majority of teenagers in our society have literally grown up with this "ideal" persona and body image.

Anorexia Nervosa

Anorexia nervosa refers to the loss of appetite due to neurotic condition (Dowling, 1991). Most anorectics (95%) are women. Most cases occur between the ages of 12 and 18, but cases in women of 40 to 50 have been reported (Brisman, 1988).

Anorexia is characterized by a significant amount of weight loss due to a purposeful attempt to stop eating and dieting. The patient starves herself and has a distorted body image. The diets of an anorexic will grow to more and more extreme measures. They use a strict diet eliminating all carbohydrate-rich food and finally eating a few vegetables a day. To stop themselves from eating, they hide the food they crave most. They also become concerned about their family's diet and they tend to prepare food for the whole family. Usually, they do not binge eat or purge the food.

A person who suffers from anorexia is intensely fearful of becoming obese, which does not stop even if the person loses weight. They consider themselves to be fat despite their thinness. Being obsessed with their body weight, even if they weigh sixty-five pounds, they will still find places on their bodies where they think they still need to lose weight. In severely advanced cases, anorectics avoid taking in all calories at all costs—even if the cost is death. A significant weight loss (at least 15% of their normal body weight) is one of the diagnostic criteria. The duration of this disorder is fifteen days or more.

Anorectics attempt to lose weight through starvation, induced vomiting, taking laxatives, using diuretics, or exercising vigorously. Finally their body becomes completely emaciated.

The body image of a person with anorexia is totally distorted. For the person who is anorexic, the dieting and weight loss take an uncontrollable, unanticipated, and unplanned course. Once dieting serves a psychological function, certain characteristics begin to surface. Patients demonstrate many compulsive behaviors such as hand-washing, preoccupation with food preparation, and selection of low-calorie foods. They tend to be perfectionists in almost every aspect of their lives. They put other people's needs ahead of their own in order to gain the approval of others. They are often referred to as approval junkies seeking love and acceptance rather than food. If this behavior becomes a pattern of their daily living, an additional diagnosis of Obsessive Compulsive Personality Disorder might be justified.

Someone who develops anorexia has not developed sufficient means of feeling competent, worthy, and effective. Despite these feelings, their school achievement is usually excellent. Anorectics tend to deny the fact that they are sick and they require medical as well as psychological treatment.

Other important features that always occur during the illness are irregularity of menstrual cycle. As illness advances, amenorrhea always is evident, often before a significant amount of weight loss has taken place related to poor nutrition. Loss of menstruation combined with attempts at dieting and an intense fear of becoming fat are clues that anorexia is the problem, even before a person's body weight has dropped below the normal range.

As mentioned earlier, when anorexics are confronted with their illness, they deny that something is wrong with them. They choose to resist help and refuse treatment vigorously. Finally, as the patient becomes profoundly underweight and experiences symptoms such as hypothermia, bradycardia, and hypotension, forced treatment becomes necessary. Additional symptoms such as edema, lanugo (nconatal-like hair), and different forms of metabolic changes also appear. At this stage, anorexia is life-threatening and hospitalization should be sought.

Anorexia is a treatable disorder. A good result can be obtained if the illness is brought to the professional's attention early. Neuroleptics and tricyclics along with psychotherapy are recommended. The response of the patient's family can be a key factor in causal relation, treatment, and prognosis. The family may criticize and ostracize the patient or be supportive during the illness and/or treatment. Frequently family counseling in combination with individual psychotherapy and medical therapy have produced good results.

An associated feature of anorexia nervosa may be bulimia. Many anorectics are bulimics since they lose control over their intended voluntary restriction of food intake and have binge eating episodes followed by vomiting.

For differential diagnosis, depressive disorder or specific physical disorder should be ruled out. If there is a distorted body image along with intense fear of obesity, then anorexia might be the right choice.

Bulimia Nervosa

Bulimia is the second major type of eating disorder. This eating disorder is defined as overeating and being terrified of getting fat (Cauwels, 1983). Onset is in adolescence or early adult life. It ordinarily begins with a reasonable attempt to lose "some weight." In a way, bulimia can affect its victims for years before it is noticed. Usually, weight loss is not dramatic enough to meet criteria for anorexia nervosa. Since bulimics can be either overweight or underweight, it is difficult to tell if someone is bulimic by their weight. Usually they do not have a distorted body image.

Bulimia is characterized by eating large quantities of food in a short period of time—binging. The binge is then followed by an attempt to get rid of the food and the calories that were consumed—purging. This is why bulimia is considered the binge-and-purge disorder.

The lack of control over eating behavior such as depriving themselves of food for a couple of days and then getting the urge to consume a large quantity of food high in carbohydrates are major features of this disorder. Bulimics eat this large amount of food in a short period of time. They can eat up to three or four meals, throwing up in between, and still feel the urge to eat again. While the binge is taking place, all feelings are blocked out and nothing matters to them. The frequency of this behavior is several times a week. In a sense, they are addicted in much the same way as drug users are hooked on drugs. Eventually, the binge/purge cycle becomes a true compulsion (Sheppard, 1989).

Bulimics tend to reduce feelings of guilt over their binge eating by induced vomiting. Their obsession with food is their worry about what they should eat for easy purging. They often go for sweet taste and a texture to help facilitate rapid eating. They eat secretly and rapidly until they feel abdominal discomfort. To comfort themselves, they induce vomiting. Bulimics usually feel guilty and depressed after binge eating and do not want to relate to other people. They hate themselves for what they have engaged in. Since binge eating and fasting is usually alternated, frequent weight fluctuation becomes evident.

Controlling the urge to eat is something the bulimic is always trying to do. The loss of control often triggers a binge. The bulimic will get the food anyway she or he knows how. Bulimics are usually aware of their eating problems but they feel rather hopeless in gaining control over it.

The purging aspect can take different forms. The most common ways to purge include induced vomiting, taking laxatives, using diuretics, enemas, colonics, diet pills, or even the use of amphetamines and cocaine to hold down the hunger on the days following the binge. The use of laxatives as a purging method begins with the bulimic taking one or two. As the body becomes tolerant to the laxatives, they keep increasing the numbers to get positive results to suit their needs (Plumber, 1994). Purging varies from person to person. Some vomit during binges while others wait until the binge is over. No matter what method of purging they use, it gives them the perfect solution. They rely so heavily on the binge/purge that it becomes a major part of their daily life. In one sense, the cycle of binging and purging provides a feeling of mastery (satisfying the urge to eat).

Psychologically, binging is a way of filling up without needing others. Food is an outlet for all of the bulimics' feelings. They don't know how to express their inner troubles so the bulimia serves as a way to let the feelings out. Dynamically, a bulimic individual is locked into a struggle between two forces; the wish for total control versus the wish to be out of control. If they can't control they take it as a personal failure. Bulimics often realize that they have a problem. They admit to their psychological distress and often are aware of the consequences of their behavior. In bulimia, the mother is usually a compulsive eater. Bulimics tend to mirror a yet more hidden crisis in the mother's life (White & White, 1987).

An affective disorder such as a major depression is often associated with bulimia. Bulimics usually use some kind of substance or alcohol to cope with their problems. In some cases, one or more personality disorders are associated with this disorder. Social life is poor and academic achievement is below average or average.

Adolescence and young adulthood are the ages when bulimia is most commonly found. However, studies have shown that young girls (as young as 11) and women as old as 50 suffer from this disorder (DMSR-IV). About 90% to 95% of all bulimics are women. However, there are reports of more and more male athletes who tend to be bulimics. They often will exercise to the point of vomiting (Plumber, 1994). The statistical data in Dunn's (1992) report revealed that 11 million women and 1 million men in the United States suffer from eating disorders—either self-induced semi-starvation (anorexia nervosa) or a cycle of binging/purging with laxatives, self-induced vomiting, or excessive exercise (bulimia nervosa). According to the American Anorexia and Bulimia Association, 150,000 women die of anorexia each year (Stephens et al., 1994).

Some of the physical problems brought about by vomiting and the abuse of laxatives are skin problems. Dryness, rashes, and pimples often form on the skin. Swelling, pain, and tenderness of the salivary glands are problems for frequent vomiters (Cauwels, 1983).

Excessive vomiting, fasting, and abuse of diuretics and laxatives lead to malnutrition, electrolyte imbalance, and heart damage. Perforation of the stomach, a possible rupturing of the esophagus, and severe tooth decay are all possible and probable physical and organ damage for a bulimic.

Death from bulimia is less common than anorexia. Because bulimics admit that there is something wrong and they are willing to cooperate with treatment, and they are more likely to seek help than someone who has anorexia.

Considerable attention has been given to the treatment of bulimia. According to White (1987), Bulimia is a learned behavior, and as such, it can be unlearned. He believes unlearning should be the focus of the treatment. The most effective treatment approach is the cognitive behavioral approach that teaches the patient self-regulation and monitoring skills. Since the patient has trouble knowing when to eat, what to eat, and how much, the cognitive behavioral approach will teach the patient skills to regulate their eating patterns. It is important to note that the earlier an eating disorder is diagnosed and treated, the more likely the sufferer will get positive treatment. The longer one goes, the more physical as well as psychological suffering they will endure.

Medical treatment, such as administration of antidepressants, began in the late 1970s. The first success was reported by Dr. Daniel Moore of Yale in 1977 using amitriptyline. By using antidepressants, bulimics lose the urge to binge and vomit. Treatment combining antidepressants and psychotherapy is said to be the most effective than only medication or psychotherapy alone.

PICA

Pica is primarily a disorder of young children and is probably unrelated to anorexia nervosa and bulimia nervosa. Pica is defined as eating nonnutritive substances, such as plasters, cloth, dirt, wood, and so on for a period of at least one month. This disorder is seen most among low socioeconomic status people. Frequently children who suffer from this disorder are seen by pediatricians rather than mental health professionals. Usually the child is screened for lead poisoning or any other physical effects that he/she might have ingested. Regardless of gender, this disorder affects both sexes.

Psychoactive medication is not recommended (Reid, 1989). However, family therapy is beneficial for increasing family's coping and supervision skills. A behavior modification program is reported to be an effective treatment method. In order to make firm diagnosis, autistic disorder, schizophrenia, or Kleine-Levin syndrome should be ruled out since eating of nonnutritive substances might be reported among these disorders.

Rumination Disorder of Infancy

As is clear from the diagnostic term, this is a disorder of infancy. During this illness, the infant regurgitates after every feeding and he or she fails to gain weight. A duration of one month or more followed by a period of normal functioning is required to make a firm diagnosis. Age unset is usually between 3 and 12 months. However, it might appear later in mentally retarded children. The predisposing factor is unknown for this rare disorder. If the illness continues, it may cause developmental delays. It is important to rule out physical problems related to gastrointestinal system. If the physiological causes are ruled out, then a behavioral program should be set up by a psychologist to work with the mother and to monitor the eating pattern of infant. A careful history and the mother's feelings toward the infant are important factors in development and the treatment of this disorder.

Feeding Disorder of Infancy or Early Childhood

This is a disorder of infancy or early childhood newly classified. There are four essential features of this disorder that results in significant failure to gain weight or lose weight. These features include:

- Persistent failure to eat adequately leading to significant failure to gain weight or significant weight loss over at least one month.
- There is no medical condition to account for the feeding disturbance.
- The feeding disturbance is not related to other mental disorders of childhood, such as rumination disorder or lack of any available food.
- The onset is before age six.

The common behavioral problems are described as irritability and the child is difficult to console during feeding. The child might appear apathetic and withdrawn. Due to poor eating, the regular growth might be delayed. Additionally, inadequate caloric intake might cause more irritability, and prolong developmental lags. Parent-child interaction problems may exist that contribute to or exacerbate the infant's eating or feeding problem. Parental psychopathology or child abuse and neglect might be another factor. Infant's responsiveness such as sleep-wake difficulties, unpredictable periods of alertness, and any other neuroregulatory difficulties may be among other associated factors in relation to this disorder. When making the diagnosis, any associated laboratory findings such as anemia should be ruled out. This disorder is equally common among males and females.

Eating Disorders Not Otherwise Specified (NOS)

These disorders are essentially variations of anorexia and bulimia, but do not meet the criteria for those diagnoses. For example, they might have the features of anorexia except for the absence of menstrual cycles. Or they might have features of bulimia except for the frequency of binge eating. However, treatment approach is chosen similarly to that of anorexia and bulimia.

REFERENCES

Arbetter, S. (1994, September 2). Eating to the extremes: The A's and B's of eating disorders. *Current Health*, pp. 6-12.

Armstrong, L., & Mallory, M. (1992, June 22). The diet business starts sweating. *Business Week*, pp. 22-23.

Birtchnell, S. A., Dolan, B. M., & Lacey, J. H. (1987). Body image distortion in non-eating disordered women. *International Journal of Eating Disorders*, 6(3), 385-391.

Bowen, D., Tomoyasu, N., & Cauoe, A. (1991, Winter). The triple threat: a discussion of gender, class, and race differences in weight. *Women & Health*, pp. 123-144.

Cain, A. (1994, August 19). Compulsive exercising often accompanies eating disorders. *Knight-Ridder/Tribune News Service*, p. 81.

Cauwels, Janice M. (1983). *Bulimia: The binge and purge compulsion*. Garden City, NY: Doubleday.

Cool, L. C. (1992, February). Mirror image. *Fitness*, pp. 24-26.

Dowling, Colette. (1988). *Perfect woman*. New York: Summit Books.

Dowling, Colette. (1991). *You Mean I Don't Have to Feel This Way?* New York: Macmillan.

Dunn, D. (1992, August 3). When thinness becomes illness. *Business Week*, pp. 74-75.

Estroff-Marano, G. (1993, January-February). Chemistry & craving: Not the same old diet story. *Psychology Today*, pp. 30-36.

Holderness, C. C., Brooks-Gunn, J., & Warren, M. (1994, July). Co-morbidity of eating disorders and substance abuse. *The International Journal of Eating Disorders, 16*, 1-33.

Kato, D. (1994, October 19). Eating disorders afflict women of all races and economic status. *Knight-Ridder/Tribune Service*, p. 101.

Kendler, K. S., MacLean, C., Neale, M., Kessler, R., Heath, A., & Eaves, L. (1991, December). The genetic epidemiology of bulimia nervosa. *American Journal of Psychiatry, 148*, 1627-1638.

Luppino, T. (1992, July-August). Yo-yo dieting: Early education is the key in the potentially fatal gain-loss weight cycle. *American Fitness*, p. 60.

Miller, L. (1994, June 6). Give them cheeseburger: Critics assail waif look in Sprite, Calvin Klein ads. *Marketing News*, pp. 1-3.

Models 'R' us; eating disorders. (1992, January-February). *Psychology Today*, p. 11.

Mosby's Medical, Nursing, and Allied Health Dictionary, (4th ed.). (1994). New York: Mosby Year Book, Inc.

Myers, P. N., & Biocca, F. A. (1992). The elastic body image. The effect of television advertising and programming on body image distortions in young women. *Journal of Communications 42*(3), 108-131.

Piirto, R. (1991, November). Food for thought. Health-consciousness among Americans; why they buy. *American Demographics, 13*, 6.

Plumber, William. (1994, August 22). Olympic dreams. *People*, August 22.

Plumber, W., Grout, P., Sandler, B., Jenkins, J., & Goulding, S. C. (1994, August 22). Dying for a medal. *People*, pp. 36-39.

Sheppard, Kay. (1989). *Food addiction*. Florida: Health Communications.

Spitzer, Robert L., & Williams, Janet B. W. (1987). *Diagnostic and statistical manual of mental disorders*, 3rd ed. rev. Washington, DC: American Psychiatric Association.

Sporkin, E. (1993, January 11). The body game. *People*, pp. 80-86.

Stephens, D. L., Hill, R. P., & Hanson, C. (1994). The beauty myth and female consumers: the controversial role of advertising. *Journal of Consumer Affairs 28*(1), 137-151.

White, Marlene B., & White, William C. (1987). *Bulimarexia: The binge/purge cycle*, 2nd ed. New York: Norton.

Yager, J. (1992, December). Has our 'healthy' life-style generated eating disorders? *The Western Journal of Medicine, 157*, 679-681.

20

Unwelcome Reflections

Suzanne Maguire Santoro

Once upon a time I was a young, tall, slender, blonde, curly-haired woman with green eyes, great Irish peaches-and-cream skin, a straight nose, and a full-lipped mouth with white, even teeth. Truck drivers and stockbrokers winked and smiled; customers always wanted to talk business over lunch and drinks; my children thought I was too good to be true.

I was a widow, my husband having died after a short bout with lung cancer. This short bout required my full-time, 24-hour attention because there was no hospital involved. It was my wish and desire to make him as comfortable as possible in our own home to the very long and exhausting, sad end. That end came without any insurance, mortgage payments still to be made, and a house and family that needed care. My children were all adults, one living at home, and two away; albeit not always on their own financially. I had embarked on a sales career almost one year before my husband became ill and immediately stopped working to attend to all his needs.

One week after the funeral, I went back to my sales career. I was selling two-way radio equipment and systems to garbage men, trucking companies, construction, security, and sewerage firms, and so on. I gave myself a time limit of three months. After that, if I had no success (working on commission only), I would go back to a job as a legal secretary in which I had many years of experience. I was good, in fact, very good. I won a top selling contest in the New York City area with a trip to Hawaii as the prize.

I have left out an important part—a very important part to this story—sometime in the months and year after my husband died, I met a soulmate—we struck sparks, made great conversations, truly liked each other; danced, laughed, and he was my companion on the trip to Hawaii.

We finally made the commitment, sold our respective condos, and bought a house together. A shack really, but my Tony had great ideas and all the skill and muscle to make them a reality. Today, it is a dream cottage, with 85-feet of dock on a canal overlooking a bird sanctuary; all black and white with glass everywhere and closets and bathrooms to die for. And so the end of the fairy tale . . .

HOW IT STARTED

Throughout my entire life, including my childhood, when I had a front tooth knocked out (and capped at 15), my pride and joy were my teeth. Unfortunately, my gums gave me great problems. I went to great expense, fear, and trembling to visit dentists and periodontists. All of this to have my teeth cleaned, scraped, and have all the latest treatments every three months.

On or about January 1991, I noticed that the area above my front capped tooth had blackened and the cap seemed to be dropping down. When this condition became quite noticeable, I began the search for a dentist and the solution.

I discussed the problem with a neighbor, who immediately recommended her own dentist as a wizard with caps, bridges, and so on. An appointment was made and the consultation held. Viola!!! It was no problem to him. He would remove all the top teeth on my left side up to and including the front dangling cap; the rest of the top teeth would be capped in order to connect it with a removable bridge he would create for the missing teeth.

It would and did take almost one year ($6,000); during most, if not all of that time, I glued in a plaster of paris top denture, and immediately stopped going out on any customer calls, refused to do or attend sales presentations, avoided most social engagements, covered my mouth with my hands, and tried to avoid smiling.

At this time, my personality began to change. I felt my looks slipping away, I was becoming a withered old lady who would someday be a toothless crone, embarrassing Tony and my children. Finally, all the caps were in and the bridge attached. It was not the panacea I had hoped for—the bridge hurt where it attached to the caps and the gums above the caps immediately started to hurt, then bleed and I had severe problems trying to talk. I consulted a speech therapist and faithfully did all her exercises and tried and tried so hard. Tony, my beloved savior, assured me that I looked as gorgeous as ever, and that my speech was very much improved. That comment went down the drain when both my brother and my first granddaughter both asked me, "Why did I talk so funny." Moving on, I told myself it was only temporary; Marilyn Monroe had a lisp and now so did I. Little did I know things were going to get much worse.

DISCOVERY

Now it was May 1992, and time for me to have a mammogram. Off to the Nassau Medical Center I went. The mammography checked out fine, but I was in so much pain that I asked a nurse to look at my mouth. She immediately made arrangements for me to see a doctor in the clinic that day. He, in turn, made immediate arrangements for me to be seen by an oral surgeon. The surgeon had me admitted on emergency status for a biopsy. I had left for the mammogram at 9 A.M. I returned home that night at 6 P.M. with blood covered pads in my mouth. Poor Tony, what now??

The odyssey begins. Two more biopsies were done. Each bigger and more invasive, but I was not overly concerned. It was going to be a fungus or some such viral thing that could and would be treated, and I was, finally, going to be on my way back.

The oral surgeon called me at my office in New York City. At this time, I had my own very successful two-way radio business going. Because of my competency and success, I had many of the top Fortune 500 companies as my customers. The oral surgeon wanted to see me at once. I explained that I was in New York City and would have to catch a train home to Seaford, pick up my car at the station, and then drive to the hospital. He said he would wait for me, and see me the moment I arrived at the hospital. He then said, "Tony was coming, too." What did that mean???? Something was wrong, but what?

Tony was waiting for me when I finally arrived at the hospital. Together we were ushered into an examining room where three oral surgeons, a nose and throat man, and the chief of the dental service, awaited me.

"THE BAD NEWS IS YOU HAVE CANCER"

At first, it didn't really sink in, I was listening, but I couldn't hear anything. Someone said something about removing all my top teeth. I remember covering my mouth and cowering, "No-not-my-teeth?" "What was I going to look like?" "What are they saying?" What cancer? Where? How? I started to sweat. I think they thought I was going to faint, but I wasn't. My body started to distract me from what they were saying. I didn't want to hear it. I knew they were mistaken. My head spun in disbelief at this macabre scene.

I did not, could not, would not have *cancer.* Tears came to my eyes, but I did not cry then, but oh, how I would cry many times after that! As a matter of fact, I cry now as I type these words. I cry for me. I became a baby again, the tears flow, my nose runs and I want it all to go away.

The rest of the day goes by in a blur. Tony and I made phone calls to my children, brothers, and sister, to his large family, a few close friends. Everyone was shocked. I looked and acted too good to have cancer. No one knew what to do or say. It was somewhat embarrassing for them to breathe a sigh of relief that I had cancer, and not them.

An appointment was made at Sloan Kettering Memorial Hospital, in New York City, with Dr. Elliot Strong, chief of oral, head, and neck surgery, the first and foremost expert in that field. Dr. Strong's office was filled with patients awaiting their turn to see him. We had to wait a half-hour or so, which gave me the opportunity to look around, consider those in the office with me, check out what their problems were, and the usual doctor's office room diversion of wondering, "What's" wrong with them?

This time that game didn't work. We knew immediately what was wrong. They were all horribly disfigured. One young woman directly across from me had her throat cut from ear to ear; she seemed to be drooling and made the most awful slurping noises. She was very thin and tired looking. Little did I know at that time that she was only out of the hospital a month or so, and was actually doing well.

I became aware that everyone had a frightening, marred, scarred, look. Some had no chins, no noses, no jawbones disfiguring lumps, holes, scars everywhere. It was a scary "Steven King" movie. That could and would never happen to me!

I had dressed very carefully for the visit. I wanted him to see that I was a successful, attractive businesswoman who knew the score, could deal with it, and just wanted him to do his very best. He should get it over with and let me get on with my life. I was scared, but I could handle it. I was strong. I had always been strong. I would face up to this and I would beat it. After all, hadn't I always?

Dr. Strong wasted no time on the biopsies, reports, and x-rays. He knew what he had to do. He did not play it up or down. He was very direct. He told me that he was going to save my life. He would operate the following Monday, June 15, 1992, remove the tumor, my top teeth, my palette, my upper jaw bone and whatever else had to be done. I would be at the hospital two weeks; there would be relatively little pain, and, oh yes, I would be fitted with an "obturator." This device would make me almost as good as new. There would be no disfigurement and from the outside no one would discern anything wrong. He did not think radiation would be in order, nor did he think the lymph nodes in my neck would have to be removed. All in all, he was very positive, cordial, and attentive. He was the "answer."

The nurse, Maura, made all the arrangements for the hospital. She was a very attractive young woman with dark curly ringlets, blue eyes, and a great smile. Suddenly, I was looking at mouths. I detected sympathetic and knowing glances, but hey, I was strong. I could do this.

We then went directly to the dental section of the hospital to meet with the chief of dental services, Dr. Ian Zatlow. Dr. Zatlow was friendly, confident and very assured. He had done this kind of job before many times. After the tumor was removed, he would enter the operating room and insert the "obturator." My first concern was that the obturator should look like teeth. Dr. Zatlow, seeing that this was my main concern, (vanity still), assured me that since I felt so strongly about it, he personally would see that the obturator had teeth and not just be a plain flesh-colored "thing." I could not imagine the "thing," but it probably would turn out to be something like false teeth and really no one had to know. All in all, I left the hospital that day feeling a little better, not good, but better.

I had to be admitted the Sunday before the Monday operation date. I had to be there for pre-testing very early, which meant I had to spend the whole day just waiting around in the hospital. By this time, I was dried up from alternate crying jags and trying to be brave for Tony, who was very concerned and worried. I polished off a whole bottle of red wine that last night. I knew pre-testing wouldn't like it, but then it just might be the last glass of wine I would ever have, and then, I did not want to spend the whole night wide awake worrying and fretting. It worked. I slept, arose very early, did my bathing, fixed my hair, applied makeup, and donned the outfit I had decided to wear coming to and going from the hospital.

I SHALL RETURN—MAYBE

The hour-long car drive was mostly silent, with a lot of handholding, hugging, soft smiles, and gentle presses. We were going to get through this. We made plans for my coming home gala two weeks hence on a Saturday, and I tried to mentally zero in on this thought.

First, I had to get through all the blood work, urine, x-rays, and that stuff, which to me was no mean matter, as I panic when I see a needle. And to get blood from me is quite a feat, what with my flinching and moving and crying. The technician was young, caring, and very capable. She worked with me through my fears. She was quick, chatty, and it went well. Now up to my room.

I was assigned a big end room on the 9th floor which was all oral, head and neck cancers. Tony and I walked in toward the far window bed which would be mine. I had to pass the other bed. There was someone in the bed, a creature, who was hooked up to some sort of pump, which was gurgling and bubbling. It had started. What was going to happen to me? What would I look like, sound like, smell like? I had to get out of there. I panicked. I wanted out of the whole thing. I wanted to go home, anything, just away from that room, that thing, that poor soul.

Quickly, Tony and I left the room, left the hospital, and started walking up and down the streets. It was a bright sunny afternoon. We stopped in for lunch at a corner cafe. I couldn't bring myself to eat, just sipped on a diet soda. My mind was going crazy. I was afraid. I couldn't do it. I was working myself up into a hysterical state, crying and feeling sick. I was going to die. I would never come out again. I would never see Tony, my children, or grandchildren. This was the last day of my life and I didn't want it to be. Tony talked and talked to me, we walked, held hands, kissed, and hugged and then more talking. We had to go back. It would be over the next day and we would laugh about it then.

Back to that "room." A special nurse came in to take more blood. By now, my nerves were jumping, she couldn't do it and hurt me terribly. My arm turned black and blue and puffed up. Another nurse came in and applied pressure to the spot and told me to squeeze the arm. She explained that I had to change into PJs (it was only 4 P.M.), and then told me the procedure for that night. The doctor and the anesthesiologist would visit me. I would take a sleeping pill and in the morning when they came for me, I would have some needles which would make me dopey, not alert, and that sounded good to me.

Nothing goes without some sort of snag, and mine was the Metro North train. Both the doctor and anesthesiologist were visiting upstate, and were delayed until almost 11 P.M. I had told Tony to go home. It had been a long day. He was beat, tired, sad, and lost and my heart felt so bad for him. He had to go through it all by himself—no Masses, angels, prayers, or well wishes. I had them all.

It was not Doctor Strong who came in that night, but his assistant, who thoroughly petrified me by announcing that they would probably remove my neck lymph nodes. Seeing my shock and fear, he backtracked by saying that he really didn't know what Dr. Strong was going to do, but not to worry and left. "Don't worry," just panic. The anesthesiologist was next in line with lots more good news. I would feel nothing and since I had asked, "No," he would not put the needle into my hand where I would see it on waking, but in my arm. A nurse came in to give me the pill and answer any questions. I had none. I just wanted to cave into the darkness of sleep until it was all over. Just before I feel asleep, my new roommate, Christine, whispered a good luck, God Bless, and goodnight.

Dr. Strong was right, I didn't feel anything. I said hello to him in the operating room and then it was, "Let's go."

BACK TO THE FUTURE

A voice somewhere said they liked the bright neon orange nailpolish on my toes. I was very warm and slept some more.

A nurse was doing something to me, and I became aware that I was back in my room. She told me it was all over. I was happy, very happy to be alive. I was warm, sleepy, and so thankful to be there in my bed. A quick thank you to God and back to sleep.

Something hurt—I felt funny—I felt sick—I was cold—it hurt to move—something was in my mouth—my nose was running—my leg was stinging—and there was something in my crotch; in fact there was something all over me, in my arms, legs, nose, mouth.

I started to cry, wiped my face with the sheet and saw blood everywhere. The bell was pinned to the pillow. I managed to ring it and a nurse appeared. Somehow, days had gone by and now I was awake, and I hurt. I was wildly afraid. It was dark, everything was quiet, I couldn't talk, my heart was beating. Everything hurt and I didn't know why—what was happening to me?

This nurse was oriental, young and very caring. She gave me a shot and stayed with me and talked to me until I found I was drifting off to sleep. She was very confident and I believed her. I went back to sleep.

On Thursday, the third day after the operation, I was alert enough to assess the situation. There was a large plastic bag on my thigh filled with blood. The catheter was in my crotch, the IV was in my hand, my nose was bleeding, and there was a horseshoe in my mouth with four white teeth dangling from it at a crazy left angle. There was also a deep line from my nose to what appeared to be my lip, but the lip wasn't there. I looked like a cleft palate person.

There was not so much pain as discomfort. My days of lounging around had ended. A nurse appeared with a latex bag with a syringe. I was advised that this contraption would be a big part of my life from here on in. She wasn't too clear as to what I had to do or maybe, I was not too clearheaded. But it sounded like I had to rinse my mouth with all that water four times a day. I appealed to her to remove the catheter and I would go to the bathroom and urinate. That deal was made. Next to go was the IV, if I would take a drink. I didn't realize it then, but that step was one of the most important steps of my life. It was too new to me to be scary. I didn't quite realize the size of the "defect," the padding, and the obturator.

I took the glass with confidence, only to find I couldn't find my mouth. Water poured down onto the bed, but some did go on my tongue and I did swallow!!! Stress had caused herpes blisters to form on top of the lip that I didn't have, and this pain distracted me from all the others. But I was alive, and on the way back. I saw Tony that night for a little, but was too tired from the getting up, washing, and hygienic instructions to do more than just hold his hand and promise to get better very soon.

THE HOSPITAL SHIFTS

Christine my roommate, and I talked. I slept, listened to Italian operas, got up each day, showered, shampooed, and dressed in my fancy summer stretch pants or shorts with long dangling earrings. I decided I wanted to lose some weight and so walked the long corridors many times during the night. I visited other people in other rooms and got to know all of the patients on that floor.

They all looked worse than me. We would all get together twice a day for special nose and mouth syringing (which I never quite got the hang of doing myself until many weeks later at Dr. Strong's office, when his nurse showed me exactly what I had to do and must do to avoid any infection). It became second nature.

I was hungry and not just for a hospital drink. I wanted food, and food I got, if I did well. First, it was ice cream, next yogurt, then jello, I was really doing good in that department. I had lost about 15 pounds and knew that my days of regular eating were over. Tony and I discussed how we would process meals and I would be able to eat anything pureed. I would never be able to "front eat." That meant no sandwiches, fruit, pizza, etc. Everything would have to be small and liquid enough to go way back to the back of the obturator where I could mash, gum, or swallow.

Dr. Strong visited every day. He seemed impressed with my recovery and explained that he had to remove more than he expected; my nose was involved, also the back of my top lip; he had inserted the implant from my thigh, but it didn't stay as expected and so my lip sort of disappeared from my face, leaving the obturator dangling crazily from my mouth. I did not look good. At that time, it was not that much of a concern to me; I was trying to feel my way around eating, talking, drooling, and spitting. I had to improve.

About the tenth day after the operation, Dr. Zatlow removed the wiring that was holding the obturator solidly in my mouth, along with yards and yards of smelly, bloody packing from my "so called" mouth and nose—it seemed to me to reach to my eyes. This procedure caused my blood pressure to soar. I was so frightened. I didn't want anyone near my mouth, especially with instruments. Dr. Zatlow and his assistant practically had to sit on my chest to cut and clip the wires. If I thought the obturator dangled before, now it was downright hanging and dropping out of my mouth. Dr. Zatlow showed me how to put it back in. He showed me and showed me. I could not do it. It was too big, I didn't know where to put it. There seemed nothing to hold on to. I just couldn't get it. That night I purposely skipped the hospital syringing call. I didn't know what to do. If I did nothing, it would get infected and then what? If I got it out, how would I put it back in? Would it ever go in? What, oh what, was I to do? By now, I realized I could not talk without it. I could not control drooling and had a problem with my tongue. My whole face caved in pitifully like the wicked witch of the west. I gave up and took a sleeping pill.

The next morning, the nurse wanted to know what happened that I wasn't at the "cleaning?" She was very sympathetic, but firm. I must learn to "do it," or else. She mentioned a male patient down the hall who couldn't or wouldn't try. She made it sound as if the end was near for him. After she left, another nurse announced that Dr. Strong was waiting for me in the "procedure room." What now?

To this day, I really don't know what he did except that he made "holes" for me in the skin graft inside my nose. It hurt, but was over quickly. He then asked me to take the obturator out for him. I got up from the examining table, sat in a chair and tried. I tried 'till sweat was running down my eyes. I couldn't get it out. Dr. Strong put his tongue depressor in and loosened it and took it out. Now, I had to put it back in. It took a long time, ten or so minutes with no one talking. I was embarrassed that I couldn't do it.

What was wrong with me? I could do anything. I had to do it for him, for me. I had to. It went in.

In the days that followed, I practiced in and out with the obturator, tried eating and drinking, each time getting cleaner and cleaner, with not so much slobbering.

Tony came each and every night. He ate with me and encouraged me on with different kinds of food (mostly soft, gucky, easy things). I even used the public phone and called my kids, family, and some friends. They were all so happy to hear from me and told me I sounded as good as ever, with maybe a little nasal quality, but then, "Everyone had some allergies or what."

VENI, VIDI, VICI

"That" day arrived. I was up, dressed, and ready to leave and Tony was right on time. It was a little strange saying, "Goodbye." Everyone had been so understanding, helpful, and used to me, my face, speech, my "defect," and now I was to go out to the real world. Would I make it? Would I be accepted? How would I look and talk? Would I ever eat out again? This was the first day of the "Rest of My Life."

The following year, running backward, I entered the hospital for plastic reconstruction. After a six-hour stint on the table, removing acres of scar tissue from my face, I recovered to find that I had a 10% return, a little lip (taken from my groin crease) which gave me a "Betty Boop" pout and scars from my eyes to the hairline.

Enough. That was it. No more. This is the final me.

TRANSCENDENCY

Since Sloan Kettering, I am on my fourth prosthesis. Remember the problem? Getting it in and out? Time passes. Now the problem is keeping it in my mouth, especially at weddings, funerals, family affairs, business outings, vacations, and all those social gatherings when you really want to be your best. I still spit when I am really into conversations; must remember to concentrate when eating; keep checking my face to make sure it is clean and try to draw on the best-looking lips my crayon can handle. Life is and continues to be good.

Politics and Culture

21

Growing Up as a Jewish Woman in a Post-Holocaust Era

Davida R. Schuman

In thinking about the Jews I have often wondered whether their survival as a distinct group was worth one single hair on the head of a single infant. Did the Jews have to survive so that six million innocent people should one day be burned in the ovens of Auschwitz?
—*Norman Podhoretz*
My Negro Problem and Ours, *1963*

When reading Podhoretz's statement I am inclined to say "Yes," the Jews had to survive, but their survival as a culture and a religious people were at a great cost. Upon a second reading of his comment, my thoughts reflect upon my experiences with anti-semitism as a child and as an adult. I was born in 1939 on the eve of World War II to parents who were first-generation Americans. In many respects, they were frightened and naive to the ways of the world. Prior to the Depression, while they were in their

mid-teens, they had both lost their fathers. Each had to find work while
completing high school. Although my father obtained a degree in law, he
practiced for just a short period of time before taking a position as a counselor with the New Jersey Rehabilitation Commission. I believe he took
the job because he knew he would be getting a paycheck on a regular
basis as compared to practicing law where the monetary rewards were
more uncertain.

My mother, on the other hand, was a housewife who bore and raised
three children. Much later on in her life, she attended college to obtain a
teaching degree. My mother kept a Jewish home, which meant she kept
kosher (dairy and meat were not eaten at the same meal and we did not
eat shellfish or pork). During the war, mother bought only kosher meat
when many women did not because of its high cost. She never questioned
whether or not she should adhere to the laws of kashrut (dietary laws). It
was just something one practiced as a Jewish homemaker. By the time I
was fourteen, I was assisting in keeping our home Jewish.

We observed the major Jewish holidays such as Rosh Hashonah, Yom
Kippur, Chanukah, Purim, and Passover. We considered ourselves to be
conservative Jews although my father worked on Saturdays. Occasionally
we would attend Sabbath services on Saturday morning. We were involved
in the synagogue and from the age of 8 my brothers and I attended Cheder
(Hebrew School) until we were 13. In addition to Sunday School, we attended Hebrew School three days a week after regular school. My brothers
were bar mitzvahed, but conservative Jews at that time did not believe girls
should be bat mitzvahed.

As a child growing up during World War II, I was not aware of anti-
semitism until I entered elementary school. I had heard my parents speak
of the atrocities that occurred in Europe, but since we had no family that
we were aware of living in Russia, Germany, or Poland, the conversations
held little meaning for me. The only recollection I have of them speaking
on a personal level was when they spoke of my father's brother who was
in the Army and fighting in Europe.

The first encounter with anti-semitism occurred in elementary school.
Although the incidents were few, they left a lasting impression. One such
incident occurred when I had stayed home from school because it was
Rosh Hashonah, and on my return I was asked by some of my peers why I
had not been in school since Ethel, who also was Jewish, had come to
school. I explained to them that it was a Jewish holiday and that I had
gone to the synagogue on the two days of Rosh Hashonah. My answer
seemed not to satisfy them and I remember one of my "interrogators" then
calling me a "dirty Jew," and screaming that the Jews had killed Jesus
Christ. Having no understanding of either accusation, and being unable to

respond, I walked away feeling completely confused and humiliated. That evening I asked my father what the children meant by these accusations. I asked him whether being a dirty Jew meant that I was bad, who Jesus Christ was, and had Jews killed him. His response was one of a parent trying to reassure and explain to a young child (I was no more than eight or nine) that neither statement was true, but that there were persons in the world who believed Jews should die because they were born Jewish. I did not learn until I was much older that there were people who may not have been Jewish themselves, but who had Jewish ancestors, who were also exterminated by Hitler's Nazis. Then he spoke to me about the Holocaust and what happened to the Jews in Europe. He told me about several Jewish families who had come to our town after the war to begin a new life. He explained that we had not killed Christ but that this idea was believed by some Christians.

I remember being confused and frightened and fearing that similar incidents would occur with my classmates each time I did not go to school because of a religious holiday. My parents decided not to speak to the school authorities because incidents such as I have described were out of the jurisdiction of the school. I believe my parents were concerned that if they did speak to the school they would be seen as making a problem where, from the school's perspective, none existed.

In Hebrew School, the Holocaust was not discussed—which I believe was a mistake. I cannot remember any time when anti-semitism as we know it today was taught or discussed during the six years I attended Hebrew School. We were taught to read and write Hebrew and we studied about the Israelites by reading and discussing the Bible stories. We learned about Palestine and its struggle as a young nation to become the Jewish homeland for all Jews.

Although I had gentile (non-Jewish) friends in school and belonged to the Brownies and the Girl Scouts, it seemed that there was a barrier that separated us. I never invited any of my non-Jewish friends to my synagogue for holiday festivities such as Chanukah and Purim, and I was never invited to their homes during Christmas. The Christmas holiday always made me feel left out and not belonging.

On the few occasions I was in a church it was because I went with my Catholic girlfriends when they went to confession. I would sit in the back pew of the church and wait for them to exit from the confessional. Since there was a particularly attractive male priest at this church, my girlfriends made sure they went to confession every two weeks and I tried to accompany them as often as I could. He was tall with dark hair and had an olive complexion and from our perspective was very handsome. After confession we would go to the park across from the church and the girls would talk about what the Father had said to them. Many times when I would pass the church on my way home from Hebrew School, he would be standing outside and would greet me. I always wondered whether he thought I was a parishioner since he would often see me with my Christian friends on Saturday afternoons.

Although both Christian and Jewish children went to the same high school, the Jewish students were always in the minority and we did not socialize very much outside of the school's activities. We attended the football and basketball games together, but we dated only within our own faith. The line was very clear-cut and to the best of my recollection no one crossed over to the other side. I never questioned it. Since there was a lack of young Jewish people to socialize with, I traveled to a nearby city where I joined a Jewish organization called B'nai Brith Girls. There I met other Jewish girls, which made my teen years more palatable. On Saturday evenings and Sunday afternoons, we would attend various functions in the Jewish Y where we met Jewish boys from another Jewish organization.

My college years were spent at a state institution which was predominantly Christian. I met several Jewish students at this college although the percentage was small. For the first time I had a few professors who were Jewish, but we never discussed anything that could be construed as particularly Jewish. If anti-semitism existed, it was hidden by the faculty and students. The only time when I felt that it may have existed is when a few instructors gave examinations during Passover. Since it was the 1950s, students did not object as they do today and Jewish students would just take a make-up exam. My parents had taught me that I was not to use my being Jewish or someone's anti-semitism as an excuse for not performing. They believed that I should be aware of a person's anti-semitism and to counteract it by achieving in school and at any job because doing well was the only avenue for Jews. They believed that although Jews lived in a predominantly Christian world, there was a boundary that separated Jews from Christians. We were not to cross over but were expected to accept this "rule" and do our best in school. I know that my father was terribly disappointed on more than one occasion when he was passed over for several positions by the New Jersey Rehabilitation Commission, but I cannot recall him ever blaming it on the fact that he was Jewish. He may have expressed it to my mother but his children were never told that he believed the reason was because he was Jewish. Affirmative action did not exist then but quotas did.

My next encounter with anti-semitism occurred when I was teaching in a public school. Since Christmas and Chanukah occurred at the same time and I had several Jewish children in my third-grade classroom, I decided to read them the story of Chanukah. Chanukah is not considered a religious holiday in the same way that Passover is. It is a minor holiday and many times it occurs about the same time as Christmas does. The day after I had read my students the story of the Maccabees, I was called to the principal's office and told that several parents had called claiming that I was teaching the children about the Jewish religion. I denied the accusation and offered to show him the book. He read the story and said that although he supported me, he was not in a position to defend me since he was only the acting principal and that my contract would not be renewed for the following year. In other words, although I had done nothing wrong, he wasn't going to go out on a limb for me because he wanted to save his own hide and become the permanent principal. I was all of 21 years old and this was the first time I had faced blatant anti-semitism. Welcome to the real world!

My father spoke to several Jewish leaders in the community, but they refused to confront the anti-semitism and were unwilling to help. I was advised to accept the situation and not to make waves (trouble) but to move on and seek another teaching position. Thus, the same feelings I had had as a child when I was called a dirty Jew were resurrected and reinforced by my parents and these Jewish politicians. As a result, I internalized my humiliation. It came as a shock that having an education was not enough for survival in the world although it was what I had been brought up to believe. Even though my father was the breadwinner in the family, he was a frightened man who hungered for security and acceptance. In comparison, my mother always seemed stronger and tougher but even she could not stand up to this situation. Both parents supported me quietly, but I learned that without the advocacy from the Jewish politicians I had nothing. There is a saying in politics that whether you are Jewish, Christian, Black, or Hispanic, you'd better have a rabbi (someone who takes a special interest in you and supports you). Well, I did not have this rabbi, and as a result I had to accept the school's decision. I was unaware of my anger because it was so deeply embedded in my psyche. It was not until years later that I was able to confront my feelings on this subject.

I began to detest being a Jewess and longed to be a white Anglo-Saxon Protestant with straight blond hair. The only physical characteristic that I had in common with Protestant females was that I was thin, had small breasts, and wore a size five dress. I had a semitic nose and dark hair which led people to think I was Italian or Spanish. But, oh, how I longed to have straight golden blond hair falling to the middle of my back. Since dyeing my hair was out of the question, I proceeded to iron it to remove the curl thinking this would help me enter the WASP world which I so dearly sought. And when ironing didn't work, I had my hair straightened so that it would lie flat down my back. Little did I know at the time that the door was closed to people like me and that there was no way to enter their space. I used to think that maybe if I had money the doors would open and I would be accepted. But it was naive of me to think that having money would make me more appealing to Anglo-Saxons. I soon realized that neither would I be accepted by the world of wealthy Jews with their caste system. It was a bitter pill to swallow, but I had no choice. I had to resign myself to the fact that I was a middle class (by then) Jewish girl from Hoboken, New Jersey, who had to work from the age of sixteen. When I look back upon those years, I realize they were the foundation of what I am today. Although my parents were unable to confront the anti-semitism, they gave me what I now know as their support and the skills to survive by telling me to go on and seek other employment. They did their best under trying circumstances.

At the next teaching position I had there were several Jewish teachers in the school who had been teaching for ten or fifteen years. They were married with growing children and had returned to teaching after having spent time at home caring for their families. I taught at the school for several years without any incident. Although the superintendent and administrators were Italian, Irish, and Jewish, the school system was gradually changing to Hispanic. The teachers would complain about the level of performance of the new students. During a discussion with several of the younger teachers concerning the Hispanic influx, one non-Jewish teacher remarked how well Jewish students performed academically. By this time, which was the early sixties, there were very few Jewish students enrolled in this particular school system. Another teacher made the remark that Jewish students are smarter and cleverer than other groups of children. The conversation continued in this manner with comments being made about how Jews make such good lawyers because they can get their clients what they want and they are very sly in business. One teacher spoke about the fur business as being controlled by Jews and that when she bought a fur hat she would "Jew the owner down" (a phrase I had never heard before). She then referred to Jews being so clever that there is a practice among Jewish businessmen referred to as "Jewish lightening." This, too, I had never heard before. She explained both statements, the first meaning that you always bargain with a Jew and that you never pay the asking price. The second phrase meant that when Jews want to have returned the money they paid for insurance for their businesses, they torch the building and collect the fire insurance. The four or five teachers who were eating lunch in my classroom all laughed while I, on the other hand, was attempting to control my anger as my religion was being assailed. I felt personally attacked by these comments, and though I tried, I was unable to make them understand that what they said was anti-semitic without my using the word. Of course, the conversation then proceeded to the next level in which comments concerning the wives of Jewish husbands were made. "Their primary concern is with spending money, wearing large diamond rings, and belonging to the right country club." There was no way for me to stop this conversation because it had taken on a life of its own. The only thing that ended it was the bell indicating that lunch was over. What was the use of my trying to explain to these women that these goals were not unique to Jewish women alone; that not all Jewish women had these desires; that Jews have been ostracized throughout the centuries and only by accruing wealth were they able to survive; and some Jews, very few in fact, had been able to buy their way out of Germany and Poland prior to the Holocaust. And lastly, that not all Jews were wealthy, most were middle and lower class, or poor, and that the reason Jews tended not to be on welfare was that there were Jewish organizations, such as the Jewish Family Service and the Hebrew Immigrant Aid Society, that subsidized Jewish families and kept them afloat until they were able to sustain themselves. Or as in the case of my father's and mother's family, every sibling went to work during and after high school and attended college at night. And in many situations, children left school in order to work to bring home money. In families where there were daughters, they were sent to work in order for their brothers to attend college. If they were fortunate, they were betrothed to someone who could help the family financially. How could I tell all this to these teachers who had no inkling about Jewish poverty but only saw the well-established Jews as those who owned businesses, and were the lawyers and the doctors whom they used or heard about? And so I kept quiet, but I was determined not to allow any situation like this one to occur again. In the future, I would be more prepared.

I can't tell you the exact date or time when I began to view myself as a spokesperson for Jews. It evolved slowly when I was in my mid-twenties. Never again would I be silent when I heard an anti-semitic remark or a joke at the expense of my people. And so, I went on a campaign to soften the prejudiced views many (it seemed to me) Christians held of Jews by presenting myself as an intelligent and affable young woman. When I was in a social environment and in the company of non-Jews, I was guarded, lest they should perceive me as one of "those Jews" who only took their money in the stores they frequented or who defended them in court. My long dark hair and svelte build allowed me the "privilege" of passing for an Italian or a Spanish woman. Even the name "Davida" lent itself to some people thinking I was something other than Jewish. I would make a point of telling them with a smile that I was Jewish of Russian and Polish descent. And frequently I would then hear from these educated and intelligent individuals a comment about how their best friend in grade school, high school, or college had been Jewish. Sometimes they would flavor their remarks with a Yiddish word or two. I would smile as I corrected their pronunciation because I knew this was their way of attempting to bond with me (and deny any bias). In my gut I knew they harbored anti-semitic feelings toward me as well as toward all Jews. In small ways I tried to alter their views of Jews. I never allowed an ethnic joke or racial slur to go by without informing them that their comments were inappropriate.

One incident I vividly recall occurred at a cocktail party. I was twenty-seven years old, an assistant professor at a private college in New Jersey, and the only Jew in the department. Several faculty were conversing when the dean of the School of Education who was Protestant, remarked that many of our female students are dark-haired Jewish girls seeking husbands with fat wallets. At the time I was unaware that his reference to dark-haired Jewish girls was not because he lusted for dark-haired women, but that he was attracted to "blond-haired girls," from his wife to his secretary (who was his mistress). His audience laughed at his remark while I stood there frozen and unable to speak. Believing that his remark was addressed to me and all Jewish women, my humiliation was overwhelming and I left the party soon after.

Again, I fell into the trap of accepting—albeit reluctantly—the dean's remark as true. I told myself, "Yes, Jewish girls are looking for rich husbands, they are stupid with nothing between the ears, and they deserve to be ridiculed." Therefore, *I* was seeking a rich husband and *I* was stupid. How utterly absurd! But at the time I was unaware of the psychological impact his statement had on me. What did surface was the realization that education does not obliterate deep-seated prejudices. This came as a shock to me. I recall thinking, what have my parents taught me? To be truthful, fair, just, charitable, to take responsibility for my actions! Jews, so I thought, were nurtured on these tenets. Why couldn't the Christian world accept and respect us for who we were? Why were they constantly degrading us? Perhaps not intending to, but doing it nevertheless. Questions are easy but answers, harder to find.

Obviously, my perceptions go back to my roots. My parents were unable to assist themselves, let alone me. They were frightened, confused people trying desperately to make sense out of their world. And they transmitted their fears to their children.

For a long time I considered my enemies the Christians whom I met both socially and professionally. As a fervent defender of the underdog and a political liberal who believed in Lyndon Johnson's Great Society, I was caught off guard by the onslaught of anti-semitism on the part of some African-Americans. Jews and African-Americans had built an

alliance together that dated back to the founding of the National Association for the Advancement of Colored People (NAACP). We had worked
and died together during the Civil Rights Movement. How could this
change towards Jews have occurred? Yes, I had read the reports concerning Louis Farrakhan's anti-semitic views as well as those of other African-
American leaders. But I was unprepared for the hate that I encountered at
the academic institution where I was a faculty member. I particularly recall the speech by a prominent African-American at the close of Black History Month in February 1992 at a college in the northeast. Specifically, he
accused Jews of playing a major role in the slave trade in England and
America. He also accused Jews of negatively portraying African Americans in films. He declared that Russian and German Jews were the major
producers in Hollywood. In their capacity as producers, during the 1920s
through the 1950s, they depicted a negative image of African-Americans
in films during this period. He and other Afro-Centrists had been speaking at colleges throughout the northeast and presenting their message of
hate, bigotry, and anti-semitic propaganda.

On a Friday, the last of February 1992 I had taken my son, who was then
ten years old, with me to the college because I wanted him to hear what an
African-American was saying about Jews. Jews and non-Jews from the faculty and administration protested outside the building where this speaker
was to address the audience. At one point, we were told that we would not
be allowed to attend his lecture. The students as well as several administrators who supported the students were informed that because the
college is a public institution, we could not be stopped from attending his
lecture. Seven faculty, Jews and non-Jews, as well as several Jews from the
community, heard his horrendous untruths about Jews and other religious,
ethnic, and racial groups. After listening to him for about an hour-and-a-
half, I left with my son to return to Brooklyn and to attend Shabbat services at my synagogue. As I was driving across the Pulaski Skyway towards
the Holland Tunnel, my son asked me why African-Americans had such a
hatred toward Jews. He asked me what had we done to warrant such an-
tipathy and venom. At the time I did not have an answer for him. I remember thinking of a similar question I had asked of my father more than forty
years ago. As I drove toward Brooklyn, I vowed that I would not stand by
silently and allow my son, or any child for that matter, to experience the
fear and humiliation that I had felt as a child.

It soon became apparent that unless this message of anti-semitism
was contained, the racial strife would worsen at the college. With this
thought in mind, I began a campaign to end the influence this speaker
had at the school. I warned the Jewish faculty and staff that unless they
spoke out we would be pushed out of the college, and that when we had

been eliminated, all white persons would be next. Most Jews did not heed my warning. They, along with my non-Jewish colleagues, believed that by conducting dialogues with minority students, the faculty, and administration, we could iron out our differences. And so the college began a series of multicultural workshops about racism, anti-semitism, and bigotry. There was a series of lectures by well-known authorities in the field of race, anti-semitism and black studies. Although I wished that my colleagues would be right, my gut feeling was that we had a long road ahead before things would change. There were times when I doubted my own sense of reality.

On April 5, 1992, a minority leader spoke in Newark, New Jersey, to an audience made up of people from the adjacent communities. In his speech, he gave animal names to various ethnic groups that had gone to Africa. For example, he referred to the big white man from England as the elephant; the big white man from Germany as the giraffe, and so on. His last animal category was the skunk and that was the Jew. "And the Jew stunk up the place." The speaker continued to denigrate Jews to his audience. "The skunk came around and stunk up everything. He stunk up the whole atmosphere." The audience applauded after each reference to Jews. The speaker told his audience that as parents with children in the schools, "You have to have peace with the skunks because they'll stink you up too. But the truth will set you free."

Throughout these three-and-a-half years since February 1992, there has been a handful of Jews and non-Jews from within the college and without that have kept up a constant campaign to rid the institution of the racial hatred permeating the campus. The battle has not yet been won. Racial and anti-semitic situations have continued to occur. I hope I have the stamina and vigilance to continue. I hope others, non-Jews as well as Jews, will join the fray. I sometimes feel that there will be no end to the disharmony and racial conflict at many of our major academic institutions. I hope that I am wrong and that the cancer of racial bigotry is removed permanently. But I realize that no threat to freedom is ever permanently removed, that "eternal vigilance (and activism) is the price of freedom," and that as long as *any* group is unfairly characterized or treated, no one is safe.

22

Cultural and
Personal Meanings

Katherine Parry

*I*n an atmosphere of both increasing interest in and increasing knowledge about the health traditions of various ethnic groups, clinicians may—out of the best of intentions—make a critical error: They may stereotype patients because of ethnic background.

Many clinicians now recognize that culture shapes the environment in every domain, from childbirth practices to rituals surrounding mourning and death. Culture shapes the response to illness by defining what illness is, who should treat it, and what the proper treatment should be.

Numerous articles and books have documented the health behaviors of ethnic groups in terms of generalizations. We may read, for example, that "Haitians in Miami tend to be Catholic in name only while still retaining their beliefs about Vodun [Voodoo]"[1] or that "Blacks have a fatalistic outlook in illness and pain."[2]

Reprinted with permission of PT Magazine.

As physical therapists learn about the health behaviors and perceptions of patients from cultures other than their own, they may begin to expect patients to follow certain "recipes" of behavior. They may assume that patients will be believers or participants in the traditional health care system to which they seem to belong: "Ms. J is Haitian; therefore she must know about Voodoo." As Kay,[3] Litterst,[4] and others have pointed out, these types of expectations and assumptions ignore the impact of other differences, such as education or social class, which might make a patient ignorant of a tradition or practice. Consider the following case example.

A Panamanian woman is referred for physical therapy. The physical therapy director assigns a Panamanian-educated female therapist to that case because she assumes that this therapist would have a better understanding and establish a better rapport than would a U.S.-educated male or female therapist. Later it is discovered that the patient is aghast that the therapist's upbringing and background are totally different from and at odds with her own more "conservative" upbringing and background. The patient is from a generation, religion, and social class different from those of the therapist, and incompatibility is the end result, as each subtly displays disdain for the other's comportment.

There are two lessons to be learned from this case. First, in U.S. culture these types of differences might have only a minimal impact on the patient-therapist relationship, whereas in other cultures, they may have a major impact. Second, although it is necessary to be informed of the norms of any particular ethnic group, it is essential in clinical practice to go beyond ethnicity to take into account all the other factors that influence the patient's behaviors and perceptions. Tools derived from anthropology can be adapted for use in clinical practice to help identify these "other factors."

CULTURAL IDENTITY SYSTEMS

One of the anthropological tools that can be used in the clinic is based on the cultural identity systems proposed by Hill et al.[5] This approach presumes that an individual's identity is made up of many distinct cultural identifications grouped under the following variables, or "systems":

- *Ethnicity/nationality.* Geography, homeland, migration, language, topography, political and economic history, heroic figures, flags, and other symbolic representations

- *Race.* Skin color, eye color and shape, hair color and texture, nose size and shape, musculoskeletal stature, political and economic history, heroic figures, and other symbolic representations
- *Age.* Physical growth, development, change in physical features, political and economic history, rites of passage, rituals, and other symbols of age
- *Gender.* Primary and secondary sexual characteristics, musculoskeletal stature, voice, gesture, political and economic history, heroic figures, and other symbolic representations
- *Family.* Residence, degree of consanguinity or affinity, economic and geographic history, heroic figures, crests, and other symbolic representations
- *Vocation.* Profession, work, business, subsistence activity, employment, political and economic history, heroic figures, rituals and other symbols of vocational persistence, boundary structure, and maintenance
- *Religion.* Beliefs; sacred texts handed down by or under divine guidance; sacred objects, rites, rituals, or places usually linked to religious origins; political and economic history; and heroic figures
- *Disability.* "Abnormal" physical or mental quality, chronic disease, limiting factors, political and economic history, heroic figures, and other symbolic representations

Some of the variables, such as gender and ethnicity, are static, whereas others, such as age and vocation, are fluid. All of the variables have a different meaning at different times of an individual's life cycle. The personal meaning of the identity of "female," for example, changes as an individual moves from prepuberty to childbearing to menopause to postmenopause. For a woman, variables such as religion or family may place constraints on identity because they define how a woman from "this" family or "this" religious background should act. If a woman also has a professional identity—such as that of a physical therapist—the values of her profession may supersede the values of her other identities.

When therapists treat patients on a long-term basis in settings such as rehabilitation centers, nursing homes, outpatient clinics, and home health, the patient's (and the family's) cooperation and carry-through are critical. Lack of knowledge about what cultural identifications are most important may result in conflict between patient and therapist. In the case described above, the patient's identification with age and the values of a more "conservative" generation—and with gender and the values involving how a woman conducts herself—produced in the patient an abhorrence for the therapist's status as a divorcee. The patient's identifications also produced an unexpected cultural clash. "Lumping together" these two people on the basis of ethnicity backfired because other cultural identifications were more salient than a shared country of origin.

Clinical Application

The cultural identity systems proposed by Hill et al.[5] offer alternative and sometimes competing opportunities for identification with and membership in an ethnic group within U.S. society. Filling in a grid can help the therapist assess (1) the personal meanings that each domain holds for the patient and (2) the intensity of the patient's involvement in those domains. In practice, this information is gathered over a period of time through informal conversation, careful listening to and observation of the patient's interactions, and other relevant data (e.g., the objects that the patient displays in his or her room).

The clinical value of the grids is in their potential to help the therapist conduct clinically relevant "cultural assessments" just as he or she would conduct physical therapy assessments such as musculoskeletal evaluation.

Case in Point. Ms. J is an unmarried Haitian woman with hemiplegia resulting from injury. She was not fully cooperative with physical therapy and left therapy 2 weeks before she was scheduled to be discharged.

The identification grid filled out after she terminated therapy reveals that Ms. J identified strongly with her Haitian upbringing and her family's emphasis on reaching "the highest level of accomplishment possible." The family, with its extended membership and support, also was of great importance, as were being employed and earning her own living. Although race was not of high personal importance to her, she disliked being "lumped together" with African Americans whose background and experiences, she believed, were diametrically opposed to her own. Gender and religion also were not of high importance to her. Although she was unable to use her left upper limb, she disregarded the effects of her disability and believed she could still realize the majority of her personal goals.

In retrospect, the therapist realized that Ms. J disagreed with the therapist's long-term goals, which "fell short" of what Ms. J felt she could accomplish. She left therapy early because returning to work and the kind of productive life to which she was accustomed were of primary importance to her. If the therapist had taken time to find out more about Ms. J's cultural identifications, goals, and opinions, could conflict have been avoided?

EXPLANATORY MODELS OF ILLNESS

In addition to understanding the patient's cultural identity systems, clinicians need to recognize that each patient has his or her own "mental map" of illness. Rather than taking for granted what a patient believes—and rather than telling the patient what he or she ought to believe according to our professional beliefs—therapists need to place the emphasis on learning about the beliefs of the patient as an individual and how those personal beliefs guide health behaviors.

Kleinman,[6] who studied healing in its cultural context, formulated the concept of "explanatory models," defined as "notions about an episode of sickness and its treatment that are employed by all those engaged in the clinical process." Information about these notions allows the therapist to understand how the patient interprets each episode of illness and what guides the patient's choice of treatment. Explanatory models address five major issues:

1. Etiology of the problem.
2. Time and mode of onset of symptoms.
3. Pathophysiology of the illness.
4. Course of illness, that is, degree of severity.
5. Type of treatment that should be sought.

Kleinman created a patient questionnaire that has been recommended for use by medical students,[7] nurses,[8] and physical therapists.[9]
It includes the questions:

1. What do you call your problem? What name does it have?
2. What do you think caused your problem?
3. Why do you think it started when it did?
4. What does your sickness do to you? How does it work?
5. How severe is your sickness? Will it have a short or long course?
6. What do you fear most about your sickness?
7. What are the chief problems your sickness has caused for you?
8. What kinds of treatments do you think you should receive? What are the most important results you hope to receive from treatment?

It can serve as a vehicle for open-ended discussion. Because some patients fear ridicule or criticism, they may not volunteer this type of information; however, they may provide the information when it is requested by a sincere, interested clinician.

When Allen and Mobley[10] used Kleinman's questionnaire in a study of folk treatment of diabetic ulcers by African Americans in Florida, they found that patients had their own rich explanations for the etiology and pathology of diabetes and diabetic ulcers. One patient, for example, reported that she believed diabetes made her blood run thick and black and that her blood was poisoned. In the context of this belief, putting uncooked fatback on a diabetic ulcer to draw out toxins—a traditional African-American remedy that may have harmful effects—can be better understood. Would asking this patient about her beliefs regarding what diabetes was doing to her body have helped health professionals intervene with more effective patient education?

Unless patients understand why and what they will gain, they may find it difficult to accept direction and instruction for taking what the clinician believes are rational steps leading to personal responsibility. The practitioner who has long been involved in giving information to patients about what they should do may have difficulty in simply asking for the patient's point of view in a nonjudgmental manner. Using a tool such as Kleinman's questionnaire can guide the practitioner in appropriate questioning.

ILLNESS COPING STYLES

Lipowski[11] suggested that individuals assign meaning to an illness using characteristic themes and that these themes are the outcome of individual coping styles, knowledge, beliefs, and cultural backgrounds. The meanings that patients may ascribe to illness—originally outlined by Lipowski, recast by Pfifferling[7] to reflect the clinician-patient interaction, and adapted here to reflect the physical therapist's clinical experience—include:

- Illness as challenge.
- Illness as God's will.
- Illness as strategy.
- Illness as value.

Illness as challenge is a coping style commonly attributed to the "Old Yankee" American. It is the style to which many U.S.-educated clinicians aspire: Illness is something to be rationally approached and "mastered." The proper authorities are consulted, advice is followed—and life goes on. This coping style follows anthropologist Kluckhohn's[12] conceptualization of the American as action-oriented and individualistic.

In contrast, *illness as God's will* emphasizes resignation. Vital events including illness may be perceived as being beyond human control. Both African-American and Hispanic-American populations have been stereotyped as "fatalistic"; however, this philosophy also is a part of a North American heritage rooted in the beliefs of early immigrant groups such as the Puritans.[13] Today, a patient's religious beliefs may have more to do with this concept than does cultural or ethnic background. When illness is perceived as God's will, the coping style may be characterized by a passive acceptance of what "cannot be changed." Patients who use this style may not be interested in aggressive procedures or even in changing their "destiny." Those who feel that illness is a result of God's punishment may feel depressed.[11]

Patients who use *illness as strategy* typically are using illness to secure attention or nurturing from parents, family—or health professionals who find them to be interesting cases. This style may need to be distinguished from the responses of members of ethnic groups such as Cuban Americans, whose culture may allow for greater demonstrations of affect and discharge of emotion during illness than do some other cultures.

Lipowski[11] believed that *illness as value* may be the "highest form" of coping. Here, illness is viewed as an opportunity that can result in important insight into the meaning of life; its occurrence may give meaning that previously had been missing. Consider the following case example:

> *An elderly Cuban woman is diagnosed with rheumatoid arthritis. A priestess in the Santeria sect, she believes that the cause of her disease was a spell—cast by another person—that she had "stepped into" by mistake. She believes that by her accidental intervention, she prevented the death of the individual for whom the spell was intended. She believes her personal power reduced the power of the spell to something less dangerous.*

This woman's way of dealing with her disease is to recast its meaning. She internalizes it as the result of a self-sacrificing, self-enhancing act. Her illness becomes something of value that both ennobles her and enables her to cope with the disease and the resulting deformities. If she were a patient in a physical therapy setting, would this information ever be collected? A consideration of cultural identity systems would identify religion as the central focus of her life. Using Kleinman's questionnaire would help health professionals understand what her illness means to her—and why she is coping so well with it.

Although all illness meanings may be influenced by culture, none of them is culture-specific. Individuals from different ethnic groups may use any one of them. Understanding these categories of meaning is important because misunderstandings and judgmental attitudes may develop when the patient's style of coping differs from that of the therapist. If the clinician responds to illness as a challenge for treatment, he or she may be puzzled or frustrated by the resigned, passive attitude of a patient who believes illness is God's will. It is important to recognize that there are a number of different illness meanings, none of which is more "valid" than the other.

THE PATIENT PERSPECTIVE

In an increasingly pluralistic society, divergent conceptualizations of health and illness increase. Although it is important to gain more knowledge of and conduct more research on the health behaviors of different ethnic groups, we should not lose sight of the beliefs of any one individual patient.

After all, in physical therapy, models of functional assessment fit the goals of treatment to what the patient wants to achieve. It is difficult to organize any systematic health education or prevention program if we are not aware of the individual patient's conceptualization of his or her illness. We can more effectively treat the patient when we understand the personal meaning of illness for him or her. Identifying the patient's distinct identity systems, explanatory model of illness, and coping styles can deepen and enrich our assessments and enhance the art of therapeutic communication.

REFERENCES

1. Scott, C. S. (1974). Health and healing practices among five ethnic groups in Miami, Florida. *Pub. Health Rep.*, 89:524-532.
2. Bloch, B. (1983). Nursing care of black patients. In M. S. Orque, B. Bloch, & L. S. Monrroy (Eds.), *Ethnic Nursing Care.* St. Louis, MO: C. V. Mosby Co.
3. Kay, M. (1983). Clinical anthropology. In E. Bauwen (Ed.), *The Anthropology of Health.* St. Louis, MO: C. V. Mosby Co.
4. Litterst, T. A. (1985). The reappraisal of anthropological field-work methods and the concept of culture in OT research. *Am J Occup Ther.*, 7:602-604.
5. Hill, R. F., Fortunberry, J. D., & Stein, H. F. (1989). Culture in clinical medicine. *South Med. J.*, 83:1071-1080.
6. Kleinman, A. (1980). *Patients and healers in the contexts of culture: An exploration of the borderland between anthropological medicine and psychiatry.* Berkeley, CA: University of California Press.

7. Pfifferling, J. H. (1981). Cultural prescription for medicocentrism. In L. Eisenberg, & A. Kleinman (Eds.), *The relevance of social science for medicine*, 197-222. Dordrecht, the Netherlands: D Reidal Publishing Co.

8. Chrisman, N. (1982). Anthropology in nursing: An exploration of adaptation. In N. Chrisman, & T. Mavetzki (Eds.), *Clinically Applied Anthropology*, 117-140. Dordrecht, the Netherlands: D Reidal Publishing Co.

9. Parry, K. K. (1984). Concepts from medical anthropology for clinicians. *Phys. Ther.*, 64:929-933.

10. Mobley, T., & Allen, O. (1994). *Folk treatment of diabetic ulcers among african americans: An Ethnographic Study.* Miami, FL: Barry University. Doctoral Thesis.

11. Lipowski, Z. J. (1970). Physical illness, stress and the coping process. *Psychology in Medicine*, 91-102.

12. Kluckholn, F., & Strodtbeck, F. (1951). Values and value-orientation in the theory of action. In: T. Parsons, & E. A. Shils (Eds.), *Towards a General Theory of Action*, Cambridge, MA: Harvard University Press.

13. Kluckholn, F. (1953). Dominant and variant value orientations. In: C. Kluckhohn, & H. A. Murray (Eds.), *Personality in Nature, Society, and Culture* (2nd ed.), 342-387. New York, NY: Alfred A. Knopf Inc.

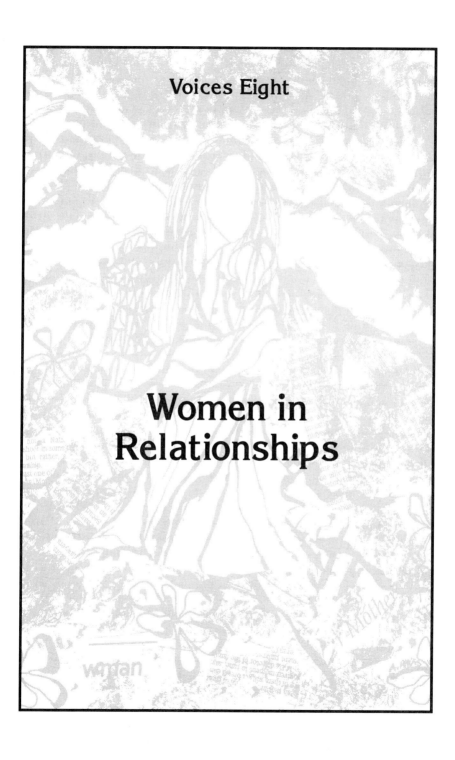

Voices Eight

Women in
Relationships

23

Reflections on a Marriage

Marcia Dombro

*F*or a woman, what is it like to be married? For me, it represents the most basic essence of being with another person. When a life is shared over a long period of time, it can't be described with one word like, "happy," "miserable," "exciting," "boring," because it is all of these. What is a successful marriage? In this era of easy divorce where more than 50% of marriages are dissolved, I suppose that an enduring marriage is an indicator of success. My comments about marriage are unique to my own experience in a relationship that has lasted since 1967.

In childhood fairy tales, frogs can be turned into princes by a lover's kiss; then the prince and princess live happily ever after. The possibility that the prince might someday return to his froggish tendencies is never mentioned. What happens then? Being in a long-term marriage, a woman must come to terms with the co-existence of both the frog and the prince. This creates constant tension, akin to what it must be like when walking a tightrope. One must proceed with a relaxed and confident attitude that it is indeed possible to accomplish this feat. On the other hand, there is the constant awareness of what will happen if equilibrium is lost, even momentarily. There is a delicate balance that must somehow be reached between the human opposites that always exist in a relationship between a man and a woman.

ROOTS/CHILDHOOD

My husband, Roy, and I came from very different backgrounds. I was the eldest child in a family of four children. Roy was an only child, born when his mother was nearly 40 years old. Her life revolved around him alone after his father died when Roy was eleven. My mother was constantly harried with so many young children. Occasional babysitting for my two younger brothers and baby sister was thrust upon me before I felt ready to accept it. I was never allowed to "act like a baby" because I was supposed to be the role model for the others. I vowed at an early age, not to have so many children that any of them would miss being a baby whenever necessary.

Like many men in the 1950s, my father focused his life on work. With so many children to support, he was often gone to one of his three jobs before I got up in the morning and was not back until after I went to sleep at night. He was a very handsome man, and as a child, I longed in vain for his attention and I don't remember having a real conversation alone with him until I was sixteen years old. He did not express his love in words to me until I was thirty-six. When I was choosing a husband, I wanted someone who would fill those gaps that I had felt as a child. I wanted someone who was willingly there for me, who would talk to me, and who would be able to say "I love you." Most of all, I looked for someone who really wanted to be involved with his children.

ENVIRONMENTAL/NEIGHBORHOOD

Roy and I grew up in totally different cultural and geographical environments. One strong memory I have is of my father spending most weekends, doing the constant repairs that needed to be made on our large old house in the Pacific Northwest. It stood on an acre of land covered with shrubs, flowers, grass, and fruit trees. My brothers and I would climb those trees to the topmost branches and survey our kingdoms, munching on apples and cherries.

Roy grew up in Brooklyn, in an apartment building. He played stickball in the streets with the neighborhood kids and his mother called the "Super" when something went wrong with the plumbing. He felt that he had the best of all possible childhoods. We had very different ideas about what childhood should be like.

CULTURAL AND RELIGIOUS BELIEF SYSTEMS

We were also different in our cultural and religious backgrounds. At an early age, I was attracted to religion by people outside of the family. I loved the storytelling, the music, the stained glass windows, and the chance to feel like more than just one of the four kids. We lived close to the church, so I was able to walk there by myself. When we moved to the "big house," the family had brief religious connections with the Presbyterian Church. We went very infrequently, since my mother did not have a driver's license and my father had to take us. He did not really enjoy church. When I grew older, I tried many different religious groups, including Lutheran, Catholic, and Unitarian.

Roy grew up as a Jew. He was not religious, but felt that being Jewish was an important cultural thing to him.

LEVEL OF EDUCATION

I was the first one on either side of my immediate family to graduate from college. One of my distant cousins had a doctorate in English literature, but was described as one of the black sheep of the family because he was a "perpetual student" and didn't seem to have a real job. I was very curious about him. When I moved to New York, I looked him up, and we became good friends. He encouraged me to go on for further education and wrote to me for many years after that.

FINDING ROY/GETTING MARRIED

In 1966, I sent in four dollars to a computer dating service called "Click." New York was not a place where one could usually know anything in advance about new acquaintances. The "Click" questionnaire asked some very important questions like: What religion should he be? How much education should he have? How concerned are you about health? What should his socioeconomic background be?

When Roy and I met, there was a feeling of inevitability. I was certain that he was the one, even though I had a migraine on our first date. He spent the evening telling me jokes, while I made smiling motions through my pain. I wanted to see him again. He seemed to be someone who would always learn and be an interesting person for the rest of his life.

Roy is Jewish, and when we decided to marry, I converted to his faith. New York rabbis were reluctant to marry Jews with converts, but we finally found one liberal soul who agreed. This was how we started.

Roy was 34 when we married and I was nearly 27. We had both worked, traveled, and experienced enough to know what we wanted. We had talked incessantly and agreed on many aspects of what our life would be like together. We decided exactly how many and when to have our children and what their religious education should be. We talked about division of labor in the household and agreed about what we then thought was fair.

Our first year of marriage was very difficult, since there were so many important details of life that we had not already worked out. These ambiguities about our roles were so troubling that I sometimes doubted the viability of our relationship. There were many days and nights when I shed bitter tears of frustration. I felt totally at a loss to know how to solve our differences.

In our first apartment, Roy had been quite comfortable. When we bought and moved into our own house, he had to make a big adjustment. There was no "Super" to fix anything. I learned to do many things myself, but sometimes I resented doing what my father would have done when I was a child. Still, part of me knew it was unreasonable to expect Roy to know about household maintenance when he had no experience with it. We eventually came to a tacit agreement that he would be the one to call repair people if any were needed. At least, though he didn't do the physical work, he had the responsibility to make sure that it was completed. As time passed, he learned to do many things around the house and he had my admiration for that.

RELATIONALITY

Emotional Expressiveness: Many men have difficulty in expressing their feelings of doubt, fear, loneliness, and love. They seem to have no trouble with anger, however. At the age of 13, I remember seeing my favorite aunt, stumbling up our back stairs, bruised and bloodied from a beating by her husband. Very early in our relationship, I made it clear to Roy that, if he ever hit me, I would leave as soon as possible. He once merely threatened me and I gave him one more warning about what I had said. "No physical violence" was part of our original contract, along with division of labor, religion, and how many children we would have.

Negativity: No one can be in a positive mood at all times. It took many years for me to finally be comfortable with this. Early in our marriage, it upset me when Roy would be angry or when I would be angry. I have always had difficulty dealing with it in myself or in others. Now I ask myself who owns the anger, instead of feeling, as I once did, that it must be my fault.

Love: When Roy and I were dating, I noticed that he did not hug me or hold hands with me as an expression of love. I did not ask for this until we had been married for more than 25 years. Now I feel that if I need this, I have a right to ask for it and to get it. Roy felt uncomfortable about it at first, but now he usually obliges without hesitation. Verbal expressions of love come more easily to him than to me.

Jealousy: The green-eyed monster has taken many forms in our marriage. I have sometimes thought that Roy wants to keep me all to himself. He used to talk about sharing me with the babies, implying that I had no time for him anymore. He would interrupt me in unpleasant ways when I talked on the telephone to friends. He said many times that I didn't need anyone else but him, that no one could love me like he did. All of this was very annoying to me and I sometimes became angry enough to think about leaving him.

I was jealous too sometimes. When we had a new baby, Roy went to lunch and other events with his lab technician. We did not want anyone else to take care of our baby, so, since I was breastfeeding, I was sometimes left alone with her, feeling trapped by my own choices.

Humor: Amusing stories have often helped us through difficult situations. Now that I know Roy better, I can use humor to say things that would be unacceptable in a serious vein. I am also trying to help him learn about my sense of humor. I read the funny papers every morning and have lately begun to cut out a favorite panel and put it on top of his pile of mail.

COMMUNICATION

Talking: This is the main thing that attracted me to Roy. He was very easy to talk to. We spent many hours talking about ourselves while we were getting to know one another. I think that we were both trying to be sure that we didn't make a mistake. Since we had already begun to witness disaster in the marriages of some of our friends.

Talking, or the lack of it, was an indicator of the health of our relationship. There were many years when we were both immersed in our careers and our children. We seemed to forget what we had together. During the last two years, in the 27th and 28th years of our relationship, we have been walking and talking just as we did when we were beginning together, but with much more comfort. Each night, we take a 3-mile hike and go over together whatever is in our minds. We talk about his work, my work, the children, what we read in the newspaper, books we have read or interesting thoughts we have. We have developed a rating system to describe each sunset. We tell each other stories, jokes, and anecdotes. We greet each dog that barks at us and compliment her on "defending the perimeter" of her property. We entertain one another. We both look forward to this experience and miss it if it doesn't happen.

Listening: We really try to listen to and understand one another. Sometimes, both of us talk about certain things just to clarify them in our own minds. The listening that goes on in this situation is to ourselves, not to one another. This is not as one-sided as it may sound, since we both get to have a turn. Perhaps not in the same conversation, but when necessary, self-talk is tolerated affectionately. At this point in our marriage, we recognize when it is happening. The talker talks and the spouse feels free to daydream since no response is really wanted or expected. This could never have happened in the early days . . . it would have been taken as a lack of attentiveness or love.

Since spending so much time together, we have developed the kind of marital ESP that one associates with long relationships. It still surprises me that he seems to know what I am thinking before I say it. I know what he is looking for before he asks me where it is. This is comforting in a way. Nothing can create this feeling but longevity and shared history. If someday we both lose half of our sanity, together we will be whole.

The Dynamics of Power: A long marriage is the quintessential arena for playing out every kind of power struggle between the sexes. We have grappled with all of them.

Personal Dynamism: Sometimes one person is more forceful than another. Perhaps this is usually the case. I have grown stronger as I have matured, but confess that I was nearly completely submissive for a number of years. Fighting about most issues was just not worth the effort. It seemed that whenever I "won" I really lost because I would be criticized and tormented for years afterward. The outcome in my favor was never "right" in Roy's eyes.

During the past few years, we have managed to make some decisions together and I have found ways to get what I want without open confrontations. I have realized that I deserve to have my needs and wants satisfied as often as he does.

Political: Roy loves to have political discussions. I am almost totally apolitical in terms of engaging in heated dialectics. I have my own opinions and make my own personal decisions about voting, which are sometimes diametrically opposed to Roy's way of thinking. We do not argue about politics.

Economic: An equal division of property and joint ownership of everything is important to a woman's security in marriage. During the times when I have not brought in a salary, I have been beset with feelings of impotence and vulnerability. This is only lately offset by the fact that I have made my own investments and retirement plans over the years. When our children were babies, I felt from Roy, an aura of condescension because I was "relaxing at home" while he was out earning money. As the years have passed, it has become clear that my wage earning potential is almost equal to his. This seems to have changed his attitude.

The power to make decisions is invested in the person who has and uses money. I have always had access to household money, but have not always chosen to be the one to use it. Doing the shopping can be a way to have economic control. Neither one of us is a big spender, and we are not dedicated to the accumulation of things, but Roy enjoys shopping more than I do. He bought most of our daughters' clothing as they were growing up and he likes to shop for groceries now. After many years of being reminded that we do not need twelve quarts of cranberry juice on hand, he has finally gotten into the habit of consulting with me before he goes to the market.

Gustatory Power: Food preparation can be a symbol of power in a relationship. The person who decides what to eat, when and how to eat it has control. Food itself has many meanings. Good food or special food can mean love. Even offering a cup of tea can mean "I care about you as much as I do about myself." Not preparing dinner at all can mean, "I am angry at you" or "I am too stressed out to eat," or "I am sick, YOU take care of me." It is important to try to be correct in the interpretation of the message.

Social: Social power carries the weight of family, old friends, social obligations from work, religious organizations, and other sources. I often felt like a "sidekick" when accompanying my husband to various family gatherings and department soirees. I went, however, because when I was growing up, husbands and wives always showed up together. When I began to have obligations too, I realized that Roy would refuse to attend some of them with me. At first, I would simply resentfully give my apologies and stay home. After about ten years of this, I began to see that, even though he did not always accompany me, he did not expect me to go to every wedding and funeral with him. Now we both feel quite comfortable in saying either yes or no to a "sidekick" request.

Friends: We have not always felt comfortable with the same people. There have been times when I would invite friends to dinner and Roy would not enter the conversation at all. Once, he even went to sleep on the couch while my friends and I were visiting. I am still trying to work this out and wonder if he is saying to me "You can't tell me who to associate with, or who my friends should be." He sometimes goes alone to see friends and I do the same.

Parental: This section was very difficult for me to write because it brought back so many feelings. When I discussed it with my 26-year-old daughter Rayna, she immediately recognized the problem. She reminded me that her father and I have very different parenting philosophies. This was reinforced on a daily basis as she grew up, leading to a great deal of frustration and conflict.

Discipline was a huge problem because Roy was much more indulgent with our daughters than I, yet he wanted to be involved in every aspect of their lives. He wanted them to have all of the privileges and material advantages that he did not have in his own childhood. This is the kind of man that I had been looking for, and yet, the reality often seemed like too much to me. The flurry of toys, books, and activities was not my idea of how to develop individuals. I wanted our daughters to have more opportunities to find their own way and to think their own thoughts. I could not seem to get him to see how I felt.

In retrospect, my daughters both help me to realize that my own influence on them was not overpowered by my husband's, although it seemed so as they were growing up. They now confide in me, woman to woman and I am delighted when they ask about what it is like to be a wife and a mother. The telling of it is for them, a revealing of their own heritage and for me, it is an adult window into their experiences as children. I cannot change the past, but in this way, we can better understand and support one another in the now.

SPATIALITY

Shared Space: Decorating a home is an expression of personal taste, which can also be an area for power struggles. I avoided trying to buy furniture for our house for several years, because I did not want to endure the conflict that would ensue. I finally hired a home decorating planner to act as mediator. This seemed to defuse the power struggle somewhat.

Another annoyance of sharing space was the ubiquitous presence of newspapers, books, and journals everywhere in the house. Both of us are avid readers and hate to throw anything away. I resented what I considered to be his messiness, but recently have begun to see my own role in the problem. I have begun to let go of my own paper and give away or shelve the books. I have bought magazine boxes and put his magazines in them, even though he resents my touching his things. He stopped complaining when he realized that it was easier to find what he wanted in the boxes. I do not accept disorder anymore, except in his own area where he can close the door.

Space at Work: When I had an office it gave me great pleasure to sit in the power seat as Roy faced me across my desk. At least here there was no argument about who would make the decisions.

Personal Space: Being able to get away from one another has always been important to us. We both need time alone and a feeling that there are some spaces in the house that belong to us as individuals, not as a couple. When we first moved into our own house, Roy claimed one of the rooms as his "den." His desk and books were there, but he never actually used the space. He would store bicycles and old boxes there. When he needed to do paperwork, he would spread out on the dining room table. I reasoned that this was a habit from childhood when he had no other place to do his homework.

When I was in graduate school, I needed a place to be away from household activity and noise. The den was the furthest room from the television set. The problem was that this had been Roy's space for many years. I knew that being able to use it would be a delicate problem. At first, I cleaned out the debris and boxes, then I began to work at Roy's desk. After a time, I needed many of my books, so, one by one, I removed his and replaced them with mine. I gradually took over the space. When he was away at a conference and our floors were being refinished, I moved his desk out too and replaced it with other furniture. I had put all of his things in an unused bedroom that had been occupied by one of our daughters. He didn't really mind, he still had a place of his own.

TEMPORALITY

Time has been an issue in our marriage because our inborn sensitivity to it has never been in synchrony. He wants to be early wherever we go. I hate to wait, there are too many other interesting things to do. Over the years, I have learned that it is easier to be ready to go on time than to fight about my right to be late. This was once a power issue, but when I recognized it as an irrational struggle, I began to change. I had to accept my own inner time clock and begin to help, rather than blame myself. It's now a personal game to estimate how long it takes to do something. I have clocks in every room and even on my computer screen as I write. I know that when I am engrossed in something creative, time loses its meaning, so I need to make allowances for this in my personal schedule. I do not claim to have gained complete control, but at least I have developed a little more understanding of myself.

CORPOREALITY

Body Image in Marriage: Being loved and accepted completely as I am is a wonderful and comfortable thing about being in a long-term relationship. The body, however, is the temple of the soul. Both Roy and I try to take care of our bodies, and we encourage one another in this. There is no greater test of body image than an intimate relationship with someone. Despite the common belief that boredom with sex occurs after many years of marriage, I do not believe that this has to happen. Avoidance of stereotypical behavior and efforts toward mutual satisfaction of needs is what has kept our interest alive.

Pregnancy and Childbirth: These were the most meaningful and profound experiences that we shared in our marriage. I was a Lamaze childbirth instructor during my pregnancies, so it gave an added dimension to the experience for my husband and I. He was not allowed in the delivery room for the first birth, but did help during labor, although he was very nervous about the whole thing. My friend Virginia Fitzsimons did the labor coaching with serenity and compassion. Another friend, Janice Waskin, effectively helped for the second birth. Roy was in the delivery room that time, and I asked the doctor to let him be the first one to hold the baby. His joy was so great, that it was the only time I have ever seen him cry.

Health: As we have grown older, both of us have experienced various health problems. We are especially concerned about one another during these times. It is important to both of us to know that someone cares and someone will help when we are ill or out of sorts. We deal with the prospect of getting old by joking about who will die first and what we will do about it. In this way, our wishes become known in a way that is not too heavy or depressing. It is comforting even to be able to discuss this with someone, in just this way.

Death: During the past few years, several of my friends have become widows. My husband is now 61 years old, one year younger than my father was when he died. I think about that a lot, and I wonder . . . if Roy was in his last hours, would he look at his life and feel that he really had love in his marriage? I wonder how much time we have left together . . . one year? twenty years? A lot has happened in our years together. We have had children and lived our lives along the same path. Some of it was happy and some of it was frustrating, constricting and miserable. For most of that time, I was very busy accomplishing things and escaping what I perceived as the "miserable." I never thought about the importance and meaning of loving. It was just something that was supposed to be part of the marriage package and something that I took for granted. If you asked whether I was "happy," I don't think that I could have answered. What does it mean to be happy? There is a description in Aldous Huxley's book, *Brave New World:*

> *Actual happiness always looks pretty squalid in comparison with the overcompensations for misery. And, of course, stability isn't nearly so spectacular as instability. And being contented has none of the glamour of a good fight against misfortune, none of the picturesqueness of a struggle with temptation, or a fatal overthrow by passion or doubt. Happiness is never grand.*

After reading this, I started to wonder if I had been overcompensating. Perhaps I really was happy and just had never stopped to realize it. If that was the case, then what does happiness in marriage look like? If it isn't grand and passionate, then it must be the appreciation and joy that can be found in everyday things. Eduard Lindemann wrote about living the "beautiful life," that everyday life itself could be a work of art. I believe that living with someone for a lifetime is a creative process. It is a struggle, sometimes filled with discord, but as the years go by a change can happen. With a great deal of work, a marriage partnership can develop into something profoundly beautiful, filled with peace, safety, security, equality of power, and most of all . . . real love.

24

A Single Woman
Adopts Catherine

Claudia Hauri

I cannot recall exactly when I decided to adopt; perhaps I was tired of
kissing frogs in hopes of finding a prince . . . so I decided to get a princess
instead. The event has been karma. Somehow Catherine was meant to be
mine and I was meant to be Catherine's mom.

I was married at 25 and divorced at 28, 2½ years of a wonderful marriage and 6 months of hell. I moved out in 1971 since my ex said he had
never had a home and my home is wherever I am because I am at home
within. I threw my energies into my career—nursing—developed as a
teacher, obtained my masters in 1974, and then became a family nurse
practitioner and faculty in a university. I did some consulting in South
America for an American school in Peru, for the Chilean Pediatric Nursing Society, and for the Red Cross Nurses in Columbia. I bought a larger
house in 1977, published, began the doctorate and settled in.

Then in 1984 I met a prince who was also divorced. We shared some
fun times and some sad times, and quite a few depressed times. Prince

eventually moved to Arizona to escape his ex-wife's wrath and I eventually healed. I guess this was the point that I thought about adoption. I remember going to a church to attend an adoption orientation program with another single friend also interested in adopting. I remember looking at the book of children available for adoption; singles, siblings, older than 3, of mixed race, and beautiful. Forms were taken home which somehow got to the bottom of the pile of things to do as I grappled and wrastled with the dissertation. During the next few years, I talked with friends and family about which gender should be a priority: first choice female/girl; age: 3 to 6 years since under two years was not my favorite stage; race: caucasian or mixed; and I would consider a handicapped child except for mental retardation. Some of my part time practice as a Nurse Practitioner is as a Consultant to the Association for Retarded Citizens (ARC) in maintaining the health of adults with developmental disabilities living in group homes and monitoring the health of children 6 months to 3 years in an early infant stimulation program. So I am well aware of the limits for some children. I eventually completed the forms and after a home visit was cleared for adoption in September 1988. I was hanging on to the end of my rope in attempting to finish the dissertation so I really did not pursue the adoption any further.

When the doctorate was obtained in 1989 I was free to be me again and was asked to be a consultant to the Public Health Department. There were an abundance of infants and children being placed in shelter and then foster care and I was to do the initial intake physical and if a court order had been obtained I was to start immunizations in anticipation that someday the child would be attending school. The summer was an eye opener as to the culture of HRS and the system that was a web of intricacies and offices that reached far and wide through something similar to going through a dense rainforest. I'll never forget the siblings that stirred again the feeling in my heart about being a mom. Susie was about 6 and her brother 4. They had travelled to this country with their parents who were apprehended at the airport for transporting cocaine into the United States. The children were placed in HRS custody and I did the physical in the shelter home where they were placed. The children had no idea what was happening, I talked to Susie and reassured her in my rusty Spanish that she would be going "home" soon, her brother looked at me with empty eyes. As I kept in touch with their status, I did intakes on children who were abandoned by parents too drunk on alcohol and high on cocaine to care about their children, left in the streets with a name tag but no other identification with a note that the parent was unable to care for the child any longer, or left at the hospital after a premature birth. Some children were "normal," others infested with lice, others full of scabies and impetigo, others developmentally delayed, others with blank stares and no ability or desire to hug and respond to human touch.

I was touched and amazed at the love, tenderness, warmth, brightness, cleanliness, teaching, caring, that the majority of the shelter and foster parents gave to each and every child. As I made the rounds, talked with the parents, and told them of my intent to adopt—to give a child a chance at life—I was advised to become a foster parent and at the appropriate time, express my intent to adopt, depending on the status of the child placed with me. In September/October 1989 I was given my license as a foster home and was assured that I would have a child by December—to go ahead and buy a ticket for the child since I was planning on spending the holidays in New Hampshire with family and doing some cross country skiing. The fall semester at the University passed. I made phone calls to the placement office but each time was told—no, there really is no child to be placed at this time. A week before flying I obtained a bogus medical letter that explained to Pan Am why "Johnny" Hauri could not fly and to please reimburse the ticket without penalty. I had fun skiing and apres ski activities and remember a conversation with my brother,

But Sis, how can you be a foster mother? What if "they" take her away?

Well, Ted, I look at it this way—HRS could take her away after a year—or a higher force could take her at 6 years to leukemia, 16 years to a drunk driver, 26 years to childbirth, or 36 years to whatever—when I lose the child is not for me to say. I just want to give her the best chance to be . . . for as long as I am allowed.

In January 1990, I was at a clinic in the center of town arranging for a clinical rotation for a student after which I found myself with some time to spare before the next appointment. Hm-mm-m I thought—HRS is around here somewhere. I found the building, found the placement office, found Carin, the placement officer and introduced myself.

Hi Carin, I'm Dr. Hauri, licensed foster status, and was assured since October that I would have a child placed with me since there was such a need.

Well, the only thing I have a need for right now is an 11-month-old girl, mixed race, hispanic I think.

Tell me yes or no.

Can I think about it?

Sure, but I really need to place her by tomorrow.

I'll call you before the end of today and give you my decision.

OK.

That was it. No identification, no nothing. I went to the University and called my mom but she didn't answer. I called my best friend at work, but she was in a meeting. A faculty member was in her office so I told Louise about the transaction so far. She was reassuring, saying things like, "if it's meant to be it's meant to be—go with your feelings—listen to your heart and your gut—you can do it." So I talked to myself, "Claudia, this is your decision, you need to make it. This is your life and you are a grown up— and if you don't try you will never know." So I called Carin and said, "I'll do it" and she said I'll call you when to pick up the child. This was Wednesday, January 18th, 1995.

The next morning I had a golf lesson with a friend at 8:30 A.M. which lasted till 9:30 after which I went to the University. Carin had already called and left a message to come to an office in the city where the child could be picked up at noon. I nearly panicked. I had nothing, not even a car seat, let alone supplies and food. So I asked Melba, a wise grandmotherly type faculty woman to come with me to get "the child." We arrived at the office and I remember seeing an infant in a stroller in an empty room with an elderly person watching her. I signed some papers and received two blue folders, and was taken to and given the child known as Maria. She was given to me with all her personal belongings: a large shopping bag containing a blanket, a bottle empty of milk (I was told she had thrown up at 10 A.M.), a change of clothing, a diaper, and a small stuffed lamb. As I held Maria I felt a warmth of heart, but her flaccid body was pale and white and noncommittal. As Melba and I walked down the stairs we said to each other how beautiful she was, and how cute, and alert and oh my gosh! am I really going to be a Mom? The memory brings back a smile and goosebumps as I sit here. Once in the garage, I put Maria on the trunk of my car and gave her the quickest, but probably most comprehensive neuromuscular and developmental physical she had ever had. And off we were!

Melba held Maria in her lap enveloped in seat belt while I drove to the nearest second-hand store. There we found a car seat, playpen, and some clothes. Next was a discount store where I purchased a playpen mattress, 2 sheets, some more clothes, and some toys. The next stop was a supermarket where I asked another shopper what size diapers I should buy, and where I bought enough staples to get me through the night and next day. The final stop was the University by 2:30 P.M. where I was greeted by faculty with open arms and champagne and lots of questions. Maria finally settled down and took a much needed nap. I reached my Mom and told her "we" were coming for dinner. Then I taught class from 4 to 5:30 and headed home with my foster daughter in the midst of rush hour traffic.

Maria cried on the way home and I sang to her to soothe her tears and discomfort. I also talked to her and reassured her that she was in good hands and I would stand beside her no matter what. My Mom was delighted and loved her from the moment she saw Maria and has been a strong support and mentor ever since. I took Friday off to find child care and buy some more supplies and order diaper service and contact friends for a crib and other items. Over the weekend, I picked up a crib, changing table, high chair, and began to put our life back together. I introduced Maria to neighbors and we began to get to know each other. From the beginning, Maria slept through the night and happily entertained herself in the morning for half an hour to 45 minutes after awakening. The shelter home in which Maria had been for 9 months was home for 6 to 8 infants under the age of 2 years. Thus Maria, already a survivor, learned to entertain herself in her own world. This was a godsend to me, because it gave me time to shower, fix breakfast, and get the morning together before I became a "mom." I soon learned not to dress until after breakfast. This way I wouldn't have to change clothes because of stains and drips and drool and crinkles in the clothing. The same rule applies six years later. That first weekend was wonderful and I shall never forget it.

Maria and I had bonded within the first month—she was such a happy, smiling, bubbling baby. She needed time getting used to being in the stroller, and a new home with new faces, and new food and tastes (during the first week she had enough garlic and parsley to last her a lifetime) and new toys and everything. Prior to this, Maria had been at the county hospital for 2 months after being born 2 months premature and septic, then the shelter home which was subsequently closed by HRS and this was where I stepped in at the Placement Office. I familiarized myself with the 2 blue folders—one was the social work record, the other the health care record. Maria was being followed at a University Affiliated Facility, a Center for Child Development, for developmental delay and I needed to maintain the appointment schedule. There were no other notations of health problems, although according to the DDST-R, Maria was delayed in physical development. Personally I thought she was on target for mental development after watching her for a month. Whatever drugs she got during her prenatal period had given her extra pizzaz as far as I was concerned!

The months passed by and we enjoyed each other and settled into a new routine for all. The first major event was a judicial review that was held in June or July of 1990. A panel of professional volunteers with legal training would hear the cases for the many children in shelter and foster care and make decisions about their future in order to relieve the burden of cases for the judges who, backlogged with cases, were months behind. The panel recommended terminating the mother's rights after hearing testimony from HRS and from me and from my Mom who was the foster grandparent (duly fingerprinted and processed for misdemeanors and felony records!). Maria's records should have been transferred directly to Adoptions, but were not and so ensued another 15 months of agony and a tug of war with the case workers and subsequent caseworkers and judges and hearings and talk of visits and commotion that would have turned me off to the process except for the fact that I reminded myself that I had earned the doctorate through tenacity and perseverance and this was another excellent opportunity to apply what I had learned about those qualities towards a worthwhile cause.

I have notes about that time in my life: the times I was trying to reach a caseworker or a supervisor and the phone rang 52 times only to be answered (?) and then a disconnect. Then the phone would be busy when I redialed. Or the time I was talking to the caseworker and he gave me the biological mother's address thinking he was talking to her—and I wondered if he had inadvertently given her my address and should I install an alarm system. There were moments of humor, when Judge Lewis asked what kind of doctor I was after I introduced myself as Dr. Hauri, and I replied a doctor of education. "Where from?" University of Florida was my reply as I made the gators jaws with my arms and the Judge laughed and smiled and wished me well in my pursuit of Maria. He once again directed HRS to obtain the signature and move the case along and to Adoptions.

That day finally came. I was nervous in many ways—this was a serious step I was taking as a single woman. I wondered briefly if I could manage, but then reminded myself that with my Mom's help and the help and support of my friends I had coped quite well so far. I had experienced many of the normal fears and doubts a biological mother has—should I take her to the doctor for an antibiotic for the cold (no); is the temperature because of teething? (yes); the tears when I was tired and wondered whether I could keep this up? (yes). Friends asked if I wasn't tired when I went to bed at night and my usual answer was "yes," but it's a nice tired. I mean I was tired before, but this is different, it's a rewarding tired. I still feel that way today, only more so because of the light and love my daughter has brought into my life and the way she shows me the world through her eyes as I lead her through the world by the hand with all the knowledge and love I have to give. Hey, sure we fight and we argue and yell at each other sometimes in the morning, but we get over it, talk it over, and give hugs and kisses and eventually say goodnight at the end of the day. In retrospect, I was 47 when I was a foster mom for Maria—she is now 6 and I will be 53 this year. I started going through menopause when I was 50 or 51 and I remember clearly one night making an entry into Maria's memory book that we were certainly on the outs that day—she was in the terrific three's and practicing being independent, and I was in a hormonal swing that left me frazzled and intolerant to the little snit saying NO! all the time. The year my career was in the pits and I was growling like a bear, I taught Maria to say "Hey Mom, stop growling like a grizzly bear" or "Chill out, mom, I love you."

It worked. I would look at her and a smile would creep across my face and I would have to admit to her that she was right and then I would give her a big teddy bear hug. And hugs have always been one of Maria's strengths. I taught her to jump up on the count of three when she wanted "uppy-uppy" and she would fit onto my body with a snugness that is uncanny—like we fit together. And she still hugs that way—morning, noon, and night. My friends will vouch for that because they are recipients of her love and hugs also. And now I really have to laugh at times because Maria will explain to me why I can't do something with the same reasons I gave her for something she wanted and the principle applies and I can't refute the logic I preached and so I admit—you're right.

And then I hear "YES!" and her thumbs are up. My frazzles are becoming less and both of us are becoming older and wiser together. Because I will be 65 when Maria is 18 I took out the Florida Prepaid Tuition Plan. That was so I don't have to work to get tuition benefits; we can go wherever Maria wants to go and room in the dorm or a trailer or a condo and Maria can be a Freshman and have her college life and I can go to Elderhostel and have my life. And then we can be together again when we want to be.

I mentioned the memory book. When I became a foster mom I joined the Foster Parents Association and I was told to start a memory book for Maria so she would have memories of the past. I did and to this day make entries although they are less often than previously. There are articles about the scandals in HRS and the children being abused and neglected because of the ills of society and the drug problem, the stories about the ups and downs I had while fostering, and times since then when I have felt the need to reflect and leave Maria a message about a time in our lives that has recently been experienced and lived in a very precious way. . . . My eyes get teary as I write this. Maria has taught me more about my life, our life, and life on earth than I would have ever learned had I not adopted. We used to look at the pictures in the memory book, but then I started pictures in albums since I knew someday that Maria would be reading and I did not want her to read certain items surrounding the foster time until she and I were ready to read and talk together. I have no record of her first 11 months except for some discharge papers from the hospital and some appointment slips for the Developmental Clinic. I wrote only what I could piece together and surmise and project from bits and pieces of information I was given. I would recommend a memory book for any mom. There are many times I would like to ask my mom about certain times or events or reflections on something, but the time is short and hurried when we are together and sometimes tense and the vibes I get are not always positive.

The adoption day came. October 20, 1991. I knew a lawyer in the neighborhood who would do the adoption for $475 which was later reimbursed by the State. I chose the name Catherine Marie so Catherine would have the same initials as mine. Her ethnicity is Hispanic/French—which ties in also with Catherine Marie. The Social Worker had done a complete job and all went smoothly in the Judge's chambers. The only testy time was when the Judge asked how much I made as a single woman—I was about to answer when the lawyer said that item had been cleared with HRS. Then I planned the party at a local restaurant so everyone who had been supportive and encouraging and helpful and worried with us could now celebrate with us. The memory book was there for signatures and an album of pictures records the good times and tears of happiness experienced.

Over the years—5 now—I have become friends with other single moms and other sets of parents through child care and now school. The support that comes through these friends is priceless. Susan and I had a real good thing going for a while . . . I would keep Jose in the morning (we had a back yard and they lived in a condo) while Susan would do her errands; that afternoon or another Saturday, Susan would keep Catherine (the condo had a real pool whereas we had a plastic one) and I could do my errands in peace. Susan's son was a year older and during the ages of 3 to 5 this worked very well. Since then Catherine is 'all knowing' that boys are yuck to girls and do boy things that aren't cool. So there. Now I have Moms and Parents that have girls and the same trade off is accomplished to the delight and sanity of both parties. That's the physical side. The mental relief is also needed and received from long standing friends I have known as long as 20 to 40 years. These are the friends that are willing to be a guardian should I die and my Mom is no longer living. And these are the friends who listen to my complaints and if they have had children they commiserate and understand very well, and if they haven't had children they still listen and give support in many different ways. I do not hesitate to ask for help if needed. Caring for myself keeps me healthy in more ways than one. Some times I pay $5.00 an hour for the same service when I get a sitter for Catherine. A long dinner and a movie with a friend can work wonders for an adult mind that has had too much 4-, 5-, 6-year-old talk and activity. When I first started with the sitters I started in the neighborhood and when those teenagers went off to college or university I asked a Mom with 3 or 4 children who she could recommend. I figured that Mom had a list for sure. I was given 4 and then some more, from the church she attended. Enough! I said, but Laz said you can never have too many. And she is right. Moms always know best. Frozen dinners come in handy on sitter nights—but I have to explain that concept. When I first got Catherine I had to practice what I taught. Over the years, I had taught parents to cook foods as naturally as possible—broil, bake, saute, steam fresh veggies, salads with fresh herbs. No salt in cooking or at the table, use lemon or garlic and parsley as my mother taught me. . . . Then blend the leftover meat with the juice from the steamed veggies and freeze in ice cube trays. When frozen transfer the cubes to plastic bags, label and freeze. This can be done when the child is an infant and first learns to eat solid foods. On 'sitter' days or 'frazzled' days I would take out 4 cubes of chicken, 4 cubes of squash, and add a dessert, usually a fresh fruit compote that my Mom had made. The Junior Oster was used quite often in those days. Today, I don't have to blend the food, but I still cook enough on the weekends to make 2 or 3 frozen dinners for the future.

I remember some weekends in the beginning when my Mom was out of town or we were on the "outs" and I was faced with caring for this much loved person. I would have moments of panic—how am I going to survive, what shall I do? 48 hours? 2 whole days? When Catherine was 2 or 3 and Deanna's son Andrew was 3 or 4 we supported each other and spent 4 or 5 hours each packing up supplies, meeting at the transit station, going for a ride, getting off, seeing the sights and the boats on the bay, and the people, and having an ice cream cone, and getting home, and both children and Moms tired enough to have a two hour nap. So 6 to 7 hours were gone already . . . Even today I think, here I am, 52 with a 6-year-old running around the house . . . life is real and this is really living.

The State provides Medicaid and a monthly stipend, both of which are invaluable. Although I have not really had to use Medicaid except for Public Health Department visits, knowing that I have insurance for my daughter is great. To have her as a dependent on my insurance through the University would cost me about $300 per month. The monthly stipend was used for child care and is now used partially for after school care and money for college. Soon I hope the balance can be used to defray the cost of a babysitter to watch Maria after school; I think the daily pick up and piano practice overseen by my Mom and 2 nights a week for dinner and to our house is taking its' toll on my Mom. And since I won round one and have had a break, I think I am ready for round two and another Princess to hold Maria's hand and mine and join us in our journey through this life on earth . . . or maybe I will get that Prince after all . . . .

25

Women Being Divorced

Sheila J. Hopkins

Separation and divorce terminate more than the social and legal contract of marriage. They signify the breakup of the family. For me, divorce not only represented the end of a particular, constant emotional suffering, it also meant an opportunity for personal growth. Yet the experience of divorce, initially, was devastating to me. I was angry, fearful, and lonely. I missed the comfort of the known daily routine. I believed I had failed.

I met my first husband in 1953, at a time when the United States had again a financial upturn. In my lifetime, we had been through nearly a decade of troubled financial times and four terrible years of the Korean war. Family values were strong, Americans desired stability in their lives, and educational opportunities were available to those who would not have been able to afford them without post-war government benefits.

Widespread alterations in divorce laws reflecting previously prevalent beliefs about matrimony and its essentials were also changing. The strains of war and associated problems that produced more divorces also made the practice more prevalent, conspicuous, and acceptable.

Simultaneously, the growth of women in the work force resulting from men leaving for war, among other reasons, afforded women an opportunity

SHEILA J. HOPKINS

for economic independence. Marriage was less essential. Life as a single individual was gradually losing its stigma. During the civil rights movement in the sixties, women struggled to shed the subordinate position of a lesser version of their male counterparts. Women resisted becoming a mirror image of men who value power, and these women fought to establish equality trying to retain the feminine qualities of tenderness and gentleness.

Challenges to institutional authority were commonplace. There were large and vocal movements challenging conventional sexual and marital norms, censorship, the war in Vietnam, and educational policies. The "no fault" divorce laws and the increasing numbers of women in the work force signaled a profound shift in the way divorce was to be handled. By the seventies, decisions about divorce were no longer the prerogative of the state and church authority was being challenged. Divorce was becoming the privilege of the married couple.

Marriage had been redefined. It was no longer primarily an economic institution, but was now outlined largely by its emotional significance. Love, companionship, and overall compatibility became the essential components. Commitment to the institution of marriage waned while the relationships between men and women became of paramount importance. But women were still held responsible for the success or failure of their marriages. Meeting such high expectations remains difficult, sustaining them is very near impossible.

MY SITUATION THEN

In the mid-fifties, I was a middle class Jewish nineteen-year-old from New England. Regardless of what was happening in the world around me, I was imbued with and acted upon the culture and mores of my family and immediate community. For me, early marriage to someone who was Jewish was the major symbol of beginning a successful life. It was anticipated that I would continue my education beyond high school and by graduation from a secondary school would be ready to be married. It was expected that one's life be patterned along a very specific timetable. In fact, a common saying, referring to young women was, "Ring by Spring or your (college tuition) money back." Also, we women who came from ethnic enclaves (which didn't begin to disappear until suburbia and civil rights flourished in the sixties) had been impassioned by an image of the prototype we would marry. He would be college educated, of a similar ethnic background, and would be involved in the rebuilding of a universal Jewish community. The horror of the Holocaust had touched and changed the lives of most American Jews. Whereas, assimilation had been the goal in previous generations, Jewish youth who were coming to adulthood after World War II were struggling with the fear of extinction. The feeling was that the only way Jews could survive was through solidarity.

So there I was. It was my first year away from home. I was living in a dorm, studying nursing in Boston, and, at nineteen (although I was not overtly aware of it), right on track and ready to "fall in love" with a nice Jewish man.

DIVORCE IN JUDAISM

Marriage is one of the corner stores of Jewish life. "No man without a wife, neither a woman without a husband, nor both of them without God" (Genesis Rabbah 8:9, Old Testament). Yet divorce is regarded as an alternative when it is "given for the sake of peace . . . and those who divorce when they must, bring good upon themselves, not evil" (Eliyahu Kitov). According to Judaic law, companionship, satisfaction of physical and emotional needs, peace, harmony, kindness, respect, and thoughtfulness are the significant tenets upon which a marriage must be built.

Judaism permits divorce and makes provision for it on grounds no more severe than simple incompatibility, but divorce must never be carried out arbitrarily or with hostility. The law of divorce is given only where every hope of healing the breach is gone and strife and bitterness prevail. Then for the peace and unity of the family divorce is granted.

It is acknowledged that the human tragedy inherent in any divorce is especially poignant when there are children. Often it is when there are children that divorce becomes a lifetime burden. Because of Judaic teachings about divorce, I did not feel encumbered by religious beliefs when contemplating my divorce.

SIGNIFICANCE OF DIVORCE

Divorce is of significance on several planes. Sociologically, it is an indicator of the stability of social systems (marriage). It is also an important transition in the life of individuals (a meaningful event in the biography of family members) and it is a microsocial descriptor of associated events such as industrialization, poverty, educational attainment, war, law, religious trends, and historical events. Although the twentieth century began with very little divorce, it draws to a close with national surveys predicting that as many as two thirds of all recent marriages will end in divorce.

It is remarkable that similar trends in divorce exist throughout the Western world despite differences in forms of government, national economics, and the role of religion.

The redefinition of marriage in the latter part of the twentieth century throughout the West, reflects profound changes in relationships between men and women. Marriage is no longer an economic institution, it is defined by its emotional significance. Love, companionship, and equality are essential to its success.

As the meaning of marriage changes so do the reasons for divorce and conversely—now that it has become more difficult to sustain a marriage it has become easier to terminate. Divorce is less costly financially, legally, and reputationally than it was in the past.

There are some documented demographic and personal characteristics that correlate with the probability of divorce. These include early age at the time of marriage, premarital births, divorce from a previous marriage, low educational attainment, and employment. I fit the profile only in terms of early age. In the 1950s, many women married young.

Consequences of divorce on children are difficult to address because longitudinal studies are just now beginning to offer evidence. It does appear that children of divorced parents feel the cumulative effect of the failing marriage and divorce at the time they enter young adulthood. They appear to have difficulty with the developmental task of establishing love and intimacy making the new families appear vulnerable to the effects of divorce. In many ways, my marital life was reflective of social, community, and family mores prevalent at the time.

FALLING IN LOVE

Falling in love at nineteen was more like a high tide crashing to shore over rocks rather than the delicate flight of a bird. It was later I learned how tenuous love can be.

Milton, my first husband, and I met in 1953. We were both in school, he studying to become a Jewish communal worker, I a nurse. I knew I had met the man who would fulfill my dreams and make my family proud. In those days, our parent's expectations shaped our plans for the future. I was in love. Part of the aura was that he appeared to be in love, too—after a whirlwind courtship (on a very limited budget), upon knowing he would have to serve in the Korean conflict, he insisted we marry before he went into the service. How romantic. I would continue my studies for the next two years while he was away. We could save from his increased allotment as a married man toward our graduate education. I was ready to "merge." In her book, *Passages,* Gail Sheehy speaks about, "The urge to merge." I not only felt, as the romantic soundtrack from the film "American Grafiti" shouts,

> *"only you can make this change in me,*
> *for it's true, you are my destiny."*

about him, I also was starry eyed about my own professional career. I felt that the need for expressing myself in a career of my own would mean growth outside of marriage. Early on I realized that it would not be simple to peruse a "destiny" outside the marriage. I was still bound by the myth that happiness, acceptance, and success was, as my mother had found, in being a good wife and mother—in subjugating myself to family needs. This meant being a super mom and wife—consistently making decisions that are best for others. Whereas to peruse an occupation was the anticipated commitment for men with the "urge to merge," women were expected to make a commitment not only to husband and children, but to cooking and baking and cleaning and handling the finances and advising. Independence was not one of the anticipated achievements. June, the mom in "Leave It to Beaver," was still the role model.

Milton and I had both planned to go to graduate school at the same time. I would work full time and study part time. He would study full time. We would live on my salary and take advantage of the many private and public scholarships available.

We married, he went to Korea, and I finished school. We were to begin our married life with all our dreams intact when he returned from the conflict. Graduate school, here we come. But, I became pregnant the first week he was home. . . . "You fear it might be silence" . . . and we began our marriage very differently than either one of us had expected.

THE MARRIAGE

Milton was furious that I had become pregnant. He was afraid that he would not be able to attend graduate school. After much cojoling and offering up plans, sacrificial to me initially, but ultimately (I thought) good for the family, Milton agreed upon one. We could live with my cousin to save rent and household expenses, I could work full time and he could go to school full time and work, if time permitted. It seemed fair that I take on the burden of solving the problem because I truly believed him when he indicated it was my fault for getting pregnant. What I hadn't expected was his continued anger at me for being pregnant. I listened and I prayed, but never did I think of leaving the marriage. My pregnancy was the first crisis in the marriage. He spoke to me only when absolutely necessary, sex became a chore, and I gained 40 pounds.

Thereafter crises occurred each time a family change or decision was to be made. We did not learn to talk to each other. In fact, whether the issue was limited finances, a new baby, imminent relocation, or as simple as who would baby sit, handling the situation was agonizing. The problem was usually resolved with my doing what I thought he wanted. There was never a question of my leaving. I believed marriage was forever. I defined myself in terms of my husband and my children. I still believed being a better wife and doing more was the only route to happiness. I felt the failure or success of the marriage was my responsibility. After all, Milton didn't drink, he didn't beat me, he didn't squander money on gambling, nor did he (to my knowledge at that time) have other women. In the 1950s, this was a portrait of a good husband. I was overwhelmed being a "modern woman" working and trying to be a perfect wife, mother, and homemaker. I shall never be able to make up the sleep lost during those years. As the years went by and my youngest child entered school, I began to, as other women were, look toward what I wanted professionally. In the 1960s, women were striving for their own identity in the work world, in relationships, in published works, and through public demonstration. Not unlike other women of the times, I ached for equality in the marriage, companionship, sexual satisfaction, and professional fulfillment. Although I never entertained the notion of relinquishing my "marital" responsibilities, or leaving the marriage, I was able to go to school part time and continue supplementing our income while caring for the family. Milton worked hard and was well-respected in his field of social work. Compared to other occupations, his salary, although adequate, was not competitive with many of his friends' incomes. Although he enjoyed the respect his position afforded, his need for more money and some semblance of fame led us to relocate several times. He was always clear that the moves focused on his career. A community with good resources, schools for the children, and opportunities for my professional advancement were secondary. I flagellated myself for having negative feelings about his self-centeredness. After all, I still believed that the process was correct. It was OK if other family members subjugate their needs to the well-being and occupational success of the husband/father. In turn, the whole family would prosper from his occupational rewards. I believed my future was totally dependent upon him. As we entered the 1970s, I began to realize that I had a responsibility to myself—I began to grow up. I no longer needed to behave as my mother had . . . I relished the idea of having a life that was part of, yet separate from, the marriage. I continued to try to be super mom and wife, but my focus was shifting. I finally embarked on a path to meet my needs, to fulfill my dreams, to shed the dormant woman I had become. I went back to school. The marriage was a prison and my relationship to Milton was largely one of inane limited conversation about operational necessities and angry exchanges about how to handle every day "crises." I was trapped. I did not want to be divorced. I wanted the family, the "marriage," not the relationship with him. Gradually the marriage became a structure not unlike a movie set where we used the empty framework to plot and act out our separate lives. My time was spent in school, at work, with the children, and with friends. Supposedly Milton was busy, busy, busy getting ahead at work. He had decided that if he did not receive the directorship of the agency where he currently worked in the next year, we would move again. I had established a life of my own and was very reluctant to go.

Once more I listened and I prayed, but what I had learned was that love can be forever or it can be fleeting, it can be nurturing or destructive, it can be happily bestowed or cruelly withheld, and that a love object can be falsely perceived, distorted by the image of our own fantasies. I did not have a good love.

We did move to Washington, DC. The older children were to remain in Connecticut. The oldest was in college already living in an apartment of her own, the middle child would finish his last year of high school living with our friends. Milton would leave in May to become acclimated to his new position. I would remain in Connecticut to sell the house, finish school, complete my work responsibilities, and allow Mike (the child who would be moving with us) to go to horseback riding camp one more time. It was during the summer that Milton met "the love of his life" in Washington. Apparently it was very difficult for him to leave the marriage, although he had become alternately angry and depressed. He did not tell me that he wanted to dissolve the marriage until several weeks after I had arrived in Washington with Mike, who was eleven. We had come to closure with all our friends and activities in Connecticut, had begun to be established in Washington, and now Mike and I were to return to Connecticut. I was furious that Milton had not said something earlier, devastated about losing my identity as a wife, frightened about finances, ashamed that I had failed, and most of all, terribly worried about the children. I felt destroyed when he told me that he had never loved me, but had married to have roots.

THE SEPARATION

I returned to Connecticut with Mike, a car in poor condition, our clothing, and five hundred dollars. It was the mid-seventies. Women had made some advances, but were not viewed as being capable of caring for themselves financially. With much humiliation, I had to have Milton sign a lease before a landlord would rent an apartment to me, a female single parent. Of course, my having a job that paid well, which I was fortunate to be able to return to, made no difference. Because of my "marital status," I was also required to pay two months rent in advance. While my daughter was hounding me to stand up for my civil rights and prosecute the landlords, I was eager to leave my friend's home where Mike and I had been staying. We needed a home of our own, more conveniently located. I wanted to return to the town we had left so the children could reestablish relationships and routines. The town was also midway between school and work for me and I had a cadre of friends waiting to welcome me back. I received no financial support from Milton during the separation. Fear of destroying any possibility of reconciliation kept me from pressuring him.

BECOMING

It was now the middle seventies and there had been multiple attitudinal changes toward women from previous decades. Society was beginning to entertain a tolerance for diversity in the role of women. Women were beginning to assert their gender in ways other than being wife and mother. We had additional opportunities to find fulfillment and earn respect. Once I was settled into a routine of children-focused activities, work, and school, I was able to spend time introspectively. What a wonderfully exhilarating time! I read about other women, I wrote poetry, I felt free. I viewed my life situation with clarity, the beauty of the world around me was breathtaking. I was exhilarated cross-country skiing with Mike, awed by the intensity of the beauty in sunsets and sunrises, I felt as though a tremendous burden had been lifted from me . . . and yet there were moments when I was overwhelmed by sadness. I mourned the probable breakup of the family (never the loss of the relationship with Milton). I worried about the effects of divorce on the children. I soared when I felt good. I was immobilized in the pits of despair when I was low, but, having been well-trained in 22 years of a bad marriage, I was able to carry on with my daily routine and reach a level of fairly consistent contentment.

My life and the lives of the children had stabilized. I wanted a legal and a Jewish divorce. Apparently, Milton was content to be with the "love of his life" and remain married to me. He agreed to the divorce with reticence and went through the process as small minded and spiteful as one could.

THE DIVORCE AND NOW

The flight of love may be quick, but some of the pain may last forever. It has been almost 20 years since my divorce. My children are successfully married and have children of their own. Each has established a relationship on their own terms with their father. I have had a wonderful second marriage, yet, whenever I remember my first marriage I'm surprised at the rancor I feel. I relish the excitement of having learned who I had been and who I have become. I remember having cried watching romantic movies because I had not had the romance I expected from my relationship with my first husband. I felt during that marriage that my days were filled with sacrifices and compromises. Everything I experienced during the separation was extraordinarily intense and poignant. I was despondent with grief, exhilarated with pleasure, I sobbed embarrassingly loudly with sadness, I wet my pants with laughter. Sunsets and sunrises were spectacular—the dam had burst. I no longer wrestled with my own private hell. This was the most profound growth period of my life. I am both grateful and proud of the way I changed. I had thought my family knew nothing about my difficulties in the marriage. After the divorce I found that was hardly the case. I am no longer ashamed of that marriage.

Slowly I began to no longer feel incomplete without a husband. I believe I was growing up and I reveled in the process, excited about the potential outcome. It was time to make my separateness complete, to complete school, to be open to romance. Unfortunately, during the divorce proceedings I had slipped into old behaviors. I had spent many hours during the separation working hard to learn about who I had been in the past and reshaping my life so that I could be who I wished to be in the future. Retrospectively, I was appalled to find that during the divorce negotiations I had regressed into the compliant, agreeable, unsure "girl" I had been in the marriage. My need to be what I considered fair, just, and honest, and 20 years of being subordinate, preempted my following my lawyer's advice and I accepted a divorce decree without provisions for alimony, with child support less than aid to dependent children payments, and with very little financial support for the children's college education. Also, in some ways, I thought this to be a show of independence. Foolish me! I am happy to admit that I weathered the financial storms and have a sense of pride that I was able to accomplish my goals and help the children accomplish theirs on my own.

The bereavement I feel about loss of the family reoccurs with weddings, birthdays, and other family occasions, but I'm largely content having had a wonderful second marriage, a fulfilling career, and a spirited social life.

Although love is a little white bird that comes to us fleetingly, there need not be disenchantment. There is strength and beauty in the song of past loves. We as women plucked from our innocence of dependence upon men can move forward toward a transformation. The trauma of divorce is a lesson in how to meet adversity. It teaches us that if the intent to bring about our own development is there, we have the ability. We learn that we can stand shoulder to shoulder with men and other women to contribute to a new world. A new world where one's style is respected and both toughness and tenderness add to peace, equality, and development. A new world where diverse logic, values, choices, and prayers are accepted with rectitude.

As we move into the post modern era, women will remain intact as total beings themselves, not as a lesser version of our male counterparts. We will have equality, married or single, in all walks of life, without forfeiting our womanliness.

26

Mother's Feelings on Kangaroo Care for Their Pre-Term Infants

Patricia R. Messmer, Joyce Wells-Gentry, Suzanne Rodriguez, and Kathy Washburn

The incidence of preterm births is rising across the United States. The use of life-support interventions has markedly improved the chance of survival and the quality of outcome for preterm infants (low birthweight, very low birthweight, or small for gestational age) in the United States and other developed countries. Approximately 50% of preterm infants are at high risk for significant morbidities during their initial neonatal hospitalization, for significant long-term neurodevelopmental sequelae, and for continued health problems requiring ongoing care and often rehospitalization (Ehrenkranz, 1994). Since charges for the initial hospitalization can range from $1,000 to $2,000 per day, the smallest, sickest infants commonly incur hospital charges well above $100,000. Many incur significant post hospitalization costs. Neonatal intensive care is costly not only to the

243

individual family, but also to society. These costs increase with decreasing birth weight and gestational age. Any attempt to limit neonatal intensive care to very low-birth-weight-infants raises important ethical questions. Moreover, neonatalogists are usually unable to determine at birth which preterm infants will survive intact and which ones will survive with significant health or neurodevelopment problems (Kenner, 1994).

Preterm infants require long periods of hospitalization and separation from their mothers. In fact, the length of stay (LOS) for preterm infants weighing 1000 gms ranges from 40 to 50 days at our institution. Physical barriers such as gowns, masks, equipment, and hospital policy, restrict close contact between mothers and preterm infants. Coffman (1993) found that the lack of close contact between mothers and their preterm infants had a negative effect on maternal-infant interaction patterns and maternal feelings. Alfonso (1993) found that mothers of preterm infants experienced anxieties or fear of the nursery environment that reduced their visits. Brooks (1993) reported that there was decreased confidence regarding parenting skills and feelings of total unpreparedness to become parents for their preterm infants. These factors may explain the findings that preterm infants are more temperamentally difficult than full-term infants and experience an increased frequency of child abuse (Hack, 1991).

To address these concerns, a pilot study of Kangaroo Care (K Care) was conducted with neonates and their families in an 8-bed NICU at Mount Sinai Medical Center, a 707-bed academic medical center in Miami Beach, Florida. K Care consists of a mother holding an unclothed, diapered preterm infant skin-to-skin and upright between her breasts or the father holding the infant against his chest. K Care, as an innovative method of care for preterm infants, has become widespread in Scandinavia; proliferating in Europe and the United States of America; occurring at numerous sites in Latin America and Africa; and beginning in Australia, Asia, and the Pacific Islands (Anderson, 1991). The method, which originated in Bogota, Columbia, represents a blend of technology and natural care. The nickname K Care was derived from its similarity to the way marsupials mother their immature young. K Care infants are reported to have less crying, longer sleep periods, greater weight gain, improved lactation, decreased oxygen requirements, and shortened hospitalization. In addition, K Care had a comforting effect on infants and their mothers. (Anderson, 1991; Brooks, 1993; de Leeuw, 1991; Ludington-Hoe, 1990; Ludington-Hoe, 1991; & Whitelaw, 1990). Ludington-Hoe (1994) reported that heart rate and abdominal skin temperature rose for K Care infants. Heat loss did not occur during K Care, and infants slept more during the K Care period as compared to the non-K Care periods. Affanso (1993) found that K Care infants were discharged at an earlier age and mothers reported confidence in their abilities to "know and monitor their babies better than the nurses or technology." K Care has a significant place in the care of high-risk neonates (Collins, 1993; Kenner, 1994).

Ourth and Brown's (1961) Continuity Hypothesis provided the conceptual framework for this study, "Since birth itself is an abrupt environmental change, it would appear that adjustment in the neonatal period can be facilitated by continuing the kinds and amount of stimulation present during the fetal period in so far as possible" (p. 288). The theory proposes that certain stimuli become familiar and salient to the fetus, and if presented repeatedly to the newborn, will have soothing and regulating effects. It has been hypothesized that one of the reasons why infant sleep is so fragmented is that infants are deprived of the regulatory influences of maternal biological rhythms. K Care provides exposure to experiences that are familiar to the neonate: the mother's voice is heard at 84 decibels through the uterine wall. In early postpartum, newborns alter their sucking patterns to be rewarded by the presence of the familiar maternal voice (DeCasper, 1980).

The maternal voice may be heard well when the infant lies against the chest in K Care; and the maternal heartbeat and cardiovascular sounds are received at the fetal ear at 72 decibels throughout pregnancy. Positioning the infant adjacent to the mother's left breast is believed to enhance reception of heartbeat sounds. When heartbeat sounds are played for newborns, crying decreases and sleep ensues (Salk, 1962). In the K Care study conducted at Mount Sinai, the mothers involved in the study reported that as a result of the four K Care episodes, their anxieties and fears of the NICU were diminished. In addition, they gained an increased confidence of their ability to care for their preterm infants and were more ready to assume the responsibility for their preterm infant's care upon discharge. The following comments are examples how the mothers expressed their feelings about participating in the K Care experience.

Mother A: "On Thursday, May 5, 1994, in the wee hours of the morning, it was determined by my doctors that my twins should be delivered three months prematurely. My husband, Michael and I had been informed two weeks earlier that the babies *might* have to be delivered early and, in preparation for that possibility, I had spoken to my cousin who had been a NICU nurse for many years. Nancy explained (in great detail) what Michael and I would encounter—from ventilators and isolettes to possible IVs in our babies heads—yet nothing could have prepared me for the first time I saw my daughter, Julia (who weighed 1 lb. 11½ ounces at birth) and son, Daniel (who weighed in at a mere 1 lb. 6 ounces).

The first time I saw them was on Mother's Day, three days after the birth. I watched in amazement as the nurses handled Julia and Daniel, changing their diapers, inserting IVs, and checking their vital signs. Intimidation was the first sensation that I experienced; at that point I couldn't imagine touching them, let alone holding them in my arms! I gradually became accustomed to the nurses and the nursery routine and, after continuous reassurance from the hospital staff, I finally felt comfortable stroking the babies while they slept in their isolettes.

Within the first few weeks, the doctors and nurses approached Michael and me about participating in the Kangaroo care study and I was extremely excited about the prospect. However, when it came down to having Julia placed on my bare chest, those nagging intimidating fears returned. She was so tiny and looked so helpless. Even more alarming were cries; her little wails were barely audible and the few that could be heard were hoarse and raspy. My 'Walter Mitty' mind went wild . . . I was certain that Julia would have an attack of apnea or bradycardia while I was holding her and that immediate life-saving measures would have to be taken.

Once Suzanne (nurse clinician) positioned Julia on my chest though, all those worries disappeared . . . actually, it was a pretty amazing transformation. I settled down into the recliner, adjusted Julia on my chest, and immediately relaxed. Initially I was afraid that the noises in the nursery might startle her or that the room might get too cold, but the nurses assured me that Julia was accustomed to the sound level and that her body temperature could adjust to mine. I slowly started to calm down and began to enjoy the experience. In fact, I got so relaxed that I fell asleep. I was somewhat upset when Suzanne came to take Julia and return her to the Isolette—I could have stayed there with her on my chest indefinitely. The first day, I participated in the Kangaroo Care study, the time seemed to fly. In fact, the time seemed to pass even more quickly on the subsequent days. After the four-day study was completed and we resumed our "watch-the-baby-in-the-isolette" routine, I felt an emptiness that I hadn't known with my first daughter, Katie. I'm anxiously looking forward to bringing both Julia and Daniel home so that we can continue our Kangaroo care uninterrupted. What an incredible experience—one that I will certainly never forget."

Mother I: "Monday 6 PM I was somewhat uncomfortable at this time because I felt not enough privacy was accorded to me (only one curtain was placed—not all around). Tuesday noon time—I was also placed on monitor and the wires prevented me from holding my baby comfortably (the wires were all messed up, the O_2 probe on my (L) thumb—the wires were not long enough to let me hold my baby in comfort). And then the alarms went on so many times, it was impossible to get relaxed. Wednesday—noon time. I felt a little bit more in control and more relaxed, except for the times when "too loud" alarms went on. "Thursday—noon time. I actually dozed off! And the alarm only went on twice. Thanks for asking me to participate in your study.

Mother L: "I felt that this was a great experience to have with the baby. Although you are permitted to share in almost every aspect of the baby's care, this allows you to go one step further and almost forget that you are in a hospital setting. I was able to forget for a short time that I was in the hospital and pretend that I was home."

Mother Y: "The Kangaroo care was a very pleasant experience. I enjoyed it just as well as the baby did and would continue doing it on the regular basis. It made me feel very close to my baby. The warmth and security was overwhelming. I especially liked the way she squeezed my hands very tight while I was holding her. She also looked very peaceful and comfortable. The most important thing about the Kangaroo Care was that it made me feel that everything is going to be allright with my baby."

Mother G: "The Kangaroo Care experience was wonderful. Having a premature baby, you miss that first touch after the baby is born—and for several days after. Even when we did get to hold him in the early days of his life, he was so wrapped up in blankets, you get no sense of his little body. Kangaroo Care, on the other hand, let me feel my baby as a living, breathing, moving human being. To feel him snuggle in to me was a feeling like no other. He was born long before I was ready to not be pregnant anymore. I was just getting used to his consistent, strong movements inside of me. After he was born, I felt a real sense of loss. Kangaroo Care brought that feeling of closeness and movement back to me. Although I did feel a connection to my baby from the start, the connection I felt between my baby and I during Kangaroo Care brought our relationship to a new level."

Mother W: "I can't begin to say how much the experience meant to me. After so many days of limited touch between me and my baby, the Kangaroo Care began a healing process for me. I was afraid to handle him and felt an emotional separation. I wasn't sure if he was my child or not! Now I'm pretty sure we belong to each other, though right now it seems like forever before I will be able to take him home. However, the therapy helped me a great deal to cope with the frustration of having so little to do with his medical treatment and even his daily needs of feeding and changing diapers. While I have no doubts that the future holds more than enough of those chores, for right now the Kangaroo Care allowed me to do something to hopefully advance my son's trip on the road to full health. And that meant a lot to me."

Mother C: "Kangaroo Care was a loving bonding experience. I felt closer to my baby. Also it was a feeling of warmth. I would suggest all mothers to share the Kangaroo Care experience. It's beautiful!"

Mother WY: "This is hard to put on paper. Prior to doing the Kangaroo Care, I was only able to hold my daughter for approximately 10 minutes. She was wrapped up in a blanket from chin to toes and usually wore a hat for warmth. Besides touching an occasional finger here and there or touching her eyebrow with my finger, that was the extent of my contact with her. With Kangaroo Care, it's incredible how your emotions kick in. Having her on my chest, touching her skin-to-skin made me feel like she was really mine. Feeling her squirm up my chest into my neck to get closer to me was just intense. I can barely think about it without crying—it just feels so good. I really feel that in the past two days her color has improved, she seems to respond to touch much more, and I honestly feel like she knows who I am. I wish I could have a small cot next to her incubator and any chance I got, she would be on *my* chest. The only draw back—it makes me crave her more. Now that I have touched her, I just can't get enough."

Mother S: "It was a great experience to finally feel my baby close, without any interference of blankets. Feeling his warm temperature and listening to him breathe was very relaxing and wonderful. It was a great experience that has encouraged me to practice it at home."

Mother N: "I feel that the experience was the best thing that I could have done for myself and my baby."

Mother AS: "I really enjoyed Kangaroo Care, so much in fact, I kind of wish I had my own pouch. In as much as I am not able to take her home with me, I really enjoyed the closeness. I feel so wonderful as a mother. I would like to thank all of the staff for the great job they do although I can't wait to the day I take their place."

Mother H: "My experience was great! When I get him home I plan to continue with K Care."

Mother AR: "The Kangaroo care was a good experience for me. Even though Aaron was fussy, I enjoyed it very much. It sure made a difference in his sleeping habits. I found that he did sleep longer and was more peaceful. I do believe the closeness helped the baby grow faster, and improves the bond between mother and child."

As a result of this K Care study, mothers of the preterm infants indicated that they and their preterm infants had greatly benefitted from this close skin-to-skin contact; thus, enhancing mother infant bonding. Providing K Care served as an opportunity for nurses to have these mothers assume responsibility and feel more confident about caring for their preterm infants at home.

REFERENCES

Alfonso, D. (1993). Reconciliation and healing for mothers through skin-skin contact provided in an American tertiary level intensive care nursery. *Neonatal Network, 12*(3), 25–32.

Anderson, G. (1991). Current knowledge about skin-to-skin care for preterm infants. *Journal of Perinatology, 11*(3), 216–226.

Brooks, F. (1993). Kangaroo care: Skin-to-skin contact in the NICU. *MCN 18,* 250–253.

Coffman, S. (1993). Mothers' stress and close relationships: Correlates with infant health status. *Pediatric Nursing, 19*(2), 135–140.

De Casper, A., & Fifer, W. (1980). Of human bonding: Newborns prefer mother's voice. *Science, 208,* 304–306.

de Leeuw, R., Colin, E., Dunnebier, E., & Mirmiran, M. (1991). Physiological effects of kangaroo care in very small preterm infants. *Biology of the Neonate, 59*(3), 149–155.

Ehrenkranz, R. (1994). Newborn intensive care. Chapter 19 in F. Olski. *Principles and Practice of Pediatrics* (308–313). 2nd ed. Philadelphia: J.B. Lippincott Company.

Hack, M., Horbar, J., Malloy, M., Tyson, J., Wright, E., & Wright, L. (1991). Very low-birth weight outcomes of the National Institute of Child Health and Human development. Neonatal Network. *Pediatrics 87,* 587.

Kenner, C., Brueggemeyer, A., & Gunderson, L. (Eds.). (1993). Comprehensive neonatal nursing: A physiologic perspective. Philadelphia: W. B. Saunders.

Ludington-Hoe, S. (1990). Energy conservation during skin-to-skin contact between prematures and their mothers. *Heart and Lung, 19*(5), 445–450.

Ludington-Hoe, S., Hadeed, A., & Anderson, G. (1991). Physiological responses to skin-to-skin contact in hospitalized premature infants. *Journal of Perinatology, XI*(1), 19–24.

250   MESSMER, WELLS-GENTRY, RODRIGUEZ, & WASHBURN

Ludington-Hoe, S., Thompson, S., Swinth, J., Hadeed, A., & Anderson, G. (1994). Kangaroo care: Research results and practice implications and guidelines. *Neonatal Network, 13*(1), 19–27.

Ourth, L., & Brown, K. (1961). Inadequate mothering and disturbance in the neonatal period. *Child Development, 32,* 287–295.

Salk, L. (1962). Mother's heartbeat as an imprinting stimulus. *Transaction of the New York Academy of Science, 24,* 753–763.

Whitelaw, A. (1990). Kangaroo baby care: Just a nice experience or an important advance for preterm infants? *Pediatrics, 85*(4), 604–605.

27

The Postlesbian

Gabriella Rosetti

The intellectual's role is no longer to place himself "somewhat ahead and to the side" in order to express the stifled truth of the collectivity; rather, it is to struggle against the forms of power that transform him into its object and instrument in the sphere of "knowledge," "truth," "consciousness," and "discourse" . . . It is not to "awaken consciousness" that we struggle . . . but to sap power, to take power.

Michel Foucault to Gilles Deleuze
"Intellectuals and Power," 207-8

I want to look at lesbian relations and, if possible, at all social relations in terms of bodies, energies, movements, and inscriptions rather than in terms of ideologies, the inculcation of ideas, the transmission of systems of belief or representations, modes of social reproduction: [I am interested in] flattening depth, reducing it to surface effects.

Elizabeth Grosz
"Refiguring Lesbian Desire," 78-79

*T*he title of this paper was appropriated from Jean Walton's "Sandra Bernhard: Lesbian Postmodern or Modern Postlesbian?" (in Doan, 244), in which Walton critiques comedienne Bernhard's public disclosure (and subsequent retraction) of her affair with pop singer Madonna as exploitation of the *Sisterhood*. Besides being a delightfully irreverent and humorous term, "postlesbian" seems a useful way to express certain problems associated with codification (a prerequisite for identity politics) and commodification (once a group of people has been codified as a discreet category of consumer, its members are subject to commercial exploitation). A "postlesbian," as Walton uses it, is a woman who appropriates a lesbian identity for short-term material gain: in Bernhard's case, to promote her career through sensationalism. As I use it, it refers to a time when the term "lesbian," laden with confusing and often negative associations, will no longer be used to identify and isolate women's bodies. Lesbian identity, visibility, and political struggles are currently and inextricably linked with the same issues of sexism, racism, classism, and homophobia[1] that face all American women and likely have been discussed in other essays in this volume. While I do not wish to dismiss issues affecting the material well-being of self-identified lesbian citizens in America as we approach the next millennium, my essay will not grapple with the efficacy of strategic essentialism, lesbian binarism, communities based on sexual preference, marginality or codification toward commodification in any of its postmodern discursive forms *except as they relate to possible ways of re-thinking lesbian desire*. As the juxtaposition of the two quotations that frame this paper suggest, I'm interested in ways to theorize lesbian desire that speak to, but do not focus on, Foucault's struggle for agency.

I am a performing artist and director currently working on a doctorate in theatre at the City University of New York with an interest in exploring theatrical self-representation by marginalized groups across America. After participating in seminars on African American, Chicano, Puerto Rican, Asian, Feminist, Southern Regional, and Native American theatres, I find myself at the end of my residency in a workshop on lesbian and gay theatre in the United States. As a bisexual woman living with another woman, I'm curious about course content and uncomfortable as I face my own internalized homophobia. I've managed to separate my private life and my work, as many other middle-class educated women have done, avoiding identification with any community based on sexual preference. I once believed that artists were exempt from settling into stable identities, a notion reinforced by experiences in artistic communities whose members seemed completely comfortable or oblivious to my sexual wayfaring. Not so in back-water academic communities, however, where I found steady work as a director and educator for many years before defecting to New York to work on the doctorate. Years in a closet have been difficult, but they could have been permanently emotionally crippling had it not been for my creative work.

As I grazed through the seminar reading list, a single essay, "Refiguring Lesbian Desire" by Elizabeth Grosz, from the same volume that published Walton's essay, resonated most deeply with my experience as an artist and educator. A highly regarded theorist in feminist psychology (her book on Lacan is an excellent road map toward re-thinking female subjectivity), Grosz finds postmodern feminist psychologic theory, at least when embracing re-configurations of Freudian and Lacanian psychic economies of lack, inadequate to address lesbian sexuality. In brief, the main points of Grosz's essay are (1) that the "lack" model of configuring human desire is a flawed discursive framework that can only lead to reproduction of commodity-based strategies (hence, an assimilationist stance that renders its proponents, no matter where they fall into the continuum of lack, as part of the problem rather than part of the solution), (2) that "unmediated" experience is impossible, so perhaps we ought to re-focus our inquiries on surface sites of desire rather than on "hidden," underlying depths, and (3) that a deconstruction of these sites, rather than revealing "underlying causes," would be better off using strategies based on Deleuze, Guattari, Lyotard, and others: that is, configuring desire as a productive process. This, she feels, might lead to a recontextualization—"a kind of 'excessive analysis' that goes beyond a well-charted terrain with Nietzschean joy" (Grosz, 69). She describes the Deleuzian approach as follows:

> Following Nietzsche and Spinoza, Deleuze understands desire as immanent, positive and productive, as inherently full. Instead of a yearning, desire is seen as an actualization, a series of practices, action, production, bringing together components, . . . creating reality. Desire is primary, not lack . . . it is primitive and given, it [does not oppose] or postdate reality, it produces reality. It does not take a particular object for itself whose attainment provides it with satisfaction; rather, it aims at nothing in particular, above and beyond its own self-expansion, its own proliferation. It assembles things out of singularities and breaks [things down] into their singularities. As production . . . it experiments . . . it is fundamentally inventive. Such a theory cannot but be of interest for feminist theorists insofar as . . . women occupy the place of men's other. Lack only makes sense to the (male) subject insofar as some other (woman) personifies and embodies it for him. Such a model . . . reveals the impossibility of understanding lesbian desire. Any model that dispenses with a reliance on lack seems to be a positive step forward and for that reason alone worthy of further investigation. (Grosz, 75-76, italics mine)

I'd like to respond to Grosz's challenge to reconfigure lesbian desire via a discussion of the Strasberg Method for actor training and a brief experimental re-reading of Holly Hughes' lesbian performance text, *The Well of Horniness*.

The evolution of Method acting in this country—based on the work of Constantin Stanislavsky, who early on in Russia was informed by Nietzschean philosophy via his youthful association with the symbolists (Carlson 1984, pp. 313-314)—was pioneered by Lee Strasberg (1901-1982). Strasberg's greatest achievements in the American theatre are generally agreed to be the establishment of the first ensemble theatre company, the Group Theatre, and the founding of the Actor's Studio, a performance space and conservatory for the training of young actors. His particular contribution to the Stanislavsky System of actor-training was the development of sense memory technique. The purpose of this technique was to allow a young artist to find a path of discovery into the body, voice, emotions, intellect, and imagination toward complete mastery of these aspects of her or his unique instrument; to "open up" the instrument. Acting teachers across the country adopted this and other Strasberg techniques because they seemed to deal directly with difficulties caused by sociocultural conditioning. It is my contention that sense memory training provides a strategy for re-thinking desire by exploring surface sites of intersection between discreet body parts, objects, and environments (using the production model) as it relates to the practice of preparing the actor for performance.

The conjunction of postmodern theory with actor training occurred to me as I re-read Grosz's poignant statement with regard to her own experience and as she develops her theme of exploring intensities and surfaces rather than latencies and depths. Stating that she cannot give "a real life illustration" of this process, instead she quotes Mary Fallon, who, in the postmodern text *Working Hot,* describes the transformative experience of surfaces and the sense of touch in terms of woman loving woman. Grosz perceives this intersection as a process that transmutes one "thing" into another through something or someone "outside." Transmutation, or "becoming," as it is commonly called in theatrical terms (also so-called by Deleuze), involves arranging fragments of sensation that produce concrete moments that are inherently evanescent, impermanent, unstable. It does not involve adherence to a fixed identity or subjectivity but instead liberates, through dis-organ-ization, an experience of "a thousand tiny sexes" to produce a multiplicity of intersections (Grosz, 79-80). This is precisely the process that occurs during the practice of sense memory technique.

In Elaine Aikin's Method-based work at the Actor's Institute in New York City, the content of a beginning class consists almost entirely of work on sense memory. I enrolled in one of her classes because I had been teaching acting myself for about ten years and I felt a review of the material from a student's standpoint would be a good idea. The class consisted of about fifteen women and men ranging in age from early twenties through late forties. We sat on folding chairs staggered throughout the re-hearsal hall, shoes off, one cheek off and one cheek on the seat of the chair, in what seemed at first to be a terribly skewed and off-center posi-tion for an initial relaxation exercise (perhaps a postmodern body posi-tion, always/already decentered, poised for change).

I remember one class in particular:

Tonight we are working on the sense memory of a ripe persimmon. We are to explore the imagined persimmon with all our senses, but we are not allowed to touch our own bodies, which we have already imagined to be naked, allowing for space between hands and bodies occupied by the ripe flesh of the persimmon. The exercise begins. The hall is silent as stu-dents concentrate on giving up their constructed "selves" to the experi-ence of becoming a machinic entity of body parts plus persimmon to release a moment of animal being. I hold out my hand and wait for the sensation of the whole persimmon to manifest. I feel its weight, its cool, smooth texture. I move it from hand to hand, I touch my face with it. I smell it. It goes away. I wait. It comes back. Pierce it with fingers and thumbs. Feel its juice dripping through fingers, over wrists; hold it up and feel juice dripping down arms, into armpits, over breasts and nip-ples. Begin to explore body parts with wet fruit. Arches, ankles, toes, be-tween toes, the exquisite viscosity, slippery, slithery, one surface eely and muscular. The persimmon is a mouth, a wound. Mud. A baby manta ray, lightly grazing the fine soft hairs on a shoulder. Feces. Inner thighs, belly, dripping, drooling, bleeding down the back. . . . Soon the room begins to fill with sighs, laughter, moans of pleasure, sobs. Something "primitive and given" in us desires this experiment, wants to give up the con-structed self to the moment of becoming. It is exciting, it is real, it is end-lessly productive of moment after moment, and it is sexual. The persimmon (or salad oil, or bubble bath, or mirror, or breakfast drink, which are imaginary objects used in other sense memory exercises) serves as the mediator, Deleuze's "third term," forming a machine of de-sire that re-engages separate "animal" components of self, other, and en-vironment. It is nonhegemonic, nonheirarchical, nonphallocentric, not composed of organisms but of a separation of wholes from parts to create new parts. Elaine brings the exercise to an end. We all talk about what we thought happened to us, when it was real. Later, we are re-minded that the art of acting consists of a continuous chain of these transformational moments experienced onstage with other actors in front of an audience.

The practice of this technique is energizing and affirming. While the production of an endless chain of sensory moments in acting class has a somewhat narrow end-product, that of creating (usually) naturalistic characters in theatrical representations, the technique of becoming itself has the effect of exploding culturally produced views of prescribed human behavior and limitation. Those who are able to apply this creative technique to their lives outside the theatre, particularly in sexual practice, will likely experience moments similar to the descriptions of sensual/sexual pleasure described in Mary Fallon's *Working Hot*. Besides providing a way to re-think desire as separate from "lack," sense memory technique introduces the notion of a multiplicity of pleasures free from the constraints of "vanilla" sex (i.e., the limitation of intersecting body parts to culturally prescribed erogenous zones). Because the practice of sensory technique involves the temporary suspension of individually constituted identity, a conscious participation in dis-organ-ization, and the mediation of a third element, it also opens the practitioner to an experience of connection with an "other" free, at least momentarily, from anxieties associated with interpretation of specific acts, from deeper or hidden meanings. I'm convinced that my early training in sensory technique was a contributing factor to the spirit of experimentation and discovery that lead to my first exploration of woman/woman love (my early training was contemporaneous with the sexual freedom and early feminist movements of the late 1960s and early 1970s, fortuitously. All signs seemed to point to "yes" for experimentation and discovery at that historical juncture).

It seems obvious that this radical strategy for reconfiguring human desire, this technique for seeing (sensing), being and becoming, a concrete, proven technique that has been available for more than sixty years in the United States, has the potential to temporarily suspend the tyrannical influence of the phallocentric order, liberating women and men alike from the dominant culture's narrow sexual prescriptives and its negative take on marginal sexual practice.

The productive model of desire cannot be owned by anyone or enforced on anyone. So far it has proven useful to performing (and other) artists in the process of creating their art. It has also proven useful to a few of us who have carried it over into our intimate lives. Of what use is it to a dominant culture based on an economy of lack (its appropriation and misuse by cult leaders notwithstanding)? If it can't be owned, controlled, or enforced, well, then it must be subversive. The conservative wing of the ruling class in America currently in power still suspects that artists are amoral, degenerate, closet-commie sociopaths; a quick review of the morning papers reveals what Republican Senator Jesse Helms has planned for the National Endowment for the Arts and public broadcasting.

Grosz does not see Deleuze's productive model of desire as a utopian vision, and the cynical part of myself agrees with her as I see the developments noted above, as I see terror motivating reactionary legislation that rescinds the small material gains gays and lesbians have made in the

last fifteen years. But part of me wants to believe that making the productive model of desire available as a choice might allow a handful of un-
happy neurotics and persecuted sexual minorities to slip through the
noose of individual or collective identity constituted on an economy and
psychology of lack, to run, skip, somersault into the uncharted terrain of
endlessly productive experience in "Nietzschean joy."

I cannot think of more appropriate artifact for the "excessive analysis"
that Grosz proposes in her challenge to re-think lesbian desire nor one
that provides an uncharted terrain of (nearly) endlessly productive experience than Holly Hughes' performance text, *The Well of Horniness*. *The
Well* is a work that creates new boundaries for what is contained in the
term "excessive." It was originally conceived as scenario for a lesbian
porn film (over too many Bloody Marys, confesses Hughes in her notes to
the published edition of the play; the writer was always/already in a state
of dis-organ-ization and intoxication, the ecstatic Dionysian state of pri-
mordial bliss that Nietzsche described), a project unabashedly conceived
out of an economy of lack (the visual commodification of lesbian sexual
practices for the lesbian spectator's consumption). Over more Bloody
Marys, Hughes crafted a text that developed into a burlesque romp: the
porn project was dropped. *The Well* opened as a live performance, was
adapted for radio, then evolved into an interesting hybrid of radio and
theatre (Shewey, *Contemporary Gay Theatre*, xxi).

The Well premiered on March 3, 1983, at the WOW Cafe, a "ghettoized"
performance space in New York's lower east side that showcases lesbian
works for audiences composed primarily of other lesbians (and some acad-
emics). The WOW's mission to limit access to aspiring (and more recently,
successful) lesbian writers/performers has led to its configuration as a producing organization more concerned with agency than art. It is significant
that this work was produced during the early years of what lesbian histo-
rian Lillian Faderman describes as the Lesbian-Feminist Sex Wars (Faderman, pp. 246–270); in fact, it appeared less than a year after the infamous
women's conference on sexuality at Barnard College (April 24, 1982). It is
speculative whether Hughes conceived this project as a response to the
narrow sexual orthodoxy posited by cultural feminists at that conference
whose organizers excluded forums on butch-femme roles, s/m, woman-
gererated porn produced for other women, and other "politically incor-
rect" sexual practices. Whether or not this is the case, in *The Well* Hughes
conveniently re-presents camp[2] constructions of the butch-femme diad, the
bisexual, the passing woman, the femme top, the bar lesbian, cutting
across boundaries of race and class . . . in short, a multiplicity of lesbian
stereotypes (caricatures, really) that could lend itself to a reading through

a grid of strategic essentialism.[3] However, approaching the work from
Grosz's suggested inquiry into surfaces, bodies, energies, movements and
inscriptions, it appears that this dis-organ-ized collective of warring lesbian
sexualities implied by bodies inscribed with a multiplicity of lesbian desires annihilates itself, from the first toilet flush to the last disclaimer that
"it was all a bad dream." It seems to me that Hughes was involved in a
moment-to-moment deconstruction of what is contained in the imaginary
organism of "the lesbian" as it is understood at an historic turning point in
twentieth century discourse on sexual practice.

As mentioned, the style of *The Well* is appropriated from the lower gen-
res of western theatre, specifically burlesque and "satire"; in a sense it
functions as a satyricon of lesbian desire (the oxymoron "satyricon of lesbian desire," with the term "satyr" attached to a celebration of phallocen-
tricity, points up the limits of language in discussing a lesbian sexuality).
It was not difficult to read the text as a collage of surfaces. Every motive,
every "subtextual" reference, is blatantly foregrounded by the structure
of the appropriated genre. The few references to "high art," including the
title of the play (from Radclyffe Hall's 1928 lesbian novel *The Well of
Loneliness*) and the title of Part Three, "In the Realm of the Senseless"
(from Nagisa Oshima's 1976 film, *In the Realm of the Senses,* considered
to be the first pornographic film for women) are assumed to be available
to most of the play's intended spectators, even if they haven't read the
book or seen the movie. On the other hand, while references to certain
sexual practices and terms referring to specific lesbian types were probably accessible to the WOW spectators, many of these terms (femme-top,
stone butch, passing woman, and ki-ki were a few) sent this scholar scur-
rying to Faderman, D'Emilio, et al., for explication. The proliferation of
pop culture images (sight and sound gags as well as spoken text), including the title of Part Two, "Victim/Victoria" (after the gender-bending
Blake Edwards film *Victor/Victoria*) prompted Don Shewey, editor of *Out
Front: Contemporary Gay and Lesbian Plays* (1987), to describe Hughes
as playwright with a "t.v.-bred instinct for savage parody and aggressive
infantilism." He suggests that *The Well* is a "pop mosaic encoded with
half-digested scraps of cultural debris and half-rejected, half embraced
stereotypes of wicked sister love (Shewey, xxi)." Hughes prefaced the
published version of the text with specific notes about production:

*The stage was linguini-shaped, with the narrowest part of the noodle fac-
ing downstage. The narrator, dressed as a cub reporter and sweating
profusely, was downstage left throughout the piece. Other actors entered
and exited through a window that led into the adjacent kitchen or into
the broken piano we neglected to remove from the stage. This sounds*

more interesting than it actually was. Staging was early sixties soap opera. All of the actors screamed on "the Well" [as in, "the Well" (scream) "of Horniness!"] . . . This is the best part of the play, so I advise all future productions to exploit it to the fullest. All the performers were, and still are as far as I know, women. I'm pretty touchy about this part. No men in The Well, *okay? . . . Occasionally the cast should break into frenetic sexual activity, such as the spaghetti dinner scene, or major catfights, as in the beginning of "The Realm of the Senseless." I have presented this play with as many as ten performers and as few as three. (Hughes in Shewey, 222)*

Although Shewey describes its first performance as a "sketch," even caricatured stereotypes imply the presence of a plot-driven text, and in *The Well* overdrawn characters are provided with an appropriately parodic overwritten plot based on the Mickey Spillane pulp detective fiction genre interspersed with commercials, news flashes, the above-mentioned catfights and wildly active sexual interludes, and asides by actors dropping their character roles. Gender-bending is omnipresent, including references to the gender-neutral narrator alternately as "sister" and "buster" and the dropping of characterizations of male roles intended to be read as "men" as when Rod (whose name clearly ostends the passing woman's possession of male power and a penis), the fiancee of victim/heroine Vicki (whose name aligns her with the Vixen's Den, the play's local lesbian bar/restaurant and also with "vixen" as a term connoting female sexual transgression), drops her/his role but maintains her/his butch masquerade during a reference to hot nights in a lesbian bar (*The Well*, p. 246). The language is spiked with explicit bawdy, and every reference to pop culture is appropriated to parody some aspect of lesbian sexuality as it is read in both straight and lesbian contexts.[4] Camp moments that seem directly appropriated from gay male performance focus on the style of dress adopted by flamboyant femme characters.[5]

The lesbian identities Hughes lampoons are "embodied" in the roles of Garnet McClit, lady dick (working class, stone butch); Babs (underclass, con artist, flamboyant femme-top . . . also the villain in the piece); Georgette (middle class, lipstick lesbian butch); Vicki (middle class, bisexual (?), homophobic and racist closet femme who falls into "the Well"); Al Dente (henchman of the ruling class, butch-to-butch loving lesbian who confesses his/her love for Rod in the "male bonding" section of the play); Rod (middle class, passing woman, a butch, like Al, who identifies completely with the male gender); a bevy of dominatrix blonde cops who frisk Vicki and the lesbian prisoners of color who promise Vicki an assortment of bondage and discipline games (working class cops, underclass prisoners, vampire s/m lesbians), and Dinette, lost twin sister of Georgette who lives separate from civilized society in the woods as a kind if Artemis archetype (lesbian-feminist-separatist, a classless category).

Of the forty scenes comprising the text, only eighteen are performed in the parodied representational style. The rest are interventions cutting into, overlapping, commenting on, and digressing from the "plot." The play's center is constantly shifting, focusing variously on parodies of consumerism, racism, sexism, homophobia, explicit lesbian sexual acts, long quotations of Marx Brothers and other classic lazzi, camp digressions on fashion, and nonsequiter recaps of previous action. Repetition of linguistic and physical tropes, a technique associated with burlesque, is one device that seems to hold the play together.

I've attempted to contextualize Hughes as a lesbian writer who by virtue of self-identification "authenticates" a lesbian camp artifact presented at a lesbian venue for the consumption and enjoyment of lesbian spectators. How does this work provide a way to re-think lesbian desire?

The conflation of stereotyped lesbian bodies with kitsch and satire, together with the self-destructive implications of the negation of those bodies in the "disappearance" of lesbians down the toilet (opening reference to the "Well") and the denial of lesbian sexual experience at the end of the play (when Vicki awakens and is reassured by Rod that her experience was "all a bad dream"), seems to dismember the collective lesbian body as it has been understood in both heterosexual and homosexual contexts to reveal what feminist theatre theorist Sue-Ellen Case posits as an explosion of culturally produced notions of the female body, the male gaze, and the structure of realism ("Towards a Butch-Femme Aesthetic" in Hart 1989, p. 297). If these constructed lesbian identities can be read as "semiotic sex toys for the lesbian couple," then masquerade, the appropriation of gender and style, sex toys such as dildoes and vibrators, and marginal sexual practices such as s/m become possible "third terms" in Deleuze's productive model of desire functioning in much the same way as the re-imagined object in the Method's sense memory exercises. The third term re-focuses lesbian sexuality through fragmented identities that transform sexual experience into potentially endless configurations of surfaces, moving energies, marked bodies that disintegrate and reappear as differently marked bodies. Like the controlled environment of the rehearsal hall that contains the practice of Method sense memory exercises, Hughes' text provides a controlled environment that makes exploration of and experimentation with lesbian discourses of desire possible. What the spectator is left with at the end of any performance is, flatly, a group of actors in costume; in this case, a group the spectators assume to be lesbian women. There isn't any proof; they could all be Sandra Bernhard clones ready to say tomorrow that they were never at the WOW Cafe. The possible recognition by lesbian spectators that masquerade, along with other options of performing lesbian desire, function as games played within signs and not ontologies opens a way to create a Deleuzian framework (or Dionysian playground) outside the theatre with no other end than to pleasure all participants engaged in a fore(grounded) play of surfaces. It gives permission to experiment, to re-think one's own sexual performance strategies, without a goal-oriented approach based on an economy of lack. I realize that this is just my reading, and that I assume a great deal when I suggest that lesbians who attended the play in 1983 saw anything more than a chance to laugh at themselves and their friends (not to diminish the value of laughing at oneself . . . it's a first step toward detachment of self from behavior).

What do the Method and *The Well* have to do with being postlesbian?

The following sprint through twentieth-century lesbian history in America is a digest of convergent facts and theories found in three gay and lesbian historical works.[6] This brief overview is intended to define and locate the postlesbian at a specific historical moment in twentieth-century discourse on sexuality.

"Lesbian" is a term used (often in a derogatory manner by non-lesbians) to define a discreet class of citizens identified as genetically tainted and scientifically abnormal by the dominant culture little more than a century ago. The first taxonomic frenzy isolating and naming the practice of women loving women as transgressive was perpetrated by late nineteenth-century sexologists who were motivated in part, no doubt, by a fear that women were capable of forming life-long relationships with other women outside of the requisite heterosexual marriage; a well-founded fear, as it happened, and a phenomenon that became increasingly alarming to men after women began entering all areas of the workforce and indeed no longer needed men to support and protect (and enslave) them. These early sexologists associated the new woman's independence with an appropriation of masculine prerogative and posited a model of sexual inversion that conflated inversion with "masculine" traits and degeneracy (Faderman, pp. 40–41). Any woman who had a masculine appearance was assumed to be an invert, even though there were many cross-dressing and passing women who did not feel desire for other women but chose to represent themselves as men for economic reasons. As the visibility of female couples increased (along with opportunities for education and work outside the home), women in relationships with other women continued to be named and marked until, by the 1920s, the sexologists' model had become part of conventional wisdom for most Americans. Although the spirit of sexual license led to an acceptance of bisexual experimentation among women during the 1920s, it was not to be confused with being a "real" lesbian, who looked and acted like a man and was "sick" or was a weak woman-child who fell prey to the sexually aggressive pseudo-male. Not surprisingly, many young women who found themselves sucked into the Well (scream) of same-sex desire internalized the sexologists' model and its stigma.

Early lesbian communities whose members accepted the sexologists' model tended to form around bar cultures and all-female environments (schools, camps, sports teams, and the military). A brief period of relief for lesbians, who had been psychologically tortured by internalized homophobia, occurred during World War II, when tolerance seemed almost attainable. It was quickly rescinded after the war when homosexuals were aggressively hunted down and exposed by HUAC, leading to a massive retreat into the closet by many lesbians. The publicly visible lesbians who continued to frequent the bars earned the dubious honor of being labeled "stone butches," so-called because they refused to shed the masquerade that defined them as sexual outlaws. Their femme counterparts could and did pass as heterosexual in the visual economy.

As HUAC witch hunts and police harassment of gay and lesbian bars continued, lesbians and gay men began to organize communities that offered alternatives to the bar scene. The Daughters of Bilitis, an underground lesbian organization, produced several publications, including *The Ladder* and *The Wishing Well* available by mail-order, that significantly extended the lesbian community to include women from smaller cities. The incipient women's gay liberation movements contemporaneous with a nationwide sexual revolution in the late sixties led to another period of bisexual experimentation for women, but it tended to be associated with swinging and other forms of group sex with men participating or looking on. The dominant visible lesbian style during this period was still the butch dressed in masculine drag.

Options for reconfiguring public lesbian identity began to open up again in the late 1960s and early 1970s with the feminist and early gay rights movements going mainstream. In 1974, the American Psychological Association removed homosexuality from its list of pathological disorders (D'Emilio 1988, p. 324). Initially shut out of the feminist movement (a result of homophobia), lesbians, who had very strong material motives for wanting to be involved with a movement whose goal was economic and social parity with white males, tried several strategies: rapprochement, assimilation, and recruitment. Of these, perhaps the last two were most successful, although the homophobia issue (along with those of race and class) splintered the movement which re-formed into liberal, cultural and material feminist factions (Dolan, 1988). It is only during the last ten years or so that the damaging effects of rejection by their straight sisters has been revealed by women who refused to be assimilated by the mainstream women's movement.[7] By the mid-1970s, there was a well-established group of lesbian-feminists who sought a utopian matriarchal social order based on cultural feminist principles, but who, like their straight counterparts in the late 1960s, continued to exclude the old-style butches, femmes and other sexual outlaws based on an assumption that they were imitating or serving the dominant culture. This exclusion led to the Lesbian Sex Wars of the 1980s mentioned above. In the meantime, continued gay rights activism, the AIDS crisis, and experiments with a new gay and lesbian activist coalition had begun to manifest. The lesbian-feminist style of visual self-representation rejected the extremes of butch-femme drag, and settled for a look that tended to make everybody resemble poverty-stricken undergraduate Health and P.E. majors. If they'd existed in the 1990s, they'd be walking advertisements for the unisex ready-to-wear drag found at the Gap or Banana Republic stores.

We now seem to be at a point where increased visibility of self-identified lesbians, particularly in positions of political power, the professions, and academic institutions in larger cities where Gay and Lesbian Studies has become an important new discipline, have produced a multiplicity of models for lesbian self-representation including but not limited to previously defined essentializing views of the lesbian as a discreet body. The inclusion in an emerging Queer Nation, for instance, of sex workers and practitioners of s/m, has already opened possibilities for new ways to explore lesbian sexuality (Dolan 1993, pp. 121–133).

Erotic desire between women certainly existed before it was codified, assigned to certain bodies, and stigmatized by the dominant culture. Erotic desire between women will certainly exist in the future. The individual's power to manipulate the visual economy, rendering biological determinism and its culturally prescribed gender roles virtually obsolete, has never been more apparent. How one is "read" in our culture becomes more and more a matter of personal choice, as lesbians have shown us. Through a reading of Hughes' performance text that deconstructs gender roles as masquerade, and the sense memory technique in Method actor training that opens a possible way to re-think lesbian (and human) desire as creative and productive rather than compensatory and need-based, the necessity for constructing a stable, consistent, visible sexual identity is significantly challenged. It is my quasi-utopian vision that discourse relating to the practice of women loving women will eventually eschew the "lesbian" body, embracing instead the notion of a self as constructed moment-to-moment, Method-style, involved in endlessly joyous production of a multiplicity of social and sexual practices and styles within a single lifetime. In this "fourth world" view, lesbianism would be just another choice, and the lesbian, for better or worse, would not exist as a discreet body: hence, postlesbian (and by extension postbisexual, postheterosexual) would be transitional terms, used in future to describe moments in the history of a culture that once labeled the bodies of its citizens in order to colonize and control them. Unfortunately, at a time when emerging theories and practices support and encourage a Deleuzian model of desire producing diverse sexualities within a single individual, social, religious and political backlash from the dominant culture (whose notions of pre-eminence and power would be undermined and leveled in the new world view) continues to grow. If they can't identify the transgressors, they can't control them. Since the transgressors can be identified at this historical moment in greater numbers than ever before, what better time to instigate a purge? In re-thinking lesbian desire, visibility politics and agency cannot be ignored (but that is another paper). These are exhilarating times, and dangerous ones.

REFERENCES

Abelove, et al., (Ed.) (1993). *The gay and lesbian reader.* New York: Routledge.

Carlson, Marvin. (1984). *Theories of the theatre.* Ithaca: Cornell University Press.

Case, Sue-Ellen. (1985). "Towards a butch-femme aesthetic." In Linda Hart (Ed.), *Making a spectacle*, pp. 284–299. Ann Arbor: University of Michigan Press.

D'Emilio, John. (1983). *Sexual politics, sexual communities.* Chicago: University of Chicago Press.

D'Emilio, John, & Estelle Freedman. (1988). *Intimate matters.* New York: Harper & Row.

Dolan, Jill. (1988). *The feminist spectator as critic.* Ann Arbor: UMI Research Press.

Dolan, Jill. (1993). "Desire cloaked in a trenchcoat?" In Dolan, *Presence and desire.* Ann Arbor: University of Michigan Press.

Faderman, Lillian. (1991). *Odd girls and twilight lovers.* New York: Columbia University Press.

Fallon, Mary. (1989). *Working hot.* Melbourne: Sybella Press.

Foucault, Michel. (1977). "Intellectuals and power: A conversation between Michel Foucault and Gilles Deleuze." In Donald F. Bouchard, (Ed.) *Language, counter-memory, practice: Selected essays and interviews*, pp. 205–217. Ithaca: Cornell University Press.

Grosz, Elizabeth. (1990). *Jacques Lacan: A feminist introduction.* New York: Routledge.

Grosz, Elizabeth. (1994). "Refiguring lesbian desire." In Laura Doan, (Ed.) *The lesbian postmodern*, pp. 67–84. New York: Columbia University Press.

Hughes, Holly. (1988). *The well of horniness.* pp. 221–263.

Hull, S. Lorraine. (1985). *Strasberg's method.* Connecticut: Ox Bow Publishing.

Nestle, Joan, (Ed.). (1992). *The persistent desire.* Boston: Alyson Publishing.

Shewey, Don, (Ed.). (1988). *Out front: Contemporary gay and lesbian plays.* New York: Grove Press.

Walton, Jean. (1994). "Lesbian postmodern or modern postlesbian?" In Laura Doan (Ed.) *The lesbian postmodern*, pp. 244–262. New York: Columbia University Press.

NOTES

1. Yes, homophobia. It is one of the weapons the dominant culture uses against all women who challenge the phallocentric order, and is particularly virulent in its internalized form. It was, after all, one of the first and most powerful wedges driven between coalitions of women during the Suffragist movement early in the century and the Feminist movement in the 1970s.

2. The term "camp" as applied to lesbian representation is a hotly debated issue in the 1990s. In this paper, "camp" is used in the sense of artifice, of a challenge to the dominant order of prescriptive gender role self-representation and behavior based on biological determinism, especially as artifice relates to personal style and irreverent exaggeration of sex-role stereotypes. Although the term has been appropriated from gay male bar culture, it has particular usefulness and resonance as "lesbian camp" since it mocks not only straight culture but also the stereotypes associated with dominant culture perception of lesbians (and internalized views of that perception by lesbians themselves).

3. Constructing a group identity for political visibility.

4. Explicitly bawdy references include seafood puns (appropriated from gay/male encoding of fish as synonymous with women), repetition of sucking action in every possible configuration (eating pasta, performing cunnilingus, the sucking of lesbian bodies into the Well, sucking carrots (read: phalloi) into a cuisinart), appropriations of old burlesque jokes ("did you sit in a puddle or are you just glad to see me?"), muff-diving Tridelta Tribads, double entendres relating to fingers, breasts, coming, shooting, and the names of characters (Garnet McClit, lady dick, is a blatant example).

5. Camp moments allude to the virtues and liabilities of hyper-feminine style: "she can't get far in those heels," "bullets of myopic snipers snagging her nylons," "in her flimsy peignoir, nipples baying at the north star," "Vicki was upset . . . she didn't realize that the prison uniforms would have horizontal stripes," "all this running around could ruin a girl's hairdo" are just a few examples.

6. These are Lillian Faderman's *Odd Girls and Twilight Lovers* (1991), D'Emilio's *Sexual Politics, Sexual Communities* (1983), and D'Emilio and Freedman's *Intimate Matters.* I will cite page numbers when opinions differed among the scholars.

7. Quite a few anthologies have been published recently that include narratives from women who did and didn't join the lesbian-feminist movement. See Rita LaPorte, "The Butch-femme question" (1971) and Jeanne Cordova, "Butch, lies and feminism" in Joan Nestle's *The Persistent Desire* and Biddy Martin, "Lesbian Identity and Autobiographical differences" in Abelove, et al. *The Gay and Lesbian Studies Reader.*

28

A Room of One's Own: Revisited

Lynne Hektor

*F*or women, unrelentingly socialized over centuries to needs of home and hearth, there continues to be far too little societal recognition and validation of the need of all women for a "room of one's own," be it a physical or psychic space. The purpose of this chapter is to revel in the delights of solitude, to sing the praises of time alone and unfettered, to cast out notions of obligations and responsibilities to others in favor of the unabashed joys of a cup of tea in the early morning, before anyone else is stirring, by oneself; in the secretive pleasure of an afternoon movie, a slip into a cool and dark cinema off an urban street to see a film no one *we* know would even want to see; that cool spring evening in the country, right before dark, when, sure that the baby is asleep, there is the furtive stroll, by oneself, down the lane, sky changing colors, wildflowers and weeds on the side of the road, riotious and collective, the crickets just beginning their June chirp.

Allusions to times alone are often conceptualized, for women, as "stolen." Stolen from whom? And for what? These are questions I pose that demand answers. For I would advocate that the capacity to be alone is vital to health and happiness. I quote Montaigne, "We must reserve a little back-shop, all our own, entirely free, wherein we establish our true liberty and principle retreat and solitude." Although I would agree that in infancy and early childhood that attachment to parents and/or parent substitutes is essential if the child is to survive, and that such secure attachments are indeed necessary for the child to develop into an adult capable of making intimate relationships with other adults on equal terms, I would speculate that intimate attachments to other human beings, while important, are nonetheless highly over-rated, especially for women. Attachment theory, a popular cornerstone of conventional, although largely unexamined, wisdom, gives shortshrift to the value of work, as well as to the emotional importance of what goes on in the mind of the individual when alone; in short, the *imagination.* In the words of Samuel Johnson, "Were it not for imagination, Sir, a man would be as happy in the arms of a chambermaid as of a Duchess." Intimate attachments are a center around which the life of the individual revolves, not necessarily *the* center.

How that center is defined will vary from person to person, culture to culture, historical time and place, inevitably the mixture of individual interaction with an ever-evolving context. I enter into this dialogue on behalf of all women; the busy young mother is as in need of a sip of the cool glass of solitude as the Ivory Tower academic—perhaps more so. And those who drink of that glass—especially those requiring long droughts, are frequently perceived as greedy, perhaps anti-social, or ultimately, mad. Women as artist, women as writer, women as poet, women as social activist— any women whose life includes risk and the desire for individual achievement in the public world, as well as, or worse yet, in place of, marital love, is often still villified, as frequently by her own cultural expectations as those of others. A collection follows of thoughts and writings of and about women who have chosen and relentlessly pursued their solitary visions and lives, as well as a celebration of choices too seldom celebrated.

I myself currently write from the perspective of a ten-year, live-in, heterosexual relationship. Perhaps my thoughts on, and memories of my single life are romanticized, sanitized, and ultimately idealized. But, I have resisted the legal sanctions of marriage, in part, I think, because of these memories, and because of my view of myself as a single and solitary being, free, unencumbered, autonomous. "Free, white, and twenty-one" as the old, racist saying used to go, implying all the perogatives of full citizenship and responsibilities, rights, and yes again, autonomy.

And so I am still single (legally, at least) and also childless. A true creature of the twenty-first, uniquely American century, replete with Planned

Parenthood and free birth control since before I was 18. And now nearing 50, birth control is no longer needed; children are a moot issue. Regrets? Not at the present. Maybe regrets will come; maybe they won't. As far as I'm concerned, we all take our chances, make our choices, cut our losses.

In actuality, I revel in my freedom, in a bath of frequent self-indulgence, and disclaim most responsibilities to my fellow creatures. Ultimately self-ish, I suppose, I arise early to savor hot coffee, alone. To enjoy the house with no one else stirring. To see the sun come up, alone. To sniff the air with my cats (Of course, there are cats in my life!) and gird myself for the coming onslaught of interaction with the rest of humanity that life in 1995 brings on a daily level. I yearn for the nineteenth century—a slower pace, time to appreciate subtleties, of texture, of food, of discourse. On the week ends, I sleep late sometimes. Or don't get out of bed at all! Wickedly—for I always *feel* wicked—I peruse the paper—or worse yet read a novel! I don't answer the phone. And I don't feel obliged to have dinner parties, either. I view attachment as highly over-rated.

I guess at a different point in time, historically, or in a different culture, I could be burned at the stake. Or stoned. Or perhaps, merely viewed as mad. At best, unabashedly anti-social. Children in restaurants disturb my sense of propriety.

I remain convinced there is a vast cultural apparatus to convince us otherwise. That a life without children is unlived. That a life without a mar-riage, for a woman, is unfulfilled. That a divorced woman is unwanted, re-jected, neglected, ultimately unlovable. That the widowed are to be pitied, forever. That their life is over. Dead and buried with their dead husband. Rubbish! Garbage! That any relationship is better than waking up alone, on sheets wet and drenched from tears, touseled and wrinkled from a night of wrestling with the devil of loneliness and need.

The "nineties" woman that I know, the one with a full-time job, and a full-time husband, and full-time children, and a full-time house is not a happy camper. The ones I know are stressed—can't find the time for any quality of life; can't find the time to enjoy the house, the husband, the kids, the job. I speak in generalities. Do I think women should just stay home and raise children? That is not my point.

My point, instead, is to say the things that are not said enough, to cele-brate an alternate choice, to say some of the things we frequently dare not say aloud because of "family values"; because of the newly elected, major-ity Republican Congress; because of the Clarence Thomas on the Supreme Court; because of "Christianity"; because of the nature of what it means to be a woman; because of the "Pro-Lifers" who shoot doctors in cold blood, planned and executed; because of our husbands and mates; because of *our* mothers and fathers; because of convention; because of all the "shoulds" in our lives; because of *notions* of feminity; because of *ideas* of love and marriage, and relationships; because of *pictures* in our heads of what our home *should* look like; because of *mental images* of what the perfect female body *should* be; because of how we *should* feel; because of encrusted and outmoded definitions of *the family*.

I write instead to acclaim a different voice, and a different life. I write to remember the delight of slipping into an afternoon movie in New York City by oneself, the cool and dark interior of the cinema like a caress. (You can do what you want. Your time is your own.) The extravagence! I write to recall staying up late at night, jazz playing on the stereo, or is it the CD (you can pick what you want, with no excuses), sipping wine and savoring old pictures. Pulling out old journals. Reading. Looking. Remembering. Musing. Dreaming. Commemorating. The time to write a letter. To write in a journal. To learn to hear one's own voice. Time to feel one's own desires. Time to dream one's own dreams.

I write instead to celebrate the lives of other women who have made the choice to be themselves. Who have made the choice, in this case, not to marry. Listen to the words of Oriana Fallaci, for starters, acclaimed, albeit controversial journalist. She claims she chose against marriage because " . . . marriage is an expression that to me suggests 'giving up,' an expression of sacrifice and regret . . . The solitude [I needed] wasn't a physical solitude . . . It was an internal solitude that comes about from the fact of being a woman—a woman with responsibilities in the world of men . . . Today, I need that kind of solitude so much—that sometimes I feel the need to be physically alone. When I am with my companion, there are moments when we are two too many. I never get bored when I'm alone, and I get easily bored when I am with others" (Heilbrun, 1988, p. 89).

I write instead to commemorate the life of scientist Barbara McClintock, noted geneticist, another woman who listened to her own voice, another woman who has lived her life alone. Her biographer, Evelyn Fox Keller, called the second chapter of her recounting of McClintock's life, *A Feeling for the Organism: The Life and Work of Barbara McClintock*, "The Capacity to Be Alone" (Keller, 1986). Keller recalls a summer many years before that she spent as a graduate student at a laboratory where McClintock was working and describes her memories of the scientist, whom she had never met. "I remembered seeing her—contained, aloof, perhaps even eccentric—going to and from her laboratory or on solitary walks in the woods or by the beach" (p. 16). Years later, when Keller approached McClintock about the proposed biography, McClintock resisted. She did not see how her life could be of interest, and certainly not of value, to other women. After all, and she was adamant on this, she was too different, too much of a "maverick" to be of any conceivable interest to other women. She had never married, never had children. She had never had any interest in what she called "decorating the torso." Keller's argument was that her story was of interest precisely for these reasons.

Keller recounts McClintock's years as an undergraduate at Cornell, in particular her relation to men. In the first two years, she had lived the life of a coed, going out on many dates. "Then," she said, "Then I finally decided I had to be more discriminating. I remember being emotionally fond of several men . . . they were not casual involvements." But she continued, these attachments could never have lasted. "I was just not adjusted," she explained, "never had been, to being closely associated with anybody, even members of my own family . . . There was not that strong necessity for a personal attachment to anybody. I just didn't feel it. And I never could understand marriage. I really do not even now . . . I never went through the experience of requiring it" (p. 34).

Keller associates McClintock's stance with the word "autonomy," with its attendant indifference to conventional expectations. Noting that McClintock has lived most of her life alone—physically, emotionally, and intellectually—Keller also states that no one who has met her could doubt that it has been a full and satisfying life, a life well-lived.

For example, in McClintock's view, conventional science fails to illuminate not only "how" you know, but also and equally, "what" you know. A true naturalist in approach, she sees the need to not press nature with leading questions but to dwell quietly and patiently in the variety and complexity of organisms. Keller speculates that this is a worldview frequently unique to a woman scientist. The recent discoveries—largely led by McClintock—of genetic liability and flexibility forces us to recognize the magnificent integration of cellular processes—a kind of integration that McClintock says is "simply incredible to old-style thinking." This major revolution in thought will completely re-organize things and the way we do research. She adds, "I can't wait. Because I think it's going to be marvelous, simply marvelous. We're going to have a completely new realization of the relationship of things to each other" (p. 207). Certainly not the words of an embittered and frustrated woman, but rather the words of a woman who has trailblazed, usually alone, to reach new heights, and certainly someone who has enjoyed the ups and downs of the journey.

Unfortunately, the single-mindedness of a Fallaci or a McClintock is all too rare. What is more common is the many voices we never get to hear— women's voices hobbled by circumstances of class, color, sex, and the times into which they are born, the cultural and political apparatus that still operates to maintain the *Silences* that writer Tillie Olsen so eloquently and poignantly describes:

Wholly surrended and dedicated lives; time as needed for the work; total-
ity of self. But women are traditionally trained to place others' needs first,
to feel these needs as their own (the "infinite capacity"); their sphere, their
satisfaction to be making it possible for others to use their abilities . . .

In the twenty years I bore and reared my children, usually had to
work at a paid job as well, the simplest circumstances for creating did
not exist. Nevertheless writing, the hope of it, was "the air I breathed, so
long as I shall breathe at all." In that hope there was conscious storing,
snatched reading, beginnings of writing, and always, "the secret rootlets
of reconnaissance." (Cahill, 1994, p. 149)

She goes onto describe her days:

A full extended family life; the world of my job; and the writing, which I
was somehow able to carry around with me through work, through
home. Time on the bus, even when I had to stand was enough; the stolen
moments at work, enough; the deep night hours for as long as I could
stay awake, after the kids were in bed, after the household tasks were
done, sometimes during. It was no accident that the first work I consid-
ered publishable began: "I stand here ironing, and what you ask me
moves tormented back and forth with the iron." (p. 149)

The above ties together the several strands, all of which impinge on the
development of women as creative, self-determined creatures in and of
their own right—the internal constraints of self-concept, and the external
constraints of economic and political circumstance. This was what Virginia Woolf addressed in 1928, when she presented two papers that ultimately became *A Room of One's Own*. She straightforwardly presented
the facts as she saw them: for a woman to write fiction she must have
money and a room of her own. And therein lies the ultimate rub of the true
question of a life lived alone even now for women in 1995. For, as we approach the next millenium, how much have things in actuality changed?

Woolf's solution came in the form of a lifelong legacy bequeathed to
her. She remembers, "The news of my legacy reached me one night about
the same time that the act was passed that gave votes to women. A solici-
tor's letter fell into the post box and when I opened it I found that she
[Woolf's aunt, who died by a fall from her horse when she was riding in
the night air of Bombay] had left me five hundred pounds a year forever.
Of the two—the vote and the money—the money, I own, seemed infi-
nitely the more important (Woolf, 1929, p. 37).

There is no doubt about it. The money, the economic freedom, is not
always available to women. But again, I write here to celebrate the victories of women, to acknowledge the ability, sometimes against all odds,

external and internal, of women to create their own, unique lives. I write
to cherish the words of the woman who chooses *against* the conventional
wisdom of attachment to others, who structures her life independent of
family obligations, the woman who honors her own sensibilities. Consider Sidonie Colette, nee Landoy, whose letter written at seventy-seven
years of age to her daughter's husband, is commemorated in that daughter, Colette's, autobiography *Earthly Pleasures* (1966):

> *Sir,*
>
>   *You ask me to come and spend a week with you, which means I would
> be near my daughter, whom I adore. You who live with her know how
> rarely I see her, how much her presence delights me, and I'm touched you
> should ask me to come and see her. All the same, I am not going to accept
> your kind invitation, for the time being at any rate. The reason is that my
> pink cactus is going to flower. It's a very rare plant I've been given, and
> I'm told that in our climate it only flowers once every four years. Now, I
> am already a very old woman, and if I went away when my pink cactus
> is about to flower, I am certain I shouldn't see it flower again.*
>
>   *So I beg you, sir, to accept my sincere thanks and my regrets, together
> with my kind regards." (p. 22-23)*

Colette's commentary on the letter is also surpassing in it's own
beauty. She writes:

> *Whenever I feel myself inferior to everything about me, threatened by
> my own mediocrity, frightened by the discovery that a muscle is losing
> its strength, a desire its power, or a pain the keen edge of its bite, I can
> still hold my head up and say to myself: "I am the daughter of the
> woman who wrote that letter. . . . Let me not forget that I am the daugh-
> ter of a woman who bent her head, trembling, between the blades of a
> cactus, her wrinkled face full of ecstasy over the promise of a flower,
> who never ceased to flower, untiringly, during three quarters of a cen-
> tury." (p. 23)*

This vignette is included to illustrate the point that I am not attempting
to hold up and validate woman who externally achieve. Again, I write instead to revere the life of the psyche, of the woman who lives her life according to her own unique vision, who flies in the face of convention, the
woman who causes trouble, the woman who doesn't conform, the woman
who lives her life in exile, in cunning, the woman rebel. Her rebellion
may come early or it may come late.
   By the nineteenth century, the single woman had lost some of her
power. Although no longer burned as witches, an unmarried and childless

woman still posed a threat to the patriarchy (Auerbach, 1982, p. 111). Auerbach (1982) cites the "old maid" figures of much of the fiction of the era as illustrative of the shape of new lives lived with no basis in family. In this sense, they were in actuality " . . . stronger than the family" (p. 115). An essay on "Old Maids" in Blackwood's *Edinburgh Magazine* in 1872 had the following to say about spinsterhood:

> *The highest type of old maid has made no sacrifice, nor is she in any sense a victim, for marriage as a state is not necessary to her idea of happiness . . . She is the woman who has never met with her ideal, and who has never been cunningly persuaded to accept anything short of it. (p. 116)*

I remember my completely single, free, and unencumbered days in New York City with longing. I especially remember my days in graduate school, working on my thesis, a piece of work that intellectually and psychically absorbed me, which my single lifestyle permitted. I re-arranged my one bedroom East side apartment to accommodate my work. I set up a large, aluminum folding picnic table to have the space on which to spread out my books and papers. It was autumn; I had visited the country and returned with drying snowball flowers. Ivory and fat, they hung over my papers, dried and drooping. Doing work on an historical figure, I papered my apartment with pictures needed for inspiration. In a conceptual and methodological daze, I worked, in relative oblivion to life around me. I remember certain Saturday nights; I would work. My respite would be a stroll to the corner deli—a purchase of hot coffee in a paper Blue Acropolis cup that all New Yorkers of certain years can recall. Crossing First Avenue to the corner Newsstand to purchase the Sunday *New York Times* on Saturday night. The pleasure of the stroll home. I remember walking home from the typist, completed thesis in hand. It was a warm New Year's evening, I recall, and nighttime, but the walk was wonderful. No manic exhilaration, but contented sense of achievement. My journal for that January 1 reads:

> *Somehow it seems fortuitous to have ended up*
> *in bed writing tonite*
> *to start tonite Anew, as my thesis winds*
> *down freeing up time & energy—*
>
> *I truly do feel a sense of achievement*
> *Janet, the typist, has been great*
> *walking down First Avenue to Hunter*
> *foggy, misty, weirdly warm January nite*

past the UN, looming in the dark
the River
a New Year, 1985

Major life changes ensued for me that year.

Despite the advancement of the status of the unmarried female at the conclusion of the nineteenth century, strong sanctions in new forms continued to emerge against those women who lived their lives as they chose—the "new woman," unmarried, and committed to political and social causes. These were the suffragettes, the women of the Settlement House movement, the fighters for fair labor practices and decent treatment of children. This was the first appearance of a new breed of distinctly American womanhood: the single, highly educated, economically autonomous New Woman. This New Woman threatened existing gender relations and challenged distributions of power (Smith-Rosenberg, 1985). And, significantly, they failed. By the 1930s, women and men alike disowned the New Woman's brave visions.

As progressive women reformers had increased their political power in the years immediately preceding the First World War, and as the suffrage movement reached its crescendo, articles complaining of lesbianism in women's colleges, clubs, prisons—wherever women gathered—became common. By the 1920s, charges of lesbianism had become a common way to discredit women professionals, reformers, and educators—as well as the institutions they had founded and run. Women's rights became divorced from their social and economic context. What was the mothers demand for political power and autonomy, was recast as the daughter's quest for heterosexual pleasures. The feminist modernists rejected an older, Victorian or Edwardian female identity, tied as it was to sexual purity and sacrifice. They wished to free themselves from considerations of gender. Victories won by earlier generations of New women in educational and professional arenas had made an androgynous world possible. However, modern women shed their primary identity as woman before the world they inhabited accepted their legitimacy (Smith-Rosenberg, 1985). It is a struggle that continues.

I currently live in tandem; I live with another. But it is not a conventional marriage. I count myself lucky. And still free, unbound, unconstrained. I attribute it to years of single living and a singularly unusual man and partner.

Ultimately, I am compelled to continue to celebrate the alternate, the other, the life as woman lived alone, childless, seemingly rootless, yet reminiscent of Tennyson's experience-hungry Ulysses, scorning family ties to take his being from his world: "I am part of all that I have met"

(Auerbach, 1982, p. 125). And moreso. All that I dream, all that I imagine, all that I touch, on this journey of a life lived alone, freely chosen.

REFERENCES

Auerbach, Nina. (1982). *Woman and the demon.* Cambridge, MA: Harvard University Press.

Heilbrun, Carolyn G. (1988). *Writing a woman's life.* New York: Norton.

Keller, Evelyn Fox. (1983). *A feeling for the organism: The life and work of Barbara McClintock.* New York: W. H. Freeman.

Olsen, Tillie. (1994). Silences (excerpt). In Susan Cahill (Ed.), *Writing women's lives.* New York: Harper Perennial, pp. 148-151.

Phelps, Robert. (1966). *Earthly paradise: Colette's autobiography drawn from the writings of her life.* New York: Farrar, Straus & Giroux. Translated by Herma Briffault, Derek Coltman, & others.

Smith-Rosenberg, Carroll. (1985). *Disorderly conduct: Visions of gender in Victorian America.* New York: Alfred A. Knopf.

Woolf, Virginia. (1957). *A room of one's own.* New York: Harcourt, Brace & World.

29

"I'm Here Too"

Agnes Fleming

Hear my voice as a 12-year-old girl, as it streams from within a grown woman, still crying from the pain of a grief and loss from 20 years ago. Life and emotional integrity are held captive until that abandonment and naked invisibility are exposed and mourned.

I am that 12-year-old girl living in a town north of Boston. I am the oldest child in an Irish Catholic family with six children. The memories of the death of my grandmother are vivid. The details of that period of time are as real as if they happened yesterday. The feelings and grief associated with that period of time remained repressed for 20 years.

I'm here too," I want to cry out. Why can't they see me? Why can't they understand my painful crushing anguish? Why don't they understand that I'm devastated too? I am holding my six-month-old sister in my arms and leaning against the doorframe in the living room. I have been kept home to take care of the baby. The other children in my family were sent to the beach to be with friends.

As I look across the room, I see my best friend, my grandmother. She is lying in a casket placed in the bay window. Her dress is pink. Pink was her favorite color. I try to express my sadness. I'm told not to upset my parents, that they are upset enough already. I withdraw into the doorframe and into my sadness and memories. No tears come. I am numb. I don't want to upset my mother and father.

I am remembering how I spent a great deal of time with my grandmother. Before we moved into this house, I stayed with her while my grandfather was sick. We shopped together, we visited my grandfather in the hospital, and we took trains and buses everywhere. I was embarrassed and awed by her ability to talk with strangers. She even asked them for rides from the hospital to the bus station. My grandmother had very weak ankles. They would turn and she fell often. I was always helping her up from the ground. We held onto each other.

My grandmother was my refuge and comforter. In her eyes I could do no wrong. I wear her wedding band. She gave it to me a short time ago. I was grown up enough to be trusted with something as valuable and meaningful as her wedding ring. She loved me.

My grandmother was my roommate. We shared a bedroom. We talked in bed at night. My grandmother spent a lot of time talking with me about becoming a young lady and how young ladies are supposed to act. I learned never to send the jacket or skirt of a suit to the cleaners separately because the colors won't match when they come back. I also learned to take off my good clothes when I came in from school to keep them in good shape. "Young ladies don't wear dungarees." she stated on numerous occasions. I don't own a pair.

I remember. It is the morning of two days ago. I heard a voice calling me. I woke up. My grandmother was falling to the floor. She was gasping for air. The doctor arrived with his black bag. The ambulance arrived. It was too late.

As I stand here now, I am looking around the living room at all of the familiar faces. They don't see me. They are comforting each other. "I'm here too," I want to cry out, "I'm here too."

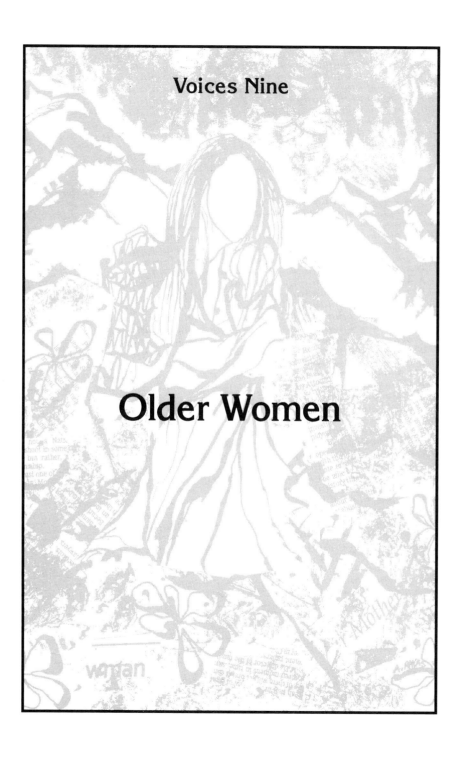

Voices Nine

Older Women

30

A Woman from the
Old World

Elizabeth J. Forbes

REMEMBERING ON PURPOSE

Reminiscence is a part of a life review as experienced by an older person. It is a natural process of unraveling events, including specific details, within various time frames of a life. In reminiscence, memories of satisfaction, sorrow, grief, nostalgia, and approval rise and fade.

When reminiscing, the older woman can assess her life and perhaps even resolve personal conflicts. Such a process is now accepted as a valuable therapeutic tool for the giver as well as the recipient. Reminiscence provides the older woman a way of reliving, reexperiencing, and/or savoring events of the past that are personally significant.

Gerontologists no longer think of reminiscence as "crazy talk" or "living in the past," but as a therapeutic communication for the human being. Topics recalled may include happy hours with family, friends, job activities, achievements and life goals, those day-to-day experiences which make up a life. Negative aspects of the past may also be verbalized and put into perspective.

Reviewing life goals, and the past life in general, provides an outlet for coping with the current stresses that must be dealt with in the present. Reminiscence of lived experiences provides the information that the gerontologist needs to help the individual relate to the aging process by constructively identifying her stresses within the framework of the past experiences. The lived experience information provides the link between the past and the present. Older women are better able to understand the present from the knowledge gained.

Reminiscence communications gives a historical perspective on the woman as an individual and adds to the understanding of the woman's perceptions of life. It is an experiential processing of memory.

Reminiscence differs from social communication in that it is goal directed and has valuable historical data. The woman doing the reminiscence becomes an unique individual. Shared human emotions, sadness, humor, fear, and historical events, bind women together across the ages and sharpens our understanding of the feminine experience. Women are the persons who live into old age: There are five women still living at age 90 for every man. Women in general live eight years longer than men. Reminiscence is an important activity for the older woman.

OLGA'S STORY

The story which follows is a very short excerpt of the taped reminiscence of a 78-year-old woman, Olga W., as told to a woman gerontologist seeking to learn from the older woman's insights and memories. The life review begins:

I am a woman of Twentieth Century; a woman of the old world. There were no airplanes, no cars, no phones, certainly no computers when I entered this world.

I was born September 2nd, 1917, at 6:00 A.M. in Wilkes-Barre, Pennsylvania, a small community in the coal mining region. Mother told me that the whistles from the foundries were blowing when I was born.

My parents came to the United States from the Ukraine fifteen years before I was born. They ran from the oncoming hoards of murdering troops of the Czar. They ran for their lives. Grandfather was the mayor of the town and took his family out the back door of his house as the troops were banging at the front door for him. They came to America with only the clothes on their backs. When I see old pictures of immigrants on the boats coming into the harbors of New York, I know that I am looking into the faces of my parents. The women wore babushkas and the children looked tired and frightened. I think of my own grandparents and what they must have been thinking as they held their children close to them and sailed past the Statue of Liberty: "Bring me your huddled masses longing to be free . . ."

Father had been a cabinetmaker apprentice in the Ukraine but worked in the mines when he arrived in Pennsylvania because of a lack of carpenter work. Mother made all of our bread, clothes, and quilts. She literally made the home; she was a homemaker.

I was one of four children, two boys and two girls; the youngest daughter and third child in line. In our home, church, and stores, Ukrainian was spoken exclusively, but I learned English from neighborhood children and at school. They were children of the Irish immigrants who themselves fled from the infamous Irish famine. I remember translating for my mother and she had to bring me to school for parent-teacher meetings. I walked 1¼ miles to school each day. I did not have to milk the cows; we had no cows—but, we did grow our vegetables in our summer garden.

I have seen poverty face-to-face. My family was poor and struggled terribly during World War I—shall I bore you with the fact that eggs were five cents a dozen? But nobody *had the five cents and so everyone was in same boat: We were all poor, economically poor so to speak, but there is a great difference between economic poverty and spiritual/cultural poverty. Family and community were the essence of our existence. We were economically poor and culturally affluent.*

Many of my friends quit school as soon as they could get working papers; they wanted to make money to help their families. Jobs cleaning offices or working in the factories paid $1.25 a week. $1.25 a week was the difference between a family eating two meals a day or nothing at all. When money is scarce, life becomes very basic. It is literally a subsistence existence of moving from meal to meal hoping that there will be enough food for the family for that night and the next day. The struggle becomes one of staving off hunger.

Consider life's hierarchy of needs; I lived them as a child. First air, food, and shelter. Our families were at that bottom rung; on the subsistence ladder. But we did learn how to subsist. My brother would be sent to the butcher shop to buy 25 cents worth of meat and to ask for a free soup bone. Because he was embarrassed, he would ask for a bone for the dog. We didn't have a dog and the butcher knew that we had no dog. Dinner consisted of soup, or a potato and mushrooms. We took leftover vegetable sandwiches to school for lunch. There were no snacks. Often, we were hungry.

We lived near the woods leading into the Appalachian flats and father taught us about how to pick mushrooms, berries, and hickory nuts. The flats are not a forest, but all greenery, and running streams. All of this made us enthusiastic and interested in nature.

I never had to write about what I did on my summer vacation because traveling was not a possibility for my family. The closest thing that I had to a vacation was to go to my godmother Mary's house two miles away. Actually, I was sent there to help my godmother with the housework. She had a daughter and two sons. One son was extremely ill and later died of a heart condition. I remember sitting next to him and he turned blue. I suppose he had some kind of heart condition and, of course, there was no treatment in those days. But I was scared of him and he certainly was visible proof of the fragility of all us.

They had an electric sweeper, a very early version of a vacuum cleaner. It was monstrous. It was a horrible looking thing compared to what we have today. But, it was "modern" and a real status symbol for that family.

My godmother's house was fun and very up-to-date. She had married a successful shopkeeper. We called it "marrying up." I used to love going there. The home was decorated beautifully. There were magnificent lamp shades with corded fringes. She had chickens and pear, plum, and apple trees. I loved to go out into the backyard, pick an apple off the ground or knock an apple off the tree. She couldn't understand why her hens weren't laying eggs. I used to walk through the fields, come upon three to four dozen eggs, and call in Ukrainian, "Naska, Naska." Now we'd call those hens "free range chickens" but what my godmother really needed was a henhouse. Then she would have had her eggs all in one basket. (She laughs at her own joke.) That was the extent of my vacation. I was homesick and looking forward to leaving. Mary said, "I'll give you bracelets and beads if you stay." I stayed for a while longer with this loot as a bribe. I guess she appreciated my housework help, but after a few weeks I left.

In those days, before Barbie dolls, a girl with my background had one little doll to play with and that was it. We didn't have piles of toys. Collecting leaves and stones was my hobby. Today, when I see all of the playthings which my grandchildren have, I feel very annoyed. I truly do feel it is too much, too much of everything. I know that I can't cope with it and I wonder does it overstimulate them? In my day, now isn't that an awful phrase? But, it is true, that, "in my day," we made up games. I'd say that we were more creative, more curious. Remember that this is before the telephone, before television, it was even before the radio. We would make mud pies, put them out in the sun to dry, play tag, throw a ball—that was my entertainment; life was much different.

Mother was smart and understood the value of education. She would not let me, my sister, or brothers quit school because education was a high priority for her. She saw the future and wanted a middle-class life for us. Education was essential for that future, it was her American dream. I had expressed a wish to be a nurse-and that was to become my vehicle out of our underclass life. Education was the driving imperative. If a woman was to work outside the home in an educated field, she had two choices. She could become a nurse or a teacher.

Mother was a wonderful role model for her children. She understood the need for literacy and the cultural arts. This woman who was my mother and who was a girl from a small rural farming village in Central Europe, understood the refinement which art, music and dancing brings to the human experience. I remember that mother wanted one of her girls to study Ukrainian dancing. Because my family could only afford to pay for one set of lessons, and my older sister did not want to learn Ukrainian dancing, I became a dancer. And how I loved the dance lessons and the socializing and opportunities to learn more about my Ukrainian culture! My colorful, authentic Ukrainian dance costume was made by women from mother's village, "back home," in the Ukraine. How I remember myself as a young 12-year-old girl in my multicolored beaded blouse, skirt, and the fancy, long-hanging hair ribbons that completed my outfit! I was beautiful and felt so proud. My Ukrainian dancing enabled me to go everywhere even before I started high school. My Ukrainian church sent us to Bucknell University Stadium for the Folk Festival. It became my middle-class passport. I learned how to eat at hotels, I think I have a picture to show you. My costume came from Europe, and my mother made certain parts of it. She made my beaded headbands. You could say that I was a professional dancer. Our troupe paid the dancers 25 cents a day and paid for our travel expenses.

My mother enjoyed my success. I'm not sure if it did her more good than it did for me. It's hard to say.

The costumes were truly works of art. They were displayed at various places including, as it happened, the General Hospital in Wilkes-Barre, Pennsylvania. Everyone appreciated the truly magnificent work. While my costume was on display at the Boston Store in Wilkes-Barre, one of the nurses at the Wilkes Hospital, who knew our family, (she was Ukrainian, also) asked if she could use my costume. She wore my glorious beaded blouse, skirt, and hair ribbons at the annual hospital festival dance and it got first prize for three years. To think that it was entirely handmade by the peasants in my mothers village and just for me. I don't know why these women were called "peasants." They were artisans with creative and skilled hands. Their ability to create beauty changed my life.

I am happy we were poor. I think it builds your character, I truly do. We learned about our own culture. We sang in the church choir and joined the Ukrainian Bandora Choir. The bandora is an Ukrainian instrument which gives a unique sound to music. It is like the mandolin but it sounds far more beautiful than the mandolin. We sang at the high school and were active in all of the other Ukrainian activities.

We might have been poor, but mother insisted that we behave like middle-class families. Discipline, reading, school work, religion, and family relationships centered us in our world. Self-esteem, pride, patience, and cleanliness were demanded of us. We grew and were dearly nurtured. Looking back now, I'd say that we were rich in many ways. Not everyone saw how rich we were, however, and I can laugh now when I tell the story of the day when President Roosevelt and other big time Washington people came touring through our town, when they wanted to tour an example of a "very poor" community.

At sixteen years old, I went to my mother and said that I was going to quit high school and take a $1.50 a week job doing housework for the factory owners' wife. I had work papers and was ready to enter the world. Mother insisted, without compromise, "No, you always said you wanted to be a nurse. You will become a nurse."

And so it happened. I graduated as a nurse 1941. I was working at Abington Hospital when war was declared—we sat around the radio listening to President Roosevelt's speech as World War II began that December.

The country was mobilized for the war effort. Everybody's life changed. My girlfriend from Maine said, "Let's join the Navy," and I said, "I think I might—but I think I want to join the Army." So Mabel went to the Navy, and I went into the Army.

My first assignment was with a station hospital in Georgia, then in New Orleans, Louisiana, then New York, and within the year, I was shipped overseas—literally shipped in a thousand-person troop carrier to Glasgow, Scotland—to a general hospital in Nottingham, England. I traveled all over England as an Army nurse during the worst periods of the German bombing. I went to a general hospital in Nottingham, then to central Wales, Sacton Sacrun Walden, then I was transferred to the Harvard Medical Unit and Army Surgical unit staffed with surgeons from Harvard University.

We saw men with terrible, mutilating wounds. Faces, hands, legs, bowels blown out with bullets and shrapnel. We witnessed the flesh of humanity being torn apart. Airmen with faces burned off as their planes went down into the English Channel in flames.

Surgeons developed new surgical techniques as they went along. We were all facing situations which were never faced before—and the tragedy of the human pain. I sat by many men as they died. Even worse was sitting with the men who awoke from their surgery to find they had no arms, or legs or even their buttocks were gone. Incredible human loss. Incredible human pain. But the women stayed by these men. The nurses' worked 24 hours a day to be with these men in their pain. We held their hands as their wounds were being debrided and they screamed in excruciating agony. We wrote letters home to their families when they had no hands to write the letters themselves. We changed dressings and let the men know that we respected them and that they were honorable and worthwhile. We saved their lives and their spirits. I felt like a woman. A woman who nurtures and heals. There were times that I could feel my healing energy move from me to the wounded "boys" (and they were boys of eighteen and nineteen). They took their wounds in battle for their country and its people. They spoke of the war and their families. Actually they spoke of their women, their mothers, girlfriends, and wives. These wounded soldiers spoke of their role in protecting the lives and freedom of their people. Valor and patriotism gave them strength and I really loved them and cried for them. And I thank them even now. Because they fought so that I might be free. I get chills now as I say this. It has been a long time since I have reflected on it.

We forget so that we can move on. But that War was real and the men were brave. And they did it for their women and families.

One physician, who was to become very famous, wrote a surgical textbook when he left the service. The Army said it was Army property, and he said it was his property. There was a nasty lawsuit and the doctor won it. The War taught the medical and nursing teams new ways of operating, new technology and new ways of caring for patients.

Of all the patients I remember most, it was the burn patients. There were land mine burns and I had this black patient, Cooper, and I'll never forget him. His skin was burned so deeply that all you could see were the bottom layers and so he was pink all over; I had to soak him twice a day. His burns wept so much that the dressings stuck onto him. Pulling them off would be far too painful and it would further injure his skin. If the dressings were not changed, infection would grow under the dressings and he would die in a purulent fever and exudate. It took four hours to soak the dressings off him. In the tub of water, his dressings would float off. And then gently, he would help me as I reapplied the sterile medicine and gauze dressings. In all of his pain, he was patient and kind toward me. I don't know how he tolerated those treatments. After a few weeks when he was stabilized, he was flown to an Army burn hospital. I never saw Cooper again but he became a part of my life, my memory.

After two years and because I now had seniority, I was sent to be a charge nurse on an orthopedic unit, and, as it happened I was to work with Captain John Mollett. The nursing unit, B17 was a hell hole and initially, I felt it was punishment. Well, everything came up roses.

Captain Mollett (his uncle is the French artist mentioned in the dictionary, Franc) would tell me about his experiences spending time in England as a child, and all that sort of thing. Anyway, he was very down-to-earth, especially after I told him he should never have been a doctor. "Captain Mollett, your progress notes are awful, your patients aren't dressed." He told me, "I said I never wanted to be a doctor"—it was his father who was a psychiatrist in Boston who insisted that John become a doctor. He was all Society—back bay. After I berated him, he said, "Let me tell you what's wrong with you?" I said, "What?" He said, "You wear too much rouge." I said, "I do?" The next day I came with rouge; he said, "Okay—let's get started. What do we do to straighten up this unit?" I said, "Let's go." And we did. John and I changed that unit, made it a clean and safe place for the men to heal and we got along fabulously. He recommended me for my first lieutenancy, and, by the way, if I had stayed in a little longer, I would have gotten a captain rank.

Let me tell you, I got around. I was in the Army three years and nine months, and I couldn't make an adjustment in civilian life when I got out. You may not believe this, but there wasn't any work for nurses in hospitals. There was no work for women outside the home after the War. Everyone of us was expected to marry and "settle down." It was terrible for me, I felt dreadful. I took one private duty case. A friend asked me to work for this doctor as a private duty nurse on a tonsil case.

A colleague with whom I used to work, Rue B. Plictard, stayed in the Army and retired as a general very young. She never married. Years later, when I read about her in a magazine, I said, "She can have it. I had my happy life with my son and husband."

My son and husband? Oh, yes, I have skipped ahead. Let me tell you that story.

After being in New York a short while, I worked with Dr. Schruell, on Fifth Avenue, behind the Frick Museum. He was a plastic surgeon with many up-scale patients. The surgeon had operated on people such as Queen Marie of Romania and the Duke and Duchess of Windsor and I felt very guilty doing that kind of work. My feet were on the ground and we had these very rich patients. I was getting tired of the tin mines of Bolivia.

One Italian patient said, "I happen to know the most wonderful person. I think he is in Washington this weekend on business. I'll have to ask my husband. But you know whoever marries him is going to be the luckiest girl in the world." I thought, "More of this silliness." Every patient had someone for me to meet—either coming off the boat or (setting) me up with someone to pair up with. It was a distress to all that I had not married yet.

Well, we had a "blind date." In walks my husband-to-be and I thought, "Oh my God, this is the man I am going to marry—what a horrible suit and he's shorter than I am."

Before going out to cocktails and dinner that night I had to run and buy a flat pair of shoes on Fifth Avenue. He was ten years older and was established. He had dated two nieces of Jimmy Walker, the Mayor of New York. Well, we fell in love and were married in June of 1947. Our son was born in March of 1948. All my friends were counting out the months on their fingers.

Olga W. had a lot more to tell me. All of the stages of an "ordinary" woman are laid out in her reminiscence exercise. But she can help us touch history. There are lessons to be learned. A mature woman has insight and experience. And she shares it with us through reminiscence, a lived experience.

REFERENCES

Burnside, I. (1990). Reminiscence: An independent nursing intervention for the elderly. *Issues in Mental Health Nursing, 11*:33.

Burnside, I., & Haight, B. K. (1992). Reminiscence and life review: Analyzing each concept. *J. Adv. Nurs., 17:*855.
Dietsche, L. (1979). Facilitating the life-review through group reminiscence. *J. Gerontol Nurs., 5:*43.
Ebersole, P. (1976). Reminiscing. *Am. J. Nurs., 76*(8):1304.
Forbes, E., & Fitzsimons, V. (1981). The older adult: A process for wellness. St. Louis: C. V. Mosby Company.
Head, P. M., Portnoy, S., & Woods, R. T. (1990). The impact of reminiscence groups in two different settings. *Int. J. Ger. Psychiatry, 5:*295.
Youssef, F. A. (1990). The impact of group reminiscence counseling on a depressed elderly population. *Nur. Pract., 15*(4):32.

31

Pain in the Golden Years

Virginia Macken Fitzsimons

*Y*ou crazy old battleax," Louise screamed at her mother Martha, "How many times have I told you that I don't care what you think. Now shut up and don't bother me." Martha, 82 years old, cried as she walked slowly up the stairs to her hot attic bedroom. The pain of her arthritis and osteoporosis was awful and she really did need a ride to her doctor, but Louise her 58-year-old daughter had no patience for her suffering. Louise had troubles of her own. In another era, it would have been Louise who was considered to be old. But in these times, Louise is still young. We have a myth of the "golden years" of untroubled retirement and relaxation. A troubled family moves the bad feelings to all of its members, including the old. Because this family is struggling with difficulties, its members feel considerable pain. Martha was filled with physical and psychological

---

Adapted from a paper presented at the United Nations, April, 1995.

pain. Instead of a life in the sheltering, loving arms of a caring family, she found herself in the middle of a conflicted, troubled family. She felt abandoned and abused. If only her two other children didn't live so far away, she could ask them for help, she thought.

Martha has been widowed for seven years now and living with Louise and her family far from the town where she had raised her own family. Louise had no patience for her. Louise had enough problems managing to cope with her own husband and three grown children. And Martha's story is far from unique.

SOCIETY'S UGLY SECRET

Behind apparently lovely closed doors is housed our society's ugly secret: violence against the elderly.

Abuse and mistreatment is something that affects up to one million elder women a year. Detection is difficult because the woman is isolated in her home. Case finding, reporting, and intervention are needed and the general members of a community, as well as its public and health-related officials are all in a position to help. Data clearly show that persons from all races, ethnic, and socioeconomic groups are included as both the abusers and the abused.

Elder abuse is the least known form of domestic violence. The entire topic is hindered by disbelief. "This can't be?" a neighbor or fellow church member thinks when confronted by a bruised or withdrawn aging person.

Misinformation prevails and underdetection is a major issue in the problem. In sharp contrast to child abuse awareness, elder mistreatment is seen in up to 4% (1 in 25) of the older female population. The overall prevalence rate of abuse in the presence of Alzheimer's Disease is a dramatic and shocking 18% (4 in 25).

Caroline sits gazing out of her 11th floor window. She remembers the days when she was an active community member, participating in her church and sending her children off to school. For all of her 70 years she cared for her house, spoke with her neighbors, and tended to her garden. Now she can hardly see the street. Few visitors come to see her in this high-rise senior citizen housing unit. Her family had convinced her to sell her home and to move here. It seemed like a good idea initially. At first it seemed to be a pleasant and safe place to live. Recently, however, the rules at this senior housing project had changed. Now in addition to seniors, "displaced" people were allowed to move in. Caroline sees men who hang around drinking and she suspects of taking drugs. There is a clear smell of urine in the room with the incinerator. Lightbulbs are broken and not replaced. Caroline feels abandoned and alone. She is right. Her family and friends have either moved away or are dead now. Like Martha, Caroline is one of the many millions of older women who are invisible in our society and who are suffering. Only 5% of all older people are in nursing homes. Many millions of seniors are safe and live independent and comfortable lives. These seniors we see in active roles, enjoying themselves, and having vacations. But, that is the visible part of our picture.

RAISING OUR CONSCIOUSNESS

Neglect and verbal mistreatment are far more common manifestations of elder abuse than are actual physical beatings. The senior women in these situations, however, feel terrified and in despair.

Psychological abuse in the form of verbal aggression, denigration, harassment, intimidation, and threats of punishment or deprivation are all abuse on a psychological level. The most common form of abuse, however, and the most open to community recognition and resolution is psychological neglect. It is a failure to provide social stimulation; it is social isolation. The family is at work and school all day and the elder person is unattended for long periods of time. In periods of family stress, verbal threatening to abandon the elderly or threats to place them in nursing homes constitute clear abuse.

Financial abuse is seen through the unauthorized use of the elderly's funds or property or taking Social Security checks or pensions or food stamps. The older person can be violated legally through violation of personal rights. The failure to allow an elderly woman to make her own decisions, depriving her of her right to privacy or self-determination or through the denial of her voting privileges constitute elder abuse. To determine if psychological abuse is present, ask:

- Can she worship where and when she wants?
- Is she receiving her mail?
- Is eviction threatened?
- Or are there threats of sending her away?

IDENTIFYING PHYSICAL ABUSE

Physical abuse can be severe. Out of 1000 older women, 32 are beaten physically and hospitalized each year. Abuse ranges from subtle and insidious to blatant. There is a lack of clear and consistent definitions. Nevertheless, we should be concerned for the safety and well-being of older women. All women will be a part of that population someday. And while there are ethnic variations of behaviors, respect for women of all ages will assist a society to value and respect its older women. As an entire nation, we must come to a place of common understanding of what is acceptable behavior toward women.

AS AN ELDER CARE PROFESSIONAL

How do I as an elder care professional, begin to address the needs of the elderly without becoming discouraged and disheartened? I have found that in my practice, my major role is to assist a community and individual families to understand the process of aging and to define the boundaries of caregiving within those communities and families.

I speak out in communities. I ask the questions and assist the community to find definitions.

- What is elder mistreatment? Elder mistreatment is an act of commission or omission that results in harm or threatened harm to the health and welfare of an older person which affects the quality of the life of that person.
- What is elder abuse? Elder abuse is a suffering imposed by means of abuse and neglect, mistreatment or related categories of abuse and neglect.

In my teaching regarding the elderly I offer facts: It is estimated that 13 cases of abuse go unreported for each case that comes to light. By law, health professionals are required to report cases. Family, friends, and community persons are morally obliged to report suspected or witnessed abuse or mistreatment.

Why the under reporting? There is a lack of recognition of cases. There is a lack of awareness of laws on reporting. There are poor expectations as to outcome. Neighbors and friends ask, "What good will it do?" There is a belief that reporting may actually harm the person. "They'll be mad." the neighbor will say, and the mistreatment and suffering continues. There is a reluctance to report abuse because of the fear of liability despite immunity provisions of the law. Always there is a fear of damage to relationships within the family.

RISK FACTORS

Knowing the risk factors and signs can assist us to be proactive to prevent elder abuse. I teach that over 75-year-old persons are most at risk. The frail or the cognitively and functionally impaired person is at risk. The person who expresses anger or commits angry acts towards caregivers is at risk.

WOMEN ABUSE OLDER WOMEN

It is women who abuse older women. The abuser is often heavily dependent on the woman being abused either financially or has housing or child-care needs from the woman. Frustration increases the anger level. The abuser often has an addiction, and lives with the woman herself. The abuser often controls access to family and friends and imposes a social isolation on the older woman. It is always an issue of control. Often, there is a history of intrafamilial violence and feelings of powerlessness.

The abuser seeks to counterbalance the situation and so strikes out with harmful acts toward the woman. Caregiver depression is often a variable. Low self-esteem is always correlated with violent feelings. A shared living situation increases tension and fatigue and can be a precipitating factor in abuse.

Mistreatment is categorized as physical violence, chronic verbal aggression, physical neglect, financial exploitation, and/or acts of omissions.

WHAT TO DO

Women are usually cast in the role of caregiver to family members. How can we protect both the caregivers and the cared for woman? What can we do?

I teach my groups these things: We can avert potentially risky situations. Plan with families of patients with dementia and Alzheimer's disease. Reduce stressors. Plan for caregiver relief. Time can be given—called respite care—when the caregiver is herself given time off.

In case finding, speak with the elder woman and caregiver separately. Be sympathetic to each. Ask the older woman: Has anyone at home ever hurt you? Has anyone ever scolded or threatened you? Have you ever signed a document you didn't understand? Are you afraid of anyone at home? Ask the caregiver: What would you like me to know about (state the woman's name)? Have you ever felt frustrated with her? How do you suppose she got the bruise on her arm? Look for unexplained delay in seeking health treatment, injuries inconsistent with medical findings, poor personal hygiene, dehydration and malnutrition. Look for fractures, falls, dislocations, or evidence of physical restraints. Be suspicious.

What skin signs will you see? There might be bruises, hematomas, welts, lacerations, and/or abrasions. Medication related signs include symptoms of over or under medication, loss of memory, dizziness, excessive sleeping, or changes in personality. Neglect is seen as decubitus ulcers, absence of needed eyeglasses, dentures, and prostheses. Is there evidence of poor hygiene? Look for signs of withdrawal, depression, agitation, low self-esteem, infantile behavior, mental status changes, and sleep disorders.

Does the caregiver refuse to let the woman see you alone? Are there unusual behavior patterns between the older woman and her caregiver. Is there a history of spousal abuse?

WHAT CAN BE DONE?

Communities and professionals from a wide range of fields can be a part of the solution. Reliable studies are needed to fully understand the problems. Anticipatory guidance for caregiver/family starts in the community. Identify caregiver depression. Encourage support groups for family members. Day care for the elder woman has great advantages. Plan for interventions to address ambivalence on the part of client and family members, refusal of services, denial, caregiver stress, and feelings of being overwhelmed.

Reduce psychological abuse. Caregiver burden is a major contributory factor. Stress and conflict may be most likely to emerge when a single relative has been designated as the primary caregiver, when there is little support from the rest of the family, when the caregiver and elder woman have had a strained relationship in the first place and when caregiving needs are great.

The stressed caregiver may have financial or other needs that keep him/her from exploring alternatives. Or the caregiver is living up to a promise never to let the elder woman go to a nursing home.

Caregivers of the chronically ill older woman have high rates of depression and low self-esteem. It is a difficult job with little recognition or appreciation. Stress increases and should not be overlooked because it is this which leads to inadequate care and then outright neglect.

Evaluate the caregiver. Ask, How many hours a day do you spend caring for her? Do you get enough sleep at night? (It is not uncommon to be disturbed 2 or 3 times a night and have sleep deprivation and the changes that go with it.) Ask, How do you feel about your caregiving responsibilities? Are there times when you feel you cannot meet her needs? Do you feel angry or frustrated? How do you deal with these feelings? Ask about the caregiver's financial status, health status, and ask are there family support systems for the caregiver? Plan for the caregiver.

Plan interventions to decompress caregiver stress, treat depression, and care for the caregiver. Acknowledge the difficulties of the overburdened caregiver. Interview therapeutically. Use community groups and resources. Use spiritual resources. Use periodic relief opportunities. Care about the caregiver. Women are usually the caregivers.

COMMUNICATE

I have witnessed conversations in families that would never be tolerated between social acquaintances or seldom in a business setting. The more control the higher the voice level. What is the communication style of the family? Is shouting common? Is name calling or berating a person permitted in the family? Do we hear monologues of complaints instead of dialogues aimed at problem solving and solution seeking? Is respect for each person the hallmark of the communication? We are only beginning to explore the issue. Family members can learn to hear each others' needs. These needs can be respected. Abuse must be replaced by new solutions.

REFERENCES

Beck, M. et al. (1990). Aging: Trading places. *Newsweek,* July 16: 48, 1990.
Elliopoulos, C. (1993). *Gerontological nursing.* Philadelphia: Lippincott.
Stanley, M. (1995). *Gerontological nursing.* Philadelphia: F. A. Davis.

32

The Quilt of Spirituality: Older Women's Experiences

Cheryl Demerath Learn

That which can not be said, conceptualized easily or explained can be made known by metaphor. (Morton, 1985, p. 210)

Quilts serve as appropriate metaphors for older women's experiences of spirituality. First, quilting is a uniquely womanly craft. Rarely is sewing textiles for clothing, household goods, or decoration a male skill while sewing is almost universally a female craft. Creative quilting allows for infinite variety (Guild, 1971). No two quilts are exactly alike as no two women's lives or spiritual experiences are alike. Quilts like older women's experiences can be gently unfolded to reveal hidden beauties. Older women's experiences of spirituality are not evident or easily apparent. Unfolding reveals complexities of pattern, design and color.

THE ESSENTIAL FEATURES

Five essential features of the experience of spirituality emerged in my study examining older women's experience of spirituality. They are (1) choosing solitude, (2) connecting with community, (3) dialoging with presence, (4) re-creating the self and (5) encountering spiritual caring.

Choosing Solitude

Loneliness is the poverty of the self; solitude is the richness of the self. (Sarton, 1966, p. 183)

The women spoke of choosing solitude in their lives. Solitude, identified by all of the women, increased in importance as they became older.

Dorothy: I lived in this apartment complex with lots of people around me all the time. I couldn't even eat a meal with someone else from outside without everyone wanting to know who, what, where, when, and why. As I became more interested in other things, I began to want quiet. Now that I have moved, I sit out in my courtyard which is so cool and shady on hot summer days. I can meditate. I've got the privacy.

Frances: Nature gives my life meaning, to get to the seashore once in a while and the mountains . . . And I guess I just enjoy it and long for it or something like that.

The women were clear on the differences between loneliness and freely chosen solitude.

Helen: I need a little time to myself everyday. I had it during my married life. I had it after everything settled down in the evening when everything was nice and quiet, and I could have a little time to myself. I could read or prop my feet up or whatever I wanted to do. I have it now. After playing pool in the early mornings with my friend, I come home and have the afternoon to myself.

Connecting With Community

In most of us there is both a spirit of community and spirit of solitariness. Sometimes they seem to war against each other. (Moore, 1992, p. 66)

Many spiritualities have emphasized dissociation from relationships and withdrawal from the world (Harris, 1989). Gilligan (1982) maintained that models based upon the male experience, were so narrow as to exclude the importance of attachment. Women value connecting with others and relationship as a source of strength and maturity (Conn, 1986; Gilligan, 1982).

Connecting with community included becoming involved with institutional communities such as a church or senior center, friendships, and nature. Ellen found her church especially important as a community of connection after her husband had died.

Ellen: When [husband] died it was during Lent and for want of something else to do or whatever it was, I was at church every night I could be there. It was just the natural place to go. I did go to a number of lectures on bereavement but I never did get much out of them but there was just something so comforting about sitting in a pew that I was used to . . . that I was just grateful.

Individual and group friendships emerged as important aspects of community for the women. Experiences of community were also remembered from the past.

Helen: I don't like this new word bonding. Everyone's using it . . . even with their dogs and I just . . . It's so ridiculous, you would think that it's something new and it's not. There was never stronger bonds than that between my parents and myself in my early life and then later with my children. Guess we just . . . love covered everything.

The search for union with nature can be seen as connecting with community. The women saw themselves as connecting or in relationship with a living environment.

Anna: At that time, the valley was very beautiful with rolling hills and grass up to your knees as far as you see. I could talk to it.

Another variation of connecting with nature as community essence was the women's relationship with their pets. Ellen described her dog as the "perfect companion." Anna and her poodle spend long summer afternoons "just being together" while Anna knits. Frances shares her twice daily walks with her dog. Georgia "minds her cat to keep her off the third floor balcony." In summarizing attitudes toward nature, Harris (1989) wrote:

> *Mysticism also teaches us that we are related to the other animals who share the Earth with us: cats and dogs, whales and whippoorwills; and that we are also in community with the Earth's elements, with wind, water, fire and soil. (pp. 41-42)*

Dialoging with Presence

So there is the Presence and we are being held there and loved. And that is an experience within the reach of anybody. (Bancroft, 1989, p. 42)

The women's narratives revealed variations of experiencing the presence of an active, invisible someone in their lives. They were not alone. The intrigue is the dialogue, the exchange of ideas and conversation which takes place between the woman and the invisible presence. Presence assumed divine and beloved familiar forms. Those women who had active religious practices sensed the presence as God. Anna, who had great losses in the deaths of three of her children, described the following experience at the time of the death of her son in World War II.

Anna: I was sick and in bed and had just heard about my son in the War. Seemed as if God was near though I didn't see or hear anything, but I felt comforted, cared for, as though God were near.

Ellen: It is just part of your being, your thinking, your acting no matter what you do, you feel as though you are not alone and you live with this presence that helps you figure things out.

Carolyn: I hear all the widows say that five or six o'clock is the loneliest time. I'm never lonely. I don't know why except that I know that I'm always in God's presence and I'm sustained by Him and I don't need anything else.

The women also experienced presence in the form of a deceased loved one in their lives. Attending to the invisible realities (James, 1900) in one's life may be a way of articulating presence.

Ellen: And I don't look upon death as a sharp line. I'm still talking to [husband], still communicating with him. The relationship still continues. So it's not anything very dramatic—just the everyday. It's just lovely to have this ongoing thing in your life that you realize is not broken up into compartments but one river going on.

Helen: Maybe that's mother kicking me from the grave. A real presence in my life. There's nobody else who even influenced me a great deal . . . except my parents.

The women reported taking an active role in seeking increased dialogue with the presence through different spiritual practices. Practices which increased the presence in their lives included consciously thinking about the presence, inviting the presence into conversation, setting aside quiet times for prayer, reading, and meditation practices.

Barbara: I consider flashes of insight in meditation. I get a flash of something valuable and I must write it down. If I feel stuck, I find meditation vitally important. It gets me into the proper state. You get an answer—it's all there but we shut it off with everyday activities and worries.

Re-Creating the Self

Re-creating the self emerged with components of integrating the past and cultivating the present. Georgia talked of the hardships in her life such as being abused by her mother after her adored and adoring father had died.

Georgia: My father died when I was twelve, and I was spoiled rotten. I was the only girl, of course being adopted and everything else. I never got a licking until after my father died, but after that I got plenty of them. But afterwards, oh boy, it wasn't so good because I always thought that she thought more of my brothers than she did of me but she didn't . . . Before she died she apologized to me and left me furniture and a car.

The women also told of the joyful, happy times in their lives and how those times have sustained them. Some of the happy times affirmed involved childhood memories while others related to their marriages.

Anna: I had a very happy childhood. Homesteading was in full swing in the Valley, and I remember running in the tall, beautiful grass. We didn't have anything to speak of and there were two more children born after me.

All of the women shared experiences of losses in their lives. As Anna put it, "You have to grieve your losses, accept them and move on into

other places of life." Dorothy described her perspective on her husband's
suicide.

Dorothy: We'd always been party people. We had so much fun and enjoyed parties and we joined the country club in [small town]. That's when
things were booming. Anyway, sadly, that drinking we both enjoyed, then
our business went kaput, and the drinking got heavier and heavier, and he
became an alcoholic. It was touch and go the last three or four years of his
life. He died ten years ago in October, but he had not had a drink for six
months. Well to me, it was his last gift and it was a gift of love, he shot
himself. Killed himself, committed suicide. But looking back on it, he
knew the bottle wasn't the answer. It was his last gift to me, to free me.

As acceptance of past events and experiences was an important part of
re-creating the self, so was cultivating the present. Barbara visualized her
present life as a time of growth.

Barbara: With spiritual and mental growth, there were so many distrac-
tions before growing old, things to do, no time to sit and think things out
when I was younger.

The women developed new interests as well as reframed their approaches to previous pursuits. Ellen finds pleasure in the physical movements of swimming and playing golf whereas years ago her score was of
primary interest. At 77-years-old, Ellen visits with family and friends, has
restarted piano lessons after fifty years and regularly attends French
movies so she can, "continue to develop my language skills and appreciation for the culture." The women talked about those things that gave
meaning to their present lives. They verbalized about moving beyond the
superficial things of their youth.

Anna: My self-worth is not based on a job. I had to get free of the externals of what I looked like or even my health. Moving life away from one
created on externals.

The last characteristic that emerged in cultivating the present was enjoying the present. Enjoying the present was expressed through sharing
incidents of humor and a sense of fun. Carolyn described an experience
she had pertaining to a decision she had made and said she would never,
never do again. Then she suddenly startled herself, sat up straight, and
her eyes flew wide open as she exclaimed, "Never? Did I say never? Did I
really say never? God help me, I better never say never again."

Georgia described one of her ex-husbands as "so lazy that she was going to get him a cat to breathe for him" and referred to herself "as like the phoenix bird, always coming back after being down."

Encountering Spiritual Caring

Spiritual caring surfaced in four variations: Awareness of divine caring, human caring, caring for others and self. Carolyn provided an excellent illustration of encountering spiritual caring retrospectively from a divine other. She related a long, involved experience about finding the right high school for her severely physically disabled yet intellectually gifted son.

Carolyn: As far as being spiritually led, it's always in the looking back. Like the school admitting [son] and the young man who drove the car for us, it was just impulse that I asked him, just plain impulse and then I thought. God did that! I didn't do that by myself. It's always in the looking back. It's not of the moment, ever. So, I'm grateful for it, extremely grateful.

As an illustration of unseen awareness of spiritual caring by human others, Barbara talked about receiving and giving spiritual caring in her prayer experiences.

Barbara: When they are, [praying for me], I feel lifted up and can't think of any reason why. Someone praying for me is the major reason. I deeply believe in prayer and I pray for a number of people daily.

The provision of spiritual caring for others involved such activities as praying for other people as well as meaningful service to others. The women perceived activities of service as spiritual caring when they were rooted in their own spiritual grounding. Barbara saw herself as spiritually caring for others in that she is a volunteer visitor in the hospital section of her retirement residence.

Spiritual caring not only emerged as a characteristic of an unseen other, a human other but also of the self, for the self. The women talked about actively seeking out those things that they knew to be spiritually caring or nurturing for themselves.

Barbara: If I feel stuck, I find meditation vitally important. It gets me into the proper state. You get an answer. It's all there but we shut it off with all the activities and worries.

Carolyn, Ellen, Dorothy, Anna, Barbara all sought spiritual growth directly through taking classes, reading helpful books, talking with interested others and using practices of prayer for themselves. Georgia reported that she grew "from Sabbath to Sabbath". Frances and Helen thought of walks outside and time alone as ways of spiritually caring for the self. Ellen, Dorothy, Frances, Helen, and Anna all thought that listening to "good" music brought them increased spiritual connections.

THE QUILT OF SPIRITUALITY

Translating the essential features of the study into the metaphor of the quilt resulted from the synthesis of the batting of solitude, borders of community, backing of presence, blocks of re-creation with the stitching of spiritual caring. Quilting, as an ancient worldwide art, originated in cold climates in the attempt to keep several layers of cloth together for warmth (Guild, 1971). Used as clothing, coverings, and armor quilts provide warmth, comfort and protection. Quilts are recognized today as artistic works and used for decoration and enrichment (Chase, 1978; Soltow, 1991). Quilts, like other crafts, have become a medium for the appreciation of skills, beauty, and, obliquely, a commentary on life (Hurst & Margetts, 1989).

Three layers constitute most quilts. The upper or top layer is frequently composed of blocks that are then sewn together in a design pleasing to the quilter. After the quilt top has been completed, it is pinned to the batting or filler layers and the backing or bottom layer. Next, these layers are then basted together to hold them in place while the quilt stitching itself is done. The quilt stitching, or quilting, holds together the layers of material and prevents the middle layer of batting from slipping in the finished quilt (Guild, 1971; Hurst & Margetts, 1989; Soltow, 1991; Wiggington, 1968).

Batting of Solitude

Just as solitude is a choice in the lives of the women in the study, choices surround the quilter's decisions about selecting batting. How thick should the batting be? Is the finished product to be a thin summer coverlet or a thick Canadian prairie quilt to ward off winter cold? How high a relief to the design does the quilter want?

Is the batting going to be a recycled older blanket, a cream colored cotton batting or a new pure white polyester batting? Whatever the case, the quilter must choose just as the women in the study chose the kinds and degrees of solitude which gave meaning to their lives. Like the quilt bat-ting, the women could not physically see solitude but were aware of its ef-fect in their lives. Solitude, like a quilt batting provided comfort, warmth, and meaning to the lives of the women in the study. The women not only valued solitude in their lives but often sought more at certain times. As high loft comforters are selected in winter seasons and low loft quilts pre-ferred in summertime, so too did the women choose to balance solitude with connecting with community.

Borders of Community

In looking at a quilt design, the elements of community and connection present themselves in that the design requires attachment among different components of the quilt. Borders or sashing or stripping separate each block from its neighbor. Even though the borders separate one block from its neighbor, they provide the connecting links among the blocks. In addi-tion, borders on the outer rim of the quilt define community boundaries.

In all of these decisions about boundaries and edging in the quilt top, the quilter freely makes her own choices. Women too, must be free to choose the circumstances of connections to community in their lives. The quilt metaphor lends itself well as a symbol for providing connection to the interior community of self. Quilts are connected not only through their designs on the decorative surface but also through the joining of the blocks of re-creation, batting of solitude and the backing of presence linked by the quilting of spiritual caring.

Backing of Presence

The bottom fabric layer of the quilt serves to contain the batting of the quilt. Without a backing of presence, the batting of solitude would have nothing to hold it to the more elaborate top of the quilt. Presence, whether divine or beloved familiar presence, does not overtly, present it-self to others. Like the back of a quilt, presence is the unseen reality (James, 1900) that operates in the lives of the women in the study. Some women chose to pay more attention to presence than did others and sought ways of increasing presence in their lives.

Just as the women thought that they could seek out presence and in-crease the dialogue with presence by attending to it, so can a quilt be turned over and the patterns of stitching sought out. The women de-scribed dialoguing with presence as everyday activity not as anything dramatic but available to them in everyday life. So, too, are quilts avail-able to us in everyday life, and it is the backing, or the quilt bottom, that touches our bodies when we wear quilted clothing or sleep under a quilt. The backing, or bottom of the quilt, remains visible to the degree that it is remembered, shared, and brought to light.

Blocks of Re-Creation

Pieced quilts are composed of blocks that are then stitched together to create the quilt top. The blocks of re-creation portrayed in textiles the narratives of the women as they re-create themselves at this particular time in their lives. The individual blocks presented some of the history and present life of each woman. Different kinds of patterns, stitchery, and quilting from a variety of traditions portrayed each woman's essential experience of spirituality.

Stitching of Spiritual Caring

As the heart of a quilt is the stitching or quilting, so is spiritual caring the heart or unifying theme of spirituality. The quilter prepares her quilt for quilting by lining up and basting the three fiber layers of the backing, the batting, and decorative top layer. The thread joins and passes through all layers of the quilt of spirituality joining the blocks of re-creation, the borders of community, the batting of solitude, and the backing of presence. Just as a keen eye is required to stitch the small, even stitches of spiritual caring, so a keen inner eye is necessary to develop the awareness of seen and unseen caring by human and divine others. The quilter may not plan in advance every detail of the quilting pattern but will see the pattern emerge as she creates it. So, too, the women noticed the emergence of spiritual caring by divine and human others in their lives.

The quilter must use a high quality thread. In the quilting process, the threaded needle passes repeatedly through the layers of the quilt causing significant tension and wear on the thread. Similarly, the women spent time in encountering spiritual caring in their lives. Whether that active stance consisted of daily times of formal spiritual caring for the self, such as prayer, meditation, or less structured experiences such as communion with nature, the women sought nurture on a regular basis.

CONCLUSION

An intelligible structure of older women's experience of spirituality can be known through the metaphor of the quilt. All the components of the quilt are present. The blocks of re-creating the self are joined by the borders of community and quilted by the stitching of spiritual caring through the batting of solitude to the backing of presence. The structural definition of older women's experience of spirituality that arose from this study is: Older women's experience of spirituality is re-creating the self by choosing solitude, connecting with community, and dialoguing with presence through encountering spiritual caring. In crafting the quilt, crafting is the process, and the completed quilt is the product. In older women's experience of spirituality, encountering spiritual caring through solitude, presence, and community is the process, and the re-created life is the product.

REFERENCES

Bancroft, A. (1989). *Weavers of wisdom: Women mystics of the twentieth century.* New York: Penguin.

Chase, P. (1978). *The contemporary quilt.* New York: E. P. Dutton.

Conn, J. W. (Ed.). (1985). *Women's spirituality: Resources for Christian development.* New York: Paulist Press.

Gilligan, C. (1982). *In a different voice.* Cambridge, MA: Harvard University Press.

Giorgi, A. (1989a). Learning and memory from the perspective of phenomenological psychology. In R. S. Valle & S. Halling (Eds.), *Existential-phenomenological perspectives in psychology* (pp. 99-112). New York: Plenum.

Giorgi, A. (1989b). One type of analysis of descriptive data: Procedures involved in following a scientific phenomenological method. *Methods, 3*(1), 39-61.

Guild, V. P. (1971). *New complete book of needle craft.* New York: Good Housekeeping Books.

Harris, M. (1989). *Dance of the spirit: The seven steps of women's spirituality.* New York: Bantam Books.

Hurst, J., & Margetts, M. (Eds.). (1989). *Classical crafts: A practical compendium of traditional skills.* New York: Simon & Schuster.

James, W. (1900). *The varieties of religious experience: A study in human nature.* New York: Penguin Books.

Moore, T. (1992). *Care of the soul: A guide for cultivating depth and sacredness in everyday life.* New York: Harper Collins.

Morton, N. (1985). *The journey is home.* Boston: Beacon Press.

Sarton, M. (1966). *Mrs. Stevens hears the mermaids singing.* New York: W. W. Norton.

Soltow, W. A. (1991). *Quilting the world over.* Radnor, PA: Chilton Book Company.

Wigginton, E. (1968). *The foxfire book.* NY: Doubleday.

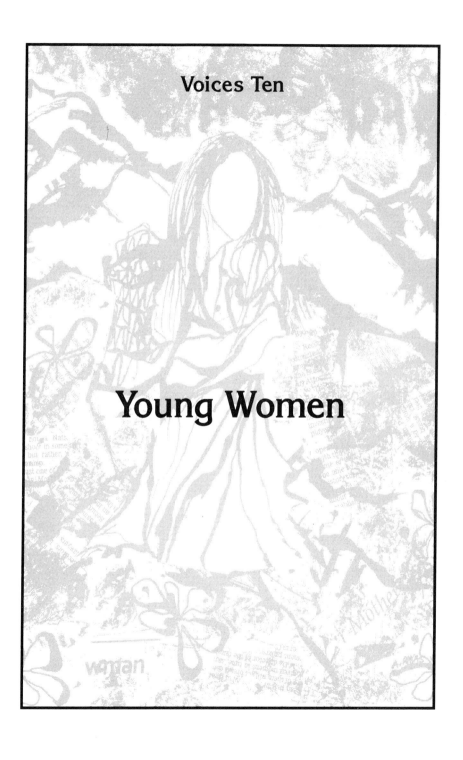

Voices Ten

Young Women

33

Reflections in
a Mirror

Suzanne G. Sitelman

*T*he typical teenage girl is often pictured as a self-absorbed egoist whose thoughts are focused exclusively either on her looks or on boys and how they might react to her. She is viewed as someone who is shallow, insufficiently aware of the external world, and its authentic problems, insensitive to others while transfixed by her own appearance. As a sixteen-year-old girl, I will confess that this stereotype of a girl in front of a mirror engrossed by her reflection is not totally without some truth. However, I do not think of myself as anything that could be called stereotypical, and yet I will admit to wasting some small amount of time worrying about whether or not I am, or that anyone, for that matter, could find me, pretty.

Instead of worrying about world starvation or international economics or my own future job prospects, I tug at my stomach and fuss with my hair, thinking my body is too big, my nose is too thick, and my eyes are too small. I admit that I probably worry a bit too much about these matters, but no more than most adult women worry about their appearance.

I remember a time when being pretty was not harder than putting on a nice dress and wearing ribbons in my hair. It was at that time that the world was small and I, of course, was the center of it. Then one day, I found the world to be much bigger than I had imagined, and I realized that not only was I not the center of the universe, but that my very existence in it might be insignificant or irrelevant. That is when the worrying began. And what better place to start than with the bathroom mirror? The truth is, we all want to succeed in this world and do not know whether or not we have the ability to do so. After all, as the fairy tale goes, "to win the prince and live happily ever after, you have to be the most beautiful girl in all the land."

Of course, we know that intelligence and character play as much a role in success as physical beauty, and yet it is very hard and especially painful to look inside oneself and pick out the weaknesses in one's own personality. Instead, we focus on our physical qualities, which are not difficult to notice since they are, after all, staring us straight in the face. Neither is it difficult to compare one's own physical appearance with the looks of others—in particular, our friends. It is an interesting conflict to see who is the most worthwhile, the most special, the most physically appealing. Even though we know how silly all of this is, we also know the pangs of painful envy we feel when we carefully examine the pretty face and body of another girl.

It is easy to mock a teenage girl's desire to be beautiful, but I compare this need to everyone's basic desire for success. Worrying about our bodies, we are also, deep inside, worrying about how we are going to turn out, and if that will end up being good enough. My concern with my looks may be a childish and hopeless vanity. However, realizing this does not change my feelings, or my frustrations, or my jealousies. It still hurts me to look in the mirror and feel a little bit cheated. My parents were very good-looking, and my older brother turns all my friends' heads. So I sometimes feel skipped over, as if there were no reason why I should not also be very attractive. It is easy to say that looks do not matter, and my parents always insist that these things are not important, but we would be fooling ourselves if we claimed that physical beauty does not make a difference in life. Physical attractiveness is important in society, and it is an extra advantage to have it.

My friends and I wonder whether we will ever find boyfriends. None of us wonder about whether we will ultimately have a career or a husband. We are convinced, after all, that this will eventually occur. We do worry, instead, whether it will be the husband and career that we want to have, and whether we will be happy. And we see our success connected to how attractive we are. So even as we despise our vanities and our shallow self-absorption, we continue to fret and stare helplessly at our reflections in the mirror.

34

The New Millennium Woman

Kathleen Mary Nugent

I will graduate from college in the year 2000. I am the new millennium woman.

You can be anything you want to be." This is how I have been raised. The whole world has been presented to me and anything is possible. The world is at my fingertips. Technology and I have grown up together, so we have become good friends. I never have a lack of knowledge or information; it is all accessible to me. The world that once seemed so overwhelming has become familiar and real to me. I can turn on my television and watch the news to find out what is happening at that moment across the ocean in a totally different country. I have the ability to use my computer in my family room to connect with a network of computers and people all around the earth. There are no limitations or restrictions to what can be done, achieved, gained if I can keep my mind open and ready to accept what comes along. Nothing is impossible and nothing is left unknown. There *is* an answer—you just have to go search for it. As a woman graduating from college at the start of the twenty-first century, it is my goal to seek and find these answers. I am determined to continue the inspiring and sometimes amazing advance of human intelligence, interaction, peace, equality, and development.

Within the short time I have lived, I have seen major, life altering global changes—the first man walked on the moon, the computer came into everyone's reach, and communism fell. We are all dependent on each other. No one can survive on her own and I have learned this well. But although I know I need others, I also know I am an individual. I can work within a team, contributing and receiving, while remaining who I am. I have been taught that I *have* a voice, and my voice cannot be pushed aside. In the past women have been submissive and quiet. Women are bolder and more forceful. Women can be a force together, unbreakable, determined. No longer is it a "man's world," but a "human's world" open to everyone no matter what gender, race, religion, or ethnicity. There is a new age approaching, with the heart of it being equality among all. My role is critical in breaking down the oppressive attitudes of the past. The color of one's skin or one's gender must no longer limit a person. One's mind, self-determination, ability, hard work, and perseverance are the only limitations. We must set our own goals and limits; no one else can do this.

This change in attitude has occurred because of the radical changes that have been taking place all around us. Countries that were once isolated are now opening to the world. The whole world is interdependent; people need each other. I see everyone around me and I see them as someone important. Everyone has a voice and their voice is significant. For too long people's voices have been muffled. Amy Tan, in her touching and powerful novel, *The Joy Luck Club,* describes the tiger, "It has two ways. The gold side leaps with its fierce heart. The black side stands still with cunning, hiding its gold between trees, seeing and not being seen, waiting patiently . . ." (p. 282). Today, women are tigers. Our black side has been shown for a long time and now with the bursting forth of the new millennium, comes the unveiling and unleashing of the woman's gold side. The woman utilizing both sides will overcome the barriers of the past and triumph.

The year 2000 brings forth a new era. Along with that new era comes a new way of thinking, living, interacting. There is no place for sexism, racism, prejudice, and discrimination. The world must become one whole functioning unit. The focus can no longer be defense, mutual protection, and war, but peace, equality, and development. The progress we have been achieving will not regress, but must surge forward. I do not have a fear of the future or any apprehensions. I see a horizon of possibilities before me and there are no restrictions on me. I am free to "be anything [I] want to be."

I am ready for this new era full of promise and hope. I have dreams and goals and a voice that will be heard. The new millennium is approaching and it will be greeted by a new generation ready to embrace the world and all it possibilities and soar.

REFERENCES

Cisneros, S. (1991). *Woman hollering creek.* New York: Vintage Contemporaries.

Helgesen, S. (1990). *The female advantage: Women's ways of leadership.* New York: Doubleday.

Tan, A. (1989). *The joy luck club.* New York: Ivy Books.

35

Studying the
Psychology of Women

Mia Rene Martin, Craig T. Munhall,
and Judith Migoya

*M*any colleges and universities in the United States have a course on the
"Psychology of Women." This program promotes understanding the experience of being a woman and challenges all gender stereotypes. The following three pieces were written by students in Francine Glick's course
at Barry University. They reflect students' own feelings about the nature
and stereotyping of females and males.

* * *

Let me start by introducing myself. My name is Mia Rene Martin and I am
a twenty-one-year-old psychology major. This essay will provide you with
information about my history and the forces that guided me in certain directions throughout my life. Also, you will read about my thoughts including some of my opinions and my basic outlook on being female. After

reading this essay, you will know something of my life and how I came to be the person that I am with the views that I have today.

On March 1st, 1974, I was born to Mr. and Mrs. Willard Martin on the island of Grand Bahama in the city of Freeport. I was the third and last child that my parents would have, the eldest being my brother Willard who is four years older than I and my sister Perdita, the middle child, who is two years older than I. My mother is my idol. She is an extremely strong and aggressive black woman who has proven throughout my life to be the best mother in the world. She has never been the housewife type, although she took care of her family with wholesome home-cooked meals and provided a clean nurturing home environment. She always worked outside our home as well. Most mothers in the Bahamas work. She has a very successful career and, as a matter of fact, she has always made more money than my father. Growing up on the island with my mother as my role model, I have learned that women were not put on this earth for making a man happy or to have some silent partnership with a man. I gained a strong sense of self from my mother. At a very young age, I was taught to believe that I could make a difference. I learned that I could be whatever I wanted to be if I was determined enough. I learned that education and hard work pays off in the long run, no matter what gender you are. I was never told that I could not do the things that my brother did. As a matter of fact, I was very active in sports up until the age of thirteen.

My father is the opposite of my mother. He is more passive, more serene. Growing up, I remember asking my father something, but my mother always having the final word on the subject. As I grow older, I am discovering that I am very much like her. Apart from the physical aspects, my mother and I have amazingly similar traits and tendencies, such as our aggressiveness, slightly dominating personalities, and our self-confidence. My mother was the head of our household without a doubt and continues to be the primary provider for her kids today. My parents provided me with a healthy and loving childhood which was fun yet supplemented with very strict discipline. My parents divorced when I was ten, but it wasn't a very bitter divorce so I was not traumatized like some children are. My adolescent years were normal, whatever normal may be. Apart from the divorce, my family was not a dysfunctional one. There was no sexual, physical, or mental abuse going on, nor was there any alcohol or drug abuse of any kind. There wasn't even cigarette smoking in my home. Basically, I did the things a teenager does: go to parties, spend way too much time talking about nothing on the phone, date boys, ditch class, but nothing drastic like drugs or alcohol. In high school I can remember always being one of the popular girls that hung out with the "in crowd." I look back on those days and conclude I have matured steadily since then. Now I have a really good idea of who I am.

A very big part of who I am is a Bahamian woman. Born and raised on the island, I am steeped in my Bahamian culture. I am proud to have come from a place so rich in culture—from the calypso music that beats in my heart to the native food (peas and rice, conch) to the goombay and junkanoo festivals where we dress up in elaborate, colorful costumes and dance in the street all night until the sun comes up, to the accent and the dialect that I speak. I am very proud of my blackness, however, I do not identify with the African-American culture. It was not until I came to this country that I encountered the African-American experience which is totally different from the Caribbean way of life. When you are raised on an island that is predominantly black, you never consider yourself a minority. When I moved to Miami, I had to accept the fact that I was now a minority because I was black. I have never felt oppressed and, for a long time, I didn't think that black Americans should have either, but after spending some time in this country I understand why African Americans are so bitter and feel like they live in a white man's world.

Religion has always been a major part of my life. Baptized as a Christian, I attended Bible school and church every Sunday as a child. Along with my strong awareness of God, my parents also instilled in me the extreme importance of education which remains with me today. I went from nursery school straight through to high school on the island where they follow the British system of education. I have always been interested in the sciences, specifically biology because I am a skeptical person who only takes something as a fact if it has been proven or is provable. I am a psychology major which helps me deal with people and the world. It fascinates me to study theories on why people behave the way they do and apply them to real life. People come to me for advice all the time and I enjoy counselling them. I try to figure people out to see what they are really like and usually I am a pretty good judge of character on the first encounter with someone. Psychology is a totally fascinating field of work and I would very much like to become a psychologist or psychiatrist. I have always been a little more mature for my age which I feel is an indirect result of having older siblings. I think that my mother and father got worn out raising my older siblings so by the time I came around they were tired. My outlook on life has always been a positive one. I am the type of person that always tries to look on the bright side. I am not saying that I never feel down or depressed because I am only human, but I will always attempt to pull the good out of a bad situation. I do believe that everything happens for a reason and that God always knows exactly what He is doing no matter how bad things may appear to be.

Now that I am older, I find myself thinking more and more about the future. I am definitely discovering what is truly important to me and what path I would like to see my life follow. I consider myself a woman of the nineties and I want everything that goes along with that. I want to be a successful psychologist who is totally independent. However, contrary to what I just mentioned is that a larger part of me is very traditional and wants to have a big family with lots of kids and a loving husband and devote my life to them. There is something about this way of life that I think is absolutely beautiful. Maybe I have just been conditioned this way, but the traditional way of living is very natural for me and it is something that I would love to have happen in my own home. I want to have dinner ready for my husband when he gets home from work each day and I want to be involved in every facet of my childrens' lives, going to all the P.T.A. meetings and participating in all the other school functions. I know that the two ideas can not coexist in reality. I cannot be a successful career woman and still be the perfect housewife who bakes cookies, but I am sure as hell going to try to make it work. But if I had to choose between my career and having a family, I would most likely choose my family because these are things that are important to me. Right now I am very happy with life, I think everyone could probably use a little more cash but I do thank God for health, daily bread, a roof over my head, and most importantly the people in my life that love me and that I love. I appreciate all that the Lord has blessed me with including the opportunity to attend university and make something of my life.

I thought that it was necessary for you to know a little of my background before I began discussing my views as a woman. What does being female mean to me? Being female is a wonderful thing. I am feminine, with gentle and elegant characteristics, much more so than a man. I menstruate every month, allowing me the ability to grow life inside of me. My body is different from the male's body. Its distinguishing features being the vagina, the ovaries which help produce life, the uterus which acts as a safe haven for the child until it is strong enough to come into the world, and the breasts which nourish the child once in the world. Because I am female, I am somebody's daughter, I am somebody's sister, I am somebody's girlfriend, I will be somebody's wife hopefully and I will be someone's mother. Each role being different, utilizing totally different relationships with members of the same and opposite sex but still being carried out by one human being simultaneously. As a daughter, I am my mother's and father's child. I have been taught to honor my parents and respect them. As a daughter, I am humble. I have learned so much from my mother. She has taught me how to cook, to sew, how to take care of a household and, most importantly, how to take care of myself. As a sister, I am my siblings' confidant. I am my sister's best friend and my brother's baby sister who he feels the need to protect. As a girlfriend or a wife, I would be someone's soulmate. I would be an equal partner in a loving and intimate relationship with a man. I would be the nurturer. And as a mother, I would be a giver of life. Again, I would be the nurturer. I will be the best mother I could possibly be. I think that having children is the most fulfilling thing that one experiences in life. I know that all that I do in my life to become someone is indirectly for my unborn children so that they may have a good life. I have the tremendous responsibility of raising my children to be good people, instilling in them morals and values as my mother and father did in me. I don't intend to do this job alone.

I don't consider myself a feminist, but I certainly do believe that a woman can do anything a man can do and better in some cases. As we learned in class, women have been plagued with myths from the beginning of time but we are finally moving toward a new way of thinking which I think has a lot to do with the woman's liberation movement in the 1960s. I think that women are finally getting the recognition and the treatment that they deserve. We are still a long way off from having total equality with men but we have certainly made progress. To contribute to this new way of thinking we, as mothers and future mothers, need to instill in our daughters the concept of equality with men, not prepare them for a life of subservience. We need to teach them to be proud of being female, not put restrictions on them because of it. Also we need to teach our sons that their sisters are not inferior beings. We need to teach our sons at an early age that mommy is special, not just someone who caters to dad. We need to teach both gender children that they are different but equal and capable of accomplishing the same goals. There are a lot of things that still need work like the fact that women don't get paid as much as men do for the same jobs or that women's haircuts cost so much more than men's haircuts. However, a lot more women are employed in jobs that were once considered male jobs.

Conflict is a good thing if each party involved is aware that there are differences between men and women and we learn to accept, deal with, and even enjoy these differences in the proper manner. This conflict is O.K. We must learn about dealing with these conflicts without blaming.

As we learn better communication between the sexes, we move toward a better future. My perception of the future is a very positive one. As I said before, we are improving in our thinking. From the beginning of time, women have been labeled with stereotypes or myths. First, women were seen as mother nature because of their ability to bleed every month and reproduce life as a tree bears fruit. Then, women were seen as enchantresses/seductresses because they were thought to enchant men with their magical charms and seduce men away from the high paths of their "holy" missions. Women were also viewed as a necessary evil. They were regarded as sex objects and child bearers but otherwise they were unimportant. Women were also regarded as a mystery because of the differences between men and women and because of the seeming perversity of a woman's behavior. Some more modern day labels that are placed on women have a negative connotation. We are seen as bimbos, airheads, and if we become successful in a career, then we must have slept our way to the top. If we become too assertive, then we are bitches. I don't know why men can't see women for what they really are. We are members of the opposite sex that have the same capabilities as men. We are capable of the same academic abilities, we can hold the same jobs as men, we can even hold positions in congress and in the senate. Yes, we take care of the children and we cook and clean, but we are capable of doing so much more than that. We are their mothers, their sisters, and their significant others. We are uniquely different from them. We are capable of bearing their children and for this we should be greatly respected, not put down. When will we be seen as the equals that we are? Or do these differences between men and women truly mean that we are not equal? Is male truly the superior gender? Are we really just put on this earth to serve men? Are these differences biological or are they environmental? Well, I am going to have to say that it is both biological and environmental. There has to be biological differences simply because of the ways in which our bodies are different. We have different amounts of different hormones. Men have more testosterone which gives them their masculine qualities. Women on the other hand have estrogen which helps develop and maintain female characteristics. We are, however, also conditioned from very young that there are specific gender roles. For example, we see mom in the kitchen and we see dad going to work and being served by mom when he is at home. The things we see growing up have profound effects on how we view life. The way our parents treat us as precious little girls is very different from the way they treat their macho boys which also plays a big part in the roles we develop. Growing up on the island, there is a very strong sense of the man being the head of the household, the king of the castle. Even though it wasn't so in my household, it is certainly true of my grandmother and grandfather and other family members. Even today my grandmother wakes up at 6 o'clock in the morning to make breakfast for my grandfather and you better believe that dinner is on the table the second he walks through the door. Even though she had nine children, it has always been obvious who her main priority was, her husband. I admire her loyalty to her husband but I wonder if she has her own identity. Does she love herself or does she really believe that her only purpose in life is to serve her man. I would like to have a balance of both worlds. I would do all of these wonderful things for my husband because I want to do it, not because I feel that it is my duty. While my husband would be a very big part of my life, he will certainly not be my whole life. I would have to be involved with my own projects so that I can feel good about myself as Mia, the person, not just as John Doe's wife.

Another thing that makes women different from men is our emotional nature. Men have never been encouraged to express their feelings, especially if they feel hurt. Some men would rather die than to let someone see them cry. Women on the other hand have been told that it's okay to express their feelings and it's okay to cry. Throughout time we have seen a woman's emotionality as a negative thing but we know now that it is actually very positive. Our vulnerability which was considered a weakness is now a strength. Because we were so emotional, Freud labelled us as hysterical, and envious of the male penis. Because women are the emotional ones, we are the nurturers. We are seen as weak and as the subordinates. While the strong ones (the men), who show very little or no emotion at all are capable of dealing with situations better than women, are the dominant ones. Today we are seeing a slight change though. Men are becoming more sensitive and more understanding of the woman's plight (at least in my experience). I think that men are realizing that the differences between men and women do not make women lesser human beings than men but are just that—differences that should first be acknowledged, then accepted, respected, and even cherished. Even though men tend to be more understanding in this area, these differences may still create some form of conflict.

The book, *Men Are from Mars, Women Are from Venus,* tells us that in a relationship, men and women desire different things. For example, the book states that a man needs to receive trust, acceptance, appreciation, admiration, approval, and encouragement from his woman. And a woman needs to receive caring, understanding, respect, devotion, validation, and reassurance from her man. For better relationships we need to learn this.

This class has been very instrumental in helping me understand why the roles of men and women are so different in society. There are such harsh double standards between men and women and I could never understand why. In taking this class I realize that these inequalities between women and men were present since the beginning of time and if there is going to be a change, it is going to take education and enlightening of both sexes. This change is not going to occur overnight.

Mia Rene Martin

*   *   *

My name is Craig Munhall and I took this class because I believe that there are differences in the way the sexes behave and have been treated throughout time, and I wanted to have a better understanding of why. A problem with my understanding of the female dilemma is that I'm growing up in the age after the movements and marches, I have very little awareness of what life was like before women's liberation, for women or for men. Also my mother raised me and my brother in a manner so as not to be sexist and not to be ultra "manly." I was raised in an emotional atmosphere with little emphasis on things like being the best football player. In the world today, I feel that there is similarity between the sexes in almost all areas of life, especially certain interests. By this I mean that women and men seem to share the same interests and goals as one another. But within this similarity, there are differences in acceptability. I chose this course to better understand these differences.

To me, being a man doesn't have much significance. If someone asked me if I would mind being a woman, I would probably say yes just because I wouldn't want to deal with a menstrual cycle. On the other hand, being a male means that I cannot give birth to children and feel a human develop inside of myself. With this amazing gift, women really are superior to men and should be treated as such. Being a man means that while growing up my parents and society conditioned me to act a certain way, mainly to act like my father. I do not think that I will ever be too much like my father because my parents divorced when I was young and I did not see too much of him. My role model as a child was mainly my mother. My mother taught me that being a man meant respecting women. My "male typical" behavior stems from my social interactions while growing up. It was there that I learned that "men can talk about everything more freely," "men are better at physical activities," and that "men have it easier because they do not have menstrual cycles."

I believe that gender labeling is dead because people now are in a different mode of thinking. Children born after the Women's Rights Movement were brought up to know what gender really means. Now women know that they can do anything they want to in the workplace, they can dress any way they want, and they have been taught that it is their abilities that will make them excel. These abilities are encouraged more and more by parents, society, and the educational/business fields. Men born after the movement were taught to be receptive of women in the workplace and, as generations pass, men won't see a difference in fe/male roles.

Now and in the future, the gender roles are becoming and will become more unified. Today there are male nurses and women construction workers, male housekeepers and women C.E.O.s. I feel that as time passes there will be no difference in gender except that one can give birth and the other cannot. I hope, however, that it doesn't go too far. We already had a society of dominant males, we do not need a society of dominant females. I hope that the two can meet somewhere in the middle.

Conflict is going to involve finding a happy medium between the sexes. Conflict is necessary in order for growth. If nothing was wrong then there would be no reason for change or conflict, and everything would be perfect. Conflict is what stirred up the women's movement and conflict will keep it alive until there is no need for it. The only time that conflict is not good is when people lose sight of what the true problem is and go overboard. In class we watched a video of some type of talk show where women hated men because of something that had happened to them. I think that is going too far, a conflict like that was not with a whole gender but with certain individuals. This is an important point because in conflict people often do lose sight of their real objectives.

The issues that women are concerned with are very crucial to creating an equal society. For some time, women have been the subordinate group of society. Getting out of that role and establishing yourself as a person is very difficult. Issues dealing with equality in every aspect of life are important because they are what stirs up the emotion and desire to make a change. Without women's issues and concerns, there would be no conflict or problem.

My part in all this is to never judge or discriminate against a person based on sex. I should also try to set an example to others that it isn't right to be sexist. If I should ever be in a situation where I had to hire or fire a person, I should do it based on a person's qualifications, not his or her gender. Also, when I become a father I should raise my children so that they will not be sexist or discriminatory in any way. All of this constitutes what I personally can do to help the unity of the sexes.

Society has been reluctant to change because men have not wanted to give up their superior position in society. Also by keeping their roles, competition from women was avoided altogether. Repressing women gave men the ability to dominate, to have power over someone else. This power felt good to those men and, like a drug, if it feels good you always want more. Men, for a long time and even today, have had the good "top" paying jobs. They would like to keep them, and do anything it takes to do so, even putting down a whole gender.

Searching for the truth means trying to get to the bottom of everything. In everything that you hear there is always something else underlying it. Personally, I believe in order to understand something, both sides of the story have to be examined. Not only both sides, but every angle of both sides. In the subject of psychology of women, it is important to find out what made women strive for equality and to put yourself in their shoes and imagine what it must have felt like to be a subordinate. It is equally as important to see the male perspective and find out where men are coming from. We were not bad, but society was. I think it is important for men and women to learn about the different roles that the sexes have played throughout history.

In searching for the truth, a person often relies on people that they deem as being knowledgeable in the area of concern. The real question is how knowledgeable are the authorities. The answer is that no one is a true authority. A scientist is not an authority because scientists make errors and enter situations with the mindset of a critical observer. A psychologist can be somewhat of an authority, but on the subject of gender the doctor's own gender is a relative factor in his or her analysis of a situation. Scientists and psychologists also bring into situations their own types of biases that would interfere with them seeing the whole picture the way it should be viewed. The authority of gender roles and gender positions throughout history has been and probably always will be within the *Zeitgeist* of the society—parents, teachers, scientists, and psychologists, all put together, the society that creates the ways we look at the world around us and live our lives.

There is an incredible relationship between learning and living. The only way for an individual to fully develop is for that person to live a full life. Education that is received in school is useless unless a person lives through it. Even reading, which is the most elementary learning, needs a purpose in order to be learned. The purpose, the reason for it, is that a person lives it. Also, living is important because every day something new and different can happen. What a person may consider as truth today could turn out to be false tomorrow. Learning is an ongoing adventure where, as time goes by, knowledge increases. Life is a learning process and people, more and more as time goes on, are realizing the potential of women.

Everything that is learned is really only remembered. Concepts are formed only when a person takes their memories and links them in a logical sequence so as to be retrieved when a similar set of stimuli are perceived. "Knowing" is a general term. Philosophically, there is no such thing as absolute truth. It seems however that in our society, knowledge is viewed as having answers to people's questions. Those are answers that coincide with current ideas about what is "truth." A person who is truly knowledgeable is a person who knows that they are not "right" or "wrong." To know that knowledge is subjective and separate for each individual is what I would consider as having insight. Most people think that education or specialized training equals knowledge. I disagree. The smartest person is a listener, someone who will accept other opinions.

My perception of women has changed considerably. My mother taught me a lot about how society has acted toward women over the last couple of decades, but in class I have learned that the stereotypes about women have always existed in different forms. I've learned that in the beginning women were seen as goddesses. This makes sense. If I was alive back then and saw the things that a woman can do, I too would have thought that they were divine. But through these classes I've learned why that changed and why the different roles developed throughout time. Men wanted to be the dominant society. According to Darwin, men should be dominant because of their strength. With being dominant, men were safe, they had the better jobs, and they were able to "own" women. Women also enjoyed their roles; they were the nurturers and the family's support leaders. However, when women desired to do things other than be Mrs. Housekeeper, society did not let them, and this is what led to the movements for equality. I understand more why these roles have changed and I agree wholeheartedly with what women have done for themselves. I sometimes imagine being a female in some of these roles and I wonder how I would behave. I don't consider myself weak, but I probably would conform with society's rules and try to be a model for the society. I don't think that I would have gone against the mold if I had lived back then. This only makes me feel more compassion and admiration for the women who stood up and fought for their rights.

Now that I have a somewhat better understanding of the gender problems, I wonder how long it will take for things to be really equal or if that is even possible. Gender roles start to be programmed into a person as soon as they are born. It is here that intervention has to take place in order to develop a neutral society. I do not believe that the conditioning of gender roles can ever be truly stopped. I believe that boys will always be told not to cry and I believe that girls will always be rewarded for looking pretty when they wear a dress and makeup. But maybe the conditioning itself isn't the problem, maybe it is the connotations that go along with the conditioning. If the attitudes about what is conditioned change, then there will be a difference in the conditioning and both sides will be respected equally. If a boy is taught not to cry and is told that it doesn't make him better than a girl, or if a girl looks pretty and is told that doesn't make her weak and that just because she wears a dress and the boy down the street wears pants doesn't make her less of a person, change can occur. Raising children to have differences is good and healthy. Teaching children that because there is difference doesn't make one better than the other is crucial in order to change attitudes toward gender. My brother and I learned this from my mother. She didn't teach us much sex type roles, but the ones that she did teach us were taught to us with our understanding that we are not superior because of this behavior but rather equal.

I believe that for these roles to change, society has to change. It takes a lot of effort by a lot of people to make any type of impact on a whole society. An example of this is the Women's Rights Movement. It took women everywhere getting up and standing up for what they believed in in order to make a change in society. Right know there are a lot of changes occurring in society which a lot of people are supporting. One person cannot change a whole society and a system of beliefs, but it takes one person to start a gathering of people that want the same freedoms. I do not think that everybody should join a cause, but I do feel that everyone has the potential to change society by just being open to what other individuals need. Personally I help this by being open and by living my life and accepting the fact that other people need to live their lives. Women have struggled for equality, some passively, some actively. Women will continue to get equality only if people are open to new avenues. Once a person's mind is closed then nothing can get accomplished.

I understand about how conditioning is responsible for prolonging stereotypes in children and I believe that the way to stop it is to teach future generations differently than the way we have been taught. I hope that one day there will be a female president, to show the world and the children that there is nothing a woman cannot do equally as well as a man. I definitely hope that this woman president would not hide her femininity, because being feminine is positive and to hide it, is to hide strength.

Craig Munhall

*   *   *

Throughout human history, women have been viewed in many different ways. Our peculiar behavior was first explained through myths because men could not explain it through reason. Therefore, they had to make up for their lack of knowledge or reasoning abilities by inventing myths. During pre-historical times, women were perceived and compared to nature because of their menstruation (symbolizing the moon cycles) and their ability to give birth (as mother earth gives its fruits and grains). We were then perceived as Goddesses by the ancient Europeans who used to praise and worship women. As European civilization advanced, women were perceived as those who enchanted and seduced men away from their holy missions. For the Christians of the western civilization, women were nothing but a necessary evil. They were inferior and an economic burden, but necessary to have children.

As science came to existence during the age of enlightenment, the way of viewing women changed from that of myths to stereotype. To account for this change was Darwin's theory of evolution which showed that we develop from monkeys. Monkeys were then analyzed and the studies showed that the mother monkey had something the scientists called "mother instinct." She was good at nurturing the baby monkeys and taking care of them. From this developed the stereotype of women as nurturer, care giver, tender, etc. Other studies conducted during the same period of time "supposedly" showed that women's brains were smaller than men's, which led men to believe that women were poor thinkers and were inhibited in their ability to reason and make good decisions.

Today, we are getting away from this image that has represented women for so long. We are in a new paradigm of thinking. The shift in paradigm that we are experiencing is due to the effort of women to improve themselves and their quality of life which, at the same time, has changed men's attitude toward women.

Women used to believe in the role that had been assigned to them: the role of care-taker. However, they started to notice that they could do a lot more than take care of babies and the house. They are intelligent human beings, and they have been proving this to all those people, including other women, who said that women were not good enough to work and produce. Nowadays one can see women in very high positions in very important companies. There are women who are doctors and even fire-fighters. They are really taking control.

Another change in attitude that has allowed for a new paradigm of thinking has taken place in men. Men used to be the ones to raise a fence between the two sexes, forcing the females to remain as subordinates. They believed women's only acceptable role was the one of nurturer, mother, and housewife. To them, women were not only unequal to men, but inferior, and were not able to reason because of their inferior brains. Men, however, are beginning to see the accomplishments of some women who go out and show their potentials in the work place without fear of being ridiculed or criticized. Men are changing the way they look at women and beginning to understand women's needs to produce, to contribute to society, to be something other than just a housewife. They are finally accepting women and even admiring them.

This era's way of viewing women can be said to be the result of society's understanding of what being a woman is all about. In my opinion, I have always thought that being a woman is a blessing from God. First of all, the bodily functions of a woman are extraordinary. We menstruate starting when we are teenagers, signaling that we are turning into young women. We are able to bear our own offspring. No man will ever come close to knowing how it feels to have a little baby growing inside of him, no matter how powerful he is. And what could be more powerful and rewarding than giving birth? Giving birth means giving life to another human being that was formed from one's own body. It must almost feel like God creating the earth.

Being a woman also involves a mixture of emotions and virtues. We are usually sensitive; however, we are also very strong during hard times. There are hundreds of women whose husbands have abandoned them or died, and they have had to make it alone. Some have to parent alone. For example, my friend's father died of a heart attack when he was very young. Walter's mother was left alone with two children: Walter and Mary. She had to work very hard to support the three of them and study at the same time to secure a better future for her kids. Walter's mother turned out to be a professional and wonderful woman. All by herself she was able to make it in a strange country (they are originally from Argentina), and even buy her own home in Surfside, Florida. What is more important, she made sure that the absence of their father would not affect her son and daughter so much. She must have done a very good job of loving them, since the two children have turned out great. Mary is graduating from high school this year. Walter is going to college and is a lifeguard at the beach. Not only is he an excellent student and worker, he is the most caring, sweet, and respectful guy I have ever met, and he learned to be this way from his mother.

Just like Walter, each person learns from his experiences and becomes what he or she has learned. In other words, learning and life go hand in hand: life is an unending learning process which begins the moment a person is born. When a person is born, he/she does not even know that he/she is an individual person apart from his/her parents and objects that surround him/her. Little by little, the baby starts recognizing faces, places, objects, and himself/herself. She/he learns about right and wrong, what later transforms into her/his morals and values. The child then learns to read and write. During adolescence, the person goes through tremendous changes, both bodily and mental, and learns what these changes mean and how they will affect his/her life. As an adult, the individual sometimes succeeds, and other times fails, and each success or failure becomes part of this learning process. Accomplishments teach him/her how to go about achieving a desired goal. Failures, on the other hand, teach him/her what not to do, so the next time he/she faces the same difficulty, he/she will at least know what not to do. Failures also teach that one cannot always get what one wants and that sometimes life is not fair. However, life, most of the time, gives one another chance to achieve one's goal and apply what one has learned from the previous mistake.

As an elderly person, when one looks back at what one's life has been, one will probably remember those events in which one learned something. All these moments add up and form what everyone calls "life." These important events affect who we are, what we are, and how we see life. People who have led a life full of suffering and deceptions will probably turn out to be cold, unemotional persons who shut everyone out because they think they have to protect themselves from those who want to hurt them and even from life itself. On the other hand, those who have had caring parents and a relatively happy life as adolescents and adults will be very happy, caring, and open to old people because this is what life has taught them.

The learning process can also be applied to explain women's perceptions of womanhood. Women learn since very little that they do not have a penis which differentiates them from little boys. They also learn as children that they should play with pretty dolls, not with little cars or airplanes. As they grow older, they see that mom stays home and cooks, while dad goes out and works. Dad is also the one who makes decisions and plans, as well as the one who punishes them when they have misbehaved. What they really learn by experiencing this at home is that men have all the power, and that women's only decisions consist of deciding what they will have for dinner at night. These young females turn into women who are totally dependent on their husbands and who are too afraid to take initiative. On the other hand, there is the little girl who sees her mother struggling in the outside world. The mother has a job, just as the father does, and they both cooperate and do the house chores. This girl will not hesitate to do things for herself when she grows up, instead of waiting around at home, and expecting the man to support her. This type of girl will also probably stand up for her gender in the future and confront anyone who tries to put women down.

Women who confront those who underestimate their abilities often find themselves involved in conflict. Conflict can be good or bad, depending on the other party in the discussion. If the person does not know how to listen and has no respect for the other person's opinion, the conflict could turn into a terrible fight. However, conflict can have very positive results if the two people respect each other and treat each other as human beings. Not only can conflict be good, but it is also sometimes necessary.

There are not two people in this world totally identical. Everyone has got his/her own way of thinking and his/her own ideas. Most people think their ideas are the correct ones, therefore they ignore or rule out any other input or contribution that another person could provide in the attempt to correct, change, or expand the person's original idea. Conflict is good because it is what exposes two different people with different opinions to each other's point of view. Only through open conflict, where two or more people express their differences without judging each other, can we learn to open up and accept some constructive criticism. It is through conflict that most people reach agreements or compromises, and most of all, grow as individuals.

In the case of women, it is conflict that has gotten us so far. If we would have just kept quiet as we did for so long, we would have never gotten respect or at least consideration from anybody. However, we were brave enough to express our points of view, our needs, and our concerns. Maybe at the beginning of the entire process of liberation we were criticized for this, but at this moment in time, our ideas are being heard and accepted. Thanks to conflict we are finally being appreciated as intelligent women.

Our ideas are also kept alive through our involvement in women's issues. Women's issues are important because there are many women in the world who are still oppressed, who are still sitting at home because their husbands do not let them go out and work. There are hundreds of women who are being discriminated against in the work place. They are getting paid a lot less than men with the same position. They are being harassed because powerful people think they have control over these women. They are being prevented from advancing in every way. Women in many countries are not even allowed to participate in politics. There are too many injustices being committed against women, and if women themselves do not take a stand to protect women's rights, then they will just continue to be stepped on.

Women's issues are also important because they give women the opportunity to be noticed, to stand out as admirable, brave persons. Women's issues emphasize the truth about women: they are intelligent, capable individuals, worthy of everyone's respect. For example, if women would not file suits when they are not promoted at their jobs because the directors do not want a woman making important decisions, even though their performance at the work place has been excellent, they would not be giving themselves the chance to prove to themselves and others that they can do the job and a lot more. They would just stay in a mediocre position, and the world would just continue to think that women do not have a place outside the home.

Everyone has the responsibility of emphasizing the importance of women's issues if we want to live in a just society. However, we cannot achieve anything by blaming or putting the other sex down, as many women in feminist groups do. Instead, we should act as if we are in a partnership, where everyone has equal rights, and no sex is better than the other, just different.

I, as does every other woman, have the responsibility to make this partnership a truly equal one. Some women go to extremes in the effort to create a bridge between males and females. They want to prove that women are as good as men are. However, they try to prove this by putting men down instead of by raising women's self-esteem, positive qualities, and potentials. This creates a bridge between both sexes, but a negative one. If we want to reach the other sex, we should not do it by force or wrong doing. The best way to reach out to someone is through communication. Communication is the basis for any partnership, including the one we are trying to create between men and women. Through communication we can approach even those who do not want to listen.

I think we must take responsibility in letting those men who we are close to get in touch with their feelings. Men have always been admired for their strength and their control of emotions. They have come to think that feeling sad, nervous, or vulnerable makes them less of a man. Therefore, they want to prove to society that they are real men by projecting a "macho" image. If we, as women, let them know how much we admire them whenever they put their pride aside and admit that they are feeling vulnerable, then they would probably feel more at ease letting their feelings show. The problem is that women, sometimes without noticing, promote this concept of manhood that we are trying to abolish. We are used to running and hiding behind our men's strength when a problem emerges, leaving it for men to solve. This leaves men with no choice but to portray a strong, non-emotional image since they have to solve their problems as well as their partner's. If we let them know that our problems are ours, and that they no longer must carry the burden of our problems, maybe they will have time and opportunity to show their feeling a little more.

We should also convey to them that it takes a very strong person to recognize his/her weaknesses. It is a lot easier to just hide behind a mask and try to forget things that make one sad or dissatisfied. Some people even avoid going out on dates because they are afraid they will end up in a steady relationship, and eventually, fall in love. As women, we should advise our brothers, friends, and love partners not to be afraid of love or any other feeling. The worst thing that could happen when one falls in love is that the other person does not reciprocate our feelings. However, when one really thinks of how bad a heartbreak can be, one realizes it cannot be so bad. It helps one mature, gain experience, and become stronger (the clue word for men).

Although seeing weaknesses as strengths may seem easy and reasonable when explained and described, it is very difficult for men to perceive it this way. Therefore, it is also hard for the society in general to see women, who are supposed to be nothing but weak, as regular human beings. Another reason for society to be so reluctant to acknowledge women as human beings vs. stereotypical labels is that these labels were created many decades ago and were never questioned before. When there is an entire society believing one thing, it is very hard to change its ways all of a sudden. Change involves a person or group of persons being strong enough to take the initiative and make the first move toward their ideals. Most people do not want to be this first person because they fear the embarrassment, criticism, and accusation of "trouble makers." Even when this person or group does take action to change society, the transition does not take place right then and there. Changes take time because it takes a long time for a society to first accept and then support a different way of thinking, perceiving, and/or doing things.

Authorities promoting erroneous stereotypes of women are also accountable for society's lack of acknowledgment of women as human beings. Big companies did not want women in their work force. Even hospitals would reject women if they attempted to reach positions any higher than nurses. Look at television commercials; who plays the role of the authority who directs us toward what to buy to satisfy our needs? What one most often sees is the woman cleaning, serving her husband, etc. Even in uncivilized tribes there is a division of roles enforced by the highest authority—the oldest man in the tribe.

Change is hard but, nevertheless, it can be achieved. The first step toward forming a new, liberated society must be taken individually. Finding the truth within myself is one of the things that I can do to change myself in order to improve society. Searching for this truth means opening up to myself and to others. It means looking deep down inside my heart and soul for the real me and telling myself: this is who I really am. Once I find this realistic, raw me, I can accept those aspects that cannot be changed, and change those that can be improved. If everyone would do this, they would be giving the best of themselves to society, and thus, have an almost perfect community in which there is no inequality and conflict. Everyone would truly respect each other. Another measure that could be taken on an individual level is trying to avoid the kind of aggressive conflict that is not productive and only serves to draw people apart from each other. Finally, as a woman, I would advise other women to work very hard at being the best of what they do, so that we can serve as examples to society, especially to those who still do not believe in the power of women.

Women can do anything they set their minds to. I have always perceived women as incredibly strong, intelligent, and determined human beings. My perception of women continues to be the same.

Women have proved that they can succeed in any role, whether it is as a parent or as a professional. They now believe in themselves and in what they are capable of doing. I do not think anyone will be able to stop them. The future holds a world full of opportunities for women as well as for men. These are the 1990s, and the man that wants to take care of the kids, cook, and do the laundry is more than welcome to do so. This is an era of choice and equal opportunity.

Judith Migoya

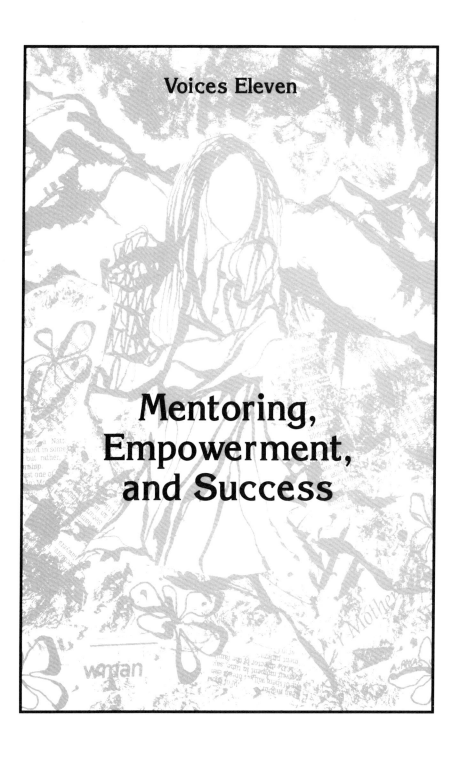

Voices Eleven

Mentoring, Empowerment, and Success

36

Woman's Work and Being a Mentor

Victoria Schoolcraft

*I*n the 1980s, women were readily accepted into the Japanese workforce due to a labor shortage. In the 1990s, women are being laid off or frozen out of major Japanese industries. This story is all too familiar, reminding me of almost any nation's days of economic growth when women are seen as competent enough to hold any position. However, as soon as the economy changes or men flood the job market, women workers are seen as dispensable by the usually male hierarchy.

One way to hold and advance women in the work place is for women who have made it into secure and influential positions to become mentors and help other women gain the stability which will make their dispensability impossible. The idea of mentoring is an ancient one. The person whose name was attached to this concept was Mentor, a character in *The Odyssey* by Homer. When the mythical Odysseus set out on his legendary trek, he asked Mentor to be the guardian and teacher of Odysseus's son, Telemakhos. Athena, the goddess of wisdom would occasionally manifest in the form of Mentor to influence the decisions of

Telemakhos. In a story about traditional male adventuring, there is some irony that such an important influence would be in the form of a woman, but this only was so because she was superhuman.

The Odyssey was first told more than 2,600 years ago in a time when roles of men and women were specifically proscribed. Women were usually the lesser characters in such stories, serving as symbols of temptation or of desire. Women were seldom portrayed as significant individuals with their own goals and wishes, other than to serve a man's objectives. Looking back over those centuries, I wonder at how durable those stereotypes of masculinity and femininity have been. The views of men and women in relation to one another and in relation to their goals have made minuscule changes compared to the vast amount of time involved.

TRADITIONAL SEX ROLES AND THE WORK WORLD

Before getting into my discussion of women and mentoring, I'd like to address some issues about women as part of the workforce. Some of the reason women have been slow to advance in the work world has been because of myths about their ability to perform the necessary tasks or even to get along appropriately with others with whom they work. My understanding of myths is that they often arise to explain something for which the myth-maker has no explanation or to provide justification for something the myth-maker wants to do.

One pervasive myth to which many women as well as men ascribe is that of the pettiness of women, especially toward one another. This is seen as a fixed quality of women which accounts for their inability to succeed in responsible positions. In some situations, women do seem petty in their competitiveness. I think this is related to the lack of significant rewards for their efforts. Any time people are in a situation where there are few available resources, they are likely to demonstrate desperate behavior as they try to garner as many of the resources as possible. Women are frequently in positions where there is very little to be gained no matter how well they do. In desperation, they may fight with one another in the nastiest ways possible over minuscule rewards. This leads to their being labeled with derisive terms and mistrusting themselves and one another. What better way to oppress a large group than to make sure they see one another as their enemies!

I don't think that even most of the men who want to oppress women think of this as a conscious strategy in keeping women down. However, it has become institutionalized by placing women in roles that have been labeled as menial and by barring them from greater opportunities. Many skills that now characterize women's jobs were at one time restricted from them as being beyond their capacities. As men found more or better things to do, these tasks somehow became achievable by women.

I'm thinking of things such as using a typewriter. Women were seen as incapable of mastering the use of such a complex machine. Men were seen as the appropriate ones to be secretaries, and the role was a valued one. In the United States government, most of the positions in the president's cabinet of advisors are called "secretaries." When that role was initiated, the role of secretary was a significant one. The responsibilities of those positions now far exceed what people would entrust to the backbone of business, the office secretary today. When men became interested in more exciting uses of their time, women were miraculously transformed into people who could learn to type and to be responsible for other aspects of the role of secretary.

Similar transformations of women's competence has occurred in my own field of nursing. In the past, only physicians (usually male, of course) monitored blood pressure with the use of sphygmomanometers. When they moved on to more challenging skills, they no longer needed to control that type of assessment equipment, and suddenly women nurses were seen as able to use such machines.

When the first intensive care units were opened, physicians were usually there around the clock, with nurses present to function only under their direct supervision. As medical and nursing knowledge advanced, physicians became no more likely to be in special care units than in any other, and nurses acquired more responsibility for maintaining the lives of the patients entrusted to them. Although this afforded slight increases in the status of nurses, they acquired very little of the prestige the physicians had who originally did this work.

In the United States, surgeons tend to be the physicians who have the highest prestige. This role is one of the oldest which physicians have fulfilled and women physicians have had difficulty finding acceptance into this field of medicine. Being a surgeon has been regarded as too challenging and difficult for women. In other countries, women have often been more readily accepted into medicine and even as surgeons. The rationale has been because of their "feminine" natures which make them "natural" care-givers. Their small hands are considered to make them more suited to performing delicate surgical procedures. Are these countries more enlightened about women? I don't think so. Usually physicians are seen more as technicians and have far from the special status accorded male physicians in the United States.

The first educators were men and formal education was first available only for male children. The first colleges for women were focused on helping young women to become appropriate wives for successful men, rather than to prepare them for their own careers. As education was made available to girls, so did the positions for teachers of children open up to women. Gradually, the male domination in education moved to the higher levels of education. Now, the younger the children, the more likely it is that their teachers will be women. In more advanced educational settings where students are engaged in professional or doctoral study, the more likely it is that the teachers will be men.

In any endeavor, it seems that as the workers become more predominantly women, their status does not improve and the status of their endeavor becomes diminished. When I was first becoming active in the women's movement, I was astonished when many supposedly enlightened women deprecated the fields which were mostly filled by women. Women struggling in business, medicine, or the law were scornful of nurses, teachers, social workers, and especially of "housewives" and secretaries. They were becoming complicit with the reigning hierarchy in labeling any work mostly done by women as being of less value than theirs.

Today, I think these attitudes are still present. If a young woman today chooses to go into a traditionally female field, men and women may think she's not capable enough to succeed in traditionally male fields, or they may think she's lazy and unwilling to accept what is seen as a greater challenge. This results in the continuing devaluation of the fields that have remained more peopled by women than men.

Even though opportunities are available for women to make more choices than ever before, the historical women's choices of mother, wife, nurse, teacher, social worker, secretary, house cleaner, and so on, are usually seen as less valuable than the newer choices. Perhaps because of that, women need mentors not only in the newly available fields, but even more in the traditional ones. In addition to helping the novice mature in the field, the mentor must help her to develop a strong self concept and self esteem for choosing an endeavor which may be minimally valued by much of society.

MENTORING

Contrary to the casual way in which the term is often used, *mentoring* is a rich and comprehensive role in which one person plays a significant part in the development of another person. Although many friends, relatives, and colleagues may influence us in our work, most do not fulfill the deep and broad role of a true mentor.

The classic definition of a true mentor in the work world comes from a group of psychologists who studied businessmen (Levinson, Darrow, Klein, Levinson, & McKee, 1976, 1978). According to their description, a mentor is a person who performs the following roles: *teacher, sponsor, host and guide, exemplar, counselor,* and *helper in the realization of the [other's] dream.* Obviously this commitment involves far more than writing a reference letter or loaning someone a book, but I have seen people describe themselves as mentors when they have done no more than that.

Although some of the terms above are self-explanatory, I think it will help if I describe each one as they are used in this context.

1. *Teacher:* [one] who enhances the skills and intellectual development of the young person.

2. *Sponsor:* [one] who uses influence to facilitate the young person's entry and advancement.

3. *Host and guide:* [one] who welcomes the initiate into the new occupational and social world, and acquaints the initiate with its values, customs, resources, and cast of characters.

4. *Exemplar:* [one] who, through his/her virtues, achievements, and way of living, serves as a model that the young person admires and seeks to emulate.

5. *Counselor:* [one] who provides advice and moral support in times of stress.

6. *Realization of the dream:* [one] who helps to define the newly emerging self by supporting and facilitating the young person's dream, by believing in the person and by giving the dream his/her blessing. (Fowler, 1980, pp. 12-13, adapted from Levinson, et al., 1978)

To be ready to serve as a mentor, a person must be experienced and advanced in her own field. We certainly provide peer support to friends and colleagues at our own level of professional development, but a mentor must be beyond the mentee in order to provide the necessary assistance.

A mentor may be useful to you no matter what field you are interested in. We usually think of mentors as people who help in the work world outside the home, and most of this essay is related to such situations. However, any endeavor will probably be more satisfying and successful with a mentor with expertise in that area. Therefore, we benefit greatly with mentors in being a spouse or a parent. All of the describers of a mentor could readily apply to helping one to be successful in intimate and personal relationships as well as work relationships. In the past, this role was usually filled by parents and other family members.

As people have become more involved in work outside and away from the family home, the skills and responsibilities of parents and spouses, sons and daughters, and siblings have become devalued. Although this paper addresses predominantly work world relationships, I want to at least recognize the vast significance of guiding and teaching that takes place within the home and family. Every day's news tells us about situations where people have lost sight of the importance of these basic relationships and of the responsibilities to one another within these settings.

To refer to the prototype of the mentor, the character of Mentor, he was charged with this responsibility because Ulysses was not going to be available to his son to function in these roles. Much of Mentor's role was to serve as a substitute father for Telemakhos. To be a good father, he provided the younger man with knowledge but also with support and caring. The human father could not overtly demonstrate the need for a father to at times behave in ways regarded as feminine. Even the human Mentor also could not seem feminine; but to fulfill all the responsibilities inherent in the parental role, Athena could inhabit Mentor to provide the necessary feminine quality.

Mentoring has much in common with healthy parenting. Mentoring also has much to do with abandoning traditional sex role behaviors.

MENTORING AND ANDROGYNY

Finding a mentor may not be an easy journey since we need to find a person who is accomplished in the field we want to pursue as well as someone who is comfortable with the variety of behaviors necessary for good mentoring. Since women have had such a difficult time rising to positions of influence and power, there aren't enough around to be able to help all of us who need their help. In addition, some women don't want to help other women because they regard other women from the same point of view as do many men. These women seem to manifest the so-called "Queen Bee Syndrome." This is the idea that some women have accomplished what they have because they are different than and better than most women.

The woman who sees herself as a queen bee probably has little appreciation for her traditionally labelled feminine qualities. She tends to over value her talents and skills that are usually seen as masculine. This results in her identifying with the male power structure and abandoning any identification with women. This point of view and subsequent behaviors make her more acceptable within many male echelons because the complicit men can also see her as a woman who is "like a man" rather than as a competent colleague who is a woman.

One of the fundamental problems in the development of respectful relationships in the work world is the pervasive use of sex role stereotypes. A sex role stereotype is a standard of behavior based on tradition and attributed only to one gender or the other. Certain qualities such as logical thinking, toughness, determination, or aggressiveness are frequently seen as male. Other qualities such as tenderness, supportiveness, indecisiveness, or emotionality are seen as female. Today I know many men and women who do not typically ascribe to these set criteria. However, these standards are so well entrenched in our collective consciousness, they often determine even the most casual attitudes of seemingly the most enlightened people!

My doctoral research was on the relationship of mentoring and androgyny (Schoolcraft, 1986). I was fascinated by the diversity in the behavior of a good mentor, especially the ability of such a person to manifest qualities which were helpful regardless of any tired notions about gender appropriateness. Just as Telemakhos's mentor was at times male and at times female, a good mentor displays either traditionally "feminine" or traditionally "masculine" characteristics as demanded by the situation. The concept of such versatile behavior is known as *androgyny,* an integration of masculine and feminine behaviors into a person's personality (Bem, 1976).

I studied college professors in nursing, education, and business. My hypotheses were that professors who act as mentors were androgynous, and those who do not act as mentors are sex-typed. I didn't find the support for my hypothesis that mentors are androgynous. However, I did find that the professors who were not mentors had strongly adopted one sex role type or the other.

In my study, mentoring was measured by *The Collegial Behaviors Inventory* which I developed for the study. This inventory asked the respondent to think of one person he or she had helped more than usual. The items were based on the qualities identified earlier as characterizing a mentor. They concerned the amount of help given by the professor in areas such as participating in research, introductions to influential people, career development, and trust. Those who scored high on 75% or more of the items were labeled as mentors for the study. The professors also responded to the *Bem Sex Role Inventory* (1981). This inventory classifies people as to gender role identification and androgyny.

Education faculty were more likely to manifest the characteristics of mentors than business or nursing professors. Education professors were much more likely than business professors to be androgynous; but they were somewhat less likely to be androgynous than nursing faculty members. Professors of business were the least likely to be mentors and tended to be sex role typed when compared to teachers of either education or nursing. Men and women mentors were equally likely to be androgynous.

From this study, I concluded that there was some support for finding a person to be your mentor who is comfortable with and manifests androgynous behavior. Other studies of androgyny have shown that people tend to become more androgynous as they age. Even our own informal observations of family and colleagues may have demonstrated that to us. This is consistent with the idea of finding someone advanced in your career field since advancement is usually related to age.

My study and others have shown that women do tend to choose to be mentors to other women. Even though there are queen bees prevalent throughout almost any endeavor, most women are actually willing to help other women. I have found no evidence that women are any more likely to be competitive with one another than are men, when other variables are equal.

STARTING A MENTORING RELATIONSHIP

Once we identify a potential mentor, we have to interest that person enough so that she will provide the guidance and other assistance we need. To work with a mentor, you initially need to be in fairly close proximity to that person. Eventually, many mentor-mentee relationships continue to flourish even though the partners are distant from one another. However, at the beginning, frequent and close contact is essential.

Look first for a mentor among the accomplished women with whom you work the most closely. Identify the women you work with who have advanced to positions similar to your own goals. Watch what they do: how they interact; how they react; and how they act in a variety of situations. Choose one whose personality is compatible to your own, but not necessarily identical to yours.

I have heard women debate whether or not to directly ask someone to be their mentor. Some people have stated that they feel a little intimidated by an overt request to become a mentor. I think that is related to the difficulty we often have as women in acknowledging our own competence. If you ask another woman to be your mentor, explain what it is you have identified that makes her your choice. Offer your service in a way that is valuable to her, such as assisting in gathering research data, or taking on less interesting chores which are part of her work.

Sometimes, a mentor will choose you. Be aware of the interest shown in you by a woman colleague. Demonstrate what you have to offer in terms of your potential to make her proud of you. I have no doubt that some women may try to exploit other women by initiating an apparent mentoring relationship. I recommend giving any colleague the benefit of a doubt. If you can see that she is accomplished in her field, she probably has been so because she has plenty of her own talent and does not need to take anything away from less experienced women. Don't be so suspicious that you pass up the opportunity to engage in a relationship which may be useful to you. There are some women who can't be trusted even in relationships with other women, but I don't think that is as prevalent as some would have us believe. Ask yourself, "Who does it serve for women to distrust each other?"

BEING A MENTOR

Using the aspects of the role as I described it earlier in this paper, I can best describe being a mentor by telling you how I do it. As a *teacher*, I help my mentees to learn what they need to know in order to succeed. Sometimes this is through a formal classroom experience, but it is often in directing them to other resources which will help them in their field. One of the most crucial things I teach is how to become a life long learner. By this I mean that I share the appreciation of learning, of never feeling that you have finished your development even though you appreciate how far you have come.

As a *sponsor*, I use my position to help my mentees to gain professional positions. I help them to understand the basics of seeking and entering the role of nurse educator. I help them to learn how to look for positions, how to interview effectively, and how to choose the best position for themselves. I write letters of recommendation for them that are enthusiastic and emphasize the mentees' strengths and potential.

In the role of *host and guide*, I help them to understand professional responsibilities that are expected even though they are sometimes unwritten. Most academic settings expect a good deal of involvement in professional and community service. I help my mentees to focus on one or two organizations and learn how to make a genuine contribution. For example, I help them to get appointed to organizational committees and choose the right times to run for office.

When we attend meetings together, I introduce them to influential or well-known leaders in the field. Students and young colleagues often are intimidated by the very thought of approaching and talking to a well known theorist or author in the field. My providing an introduction and getting a conversation started between such people and my mentees helps them to see that these people are usually gratified to talk to a young person interested in their work.

As an *exemplar*, I let my mentees know how I am involved in my professional endeavors. I discuss meetings I have attended or articles I have read. I explain my motives and strategies when I make career choices. I don't want them to copy the exact things I do, but to use their own gifts to make their own contributions. Even if I have made a mistake, I will share my reasons for doing what I did and share my analysis of what went wrong. One of the differences between a novice and an expert is not that the expert necessarily makes fewer mistakes, but that the expert knows better how to recover from a mistake. I share this with my mentees so that they will learn to be ethical and responsible even when they make errors and must take responsibility for them.

I invite my mentees to work with me on projects so that they can experience the process first-hand. For example, I may ask a mentee to work with me as a co-presenter or a co-author. My experience and reputation makes the acceptance of our presentation or manuscript more likely and the mentee gets the opportunity to learn how to prepare and make a presentation or to write for publication. The mentee earns a credit on a newly developing list of accomplishments. This helps to increase my productivity by having someone to share the work. This makes it clear why you need to be careful in choosing mentees so that you can spend time teaching them how to do things, not correcting their work.

One especially important aspect of being an exemplar is teaching my mentees how to take criticism and make it constructive. When I first wrote a manuscript for a book, I was somewhat threatened by my editor's and the copy editor's comments and changes to my writing. However, I learned a great deal from their expertise. The most important thing I learned was to use the criticism and to improve my work. I share this experience with my mentees and help them to learn to accept criticism with less defensiveness than they might otherwise have.

One of my mentees told me that at first it was hard when she read my responses to her work on her thesis. She said, "You don't butter it up, do you?" I told her that I found that "buttering it up" often makes it slip out of the writer's memory. She laughed and acknowledged that it was easier to correct things because I told her exactly what was wrong and offered ideas of how to fix it. When we met each time to discuss her progress, I used my encouraging skills to reinforce what she was doing right.

At times, mentees need my help as a *counselor*. Although this is usually about professional concerns, they sometimes need to discuss more personal things which impinge on their professional lives. I help them to examine their options and make their own choices. Although my background is in mental health and I am qualified to provide more intense counseling, I refer my mentees to other professionals if they need more extensive therapy. I believe that becoming a therapist is outside the limits of the counseling role of a mentor.

I am supportive of my mentees and comfort them when they are stressed. Sometimes a mentee needs a push or even a figurative "kick in the pants" to get moving. For example, I was working with one mentee on her thesis. She is very bright and had wonderful, expansive ideas for the research she wanted to do. After she had spent more than enough time trying to narrow the focus of her study, I finally said, "This is not your life's work. This is a thesis. It's time to get it done." To a student, a thesis is a major activity; as a mentor, I can help put it into the proper perspective.

The final component of the role is to help the mentee in *the realization of the dream*. This means that I help my mentees to define their goals, to identify their plans, and to implement their plans. Although one aspect of this component is to give my blessing, I find that is usually a covert process rather than an overt one. I have never literally said, "You have my blessing." In the things I do, my willingness to help, and my encouragement, I think I convey that I support the choices of my mentees.

CONCLUSION

Although I have never been a parent, I try to incorporate the same things into being a mentor which I think are part of being a healthy parent. I try to care more about my mentees when I'm trying to help them than I am concerned about myself at those moments. I try to help my mentees avoid obvious pitfalls, and help them to learn how to detect problems I couldn't predict. I try to help them to learn to love learning rather than to just value the facts they may learn. I try to help them to strive for success, but to be able to cope with disappointments. I try to help them to be hopeful and imaginative even in the face of painful reality and dreadful ordinariness. My fondest wish is for each mentee to turn out uniquely different than me or any other mentee, and to be happy and successful at whatever she has become.

REFERENCES

Bem, S. L. (1981). *Bem Sex Role Inventory*. Palo Alto, CA: Consulting Psychologists Press.
Fowler, D. L. (1980). An analysis of sex and departmental differences in the perceptions of assistant professors regarding work environments, mentoring, and academic employment. *Dissertation Abstracts International, 41,* 2511A–2512A. (University Microfilms No. 8026494).

Levinson, D. J., Darrow, C. N., Klein, E. B., Levinson, M., & McKee, B. (1976). Periods in the development of men: Ages 18 to 45. *The Counseling Psychologist, 6*, 21-25.

Levinson, D. J., Darrow, C. N., Klein, E. B., Levinson, M., & McKee, B. (1978). *The seasons of a man's life.* New York: Ballantine Books.

Ms. Staff (January/February, 1995). Forced out of the workforce, *Ms., V*(1), 16.

Schoolcraft, V. (1986). The relationship between mentoring and androgyny (Unpublished dissertation). Norman, OK: University of Oklahoma.

Schoolcraft, V. (1994). *A down-to-earth approach to being a nurse educator.* New York: Springer.

37

Peace, Equality, and Development of the Elementary School Child

Noreen O'Callaghan Jenott

*A*n urgent knock on the door distracts me from my phone conference with a parent. Through the window, I see an exasperated playground monitor standing between two red-faced, sixth-grade girls. The monitor's body is rigid as she physically forms a barrier between the two. Rosa is angry and glares intensely; Sarah looks scared. I respond immediately and am informed that the girls were on the verge of a fist fight when the monitor intervened. Given a choice between being sent to the principal's office for discipline or to the counselor's office for mediation they choose the latter. The mediation begins and it is soon revealed that Rosa's anger is due to the fact that Sarah had been spreading rumors about Rosa and her boyfriend. In mediation, each girl is allowed to express her perceptions and her feelings. They are allowed to express their desires and also to propose possible solutions. I act only as a facilitator; I listen without judgment and offer no advice. Within minutes, the situation has defused itself. The girls have agreed to be friends and not to talk about each other's business. As it empowers students, the mediation process has once again fostered a peaceful solution in the school environment.

TEACHING PEACE AND ALL THAT FOLLOWS

I am currently completing my first year as an elementary school counselor. I obtained my Master's Degree in Educational Counseling while teaching full time at the school where I currently hold my position. As a woman, I find myself operating as a role-model for many of the girls in school. My days are spent developing the language needed for improved relationships, cultivating assertive communication styles, and empowering girls to utilize negotiation techniques. From instruction in organizational study skills to effecting the awareness of a schoolgirl's personal power and control, the elementary school counselor plays a vital role in the development of the young girl. These skills, along with other life skills, help ready the girl child for healthy relationships, both professionally and interpersonally. They also pave an avenue to professional choice and success.

TEACHING EQUALITY

A sixth-grade classroom guidance lesson focuses on career choices. Given a list of possible employment opportunities, the students indicate whether they would be more likely performed by men or women. I am surprised that several boys and girls see choices limited and predetermined based on their sex. A lively conversation ensues as classmates argue vehemently for their stands. The girl whose mother is a lawyer sees her opportunities as unlimited. The daughter of a homemaker holds firm to the belief that a man should always make more money than his wife. That this discussion is being held in a classroom, in the United States, in 1995, startles me. With skyrocketing divorce rates and few families able to maintain a middle-class lifestyle on one income, I am taken aback by the view held by a few of these young girls. It seems archaic and most unpragmatic. I am concerned that the dream of Prince Charming lives. Equality of choices and development of options remain issues which need to be fully developed in the school environment if we are to see all girls reach their potential.

Erica met me at my office door nearly every day for the first two months of the school year. She would return again at lunchtime. If I was unavailable, she would hover in the corner of the hallway. She was friendless. She is different. It takes only slight and sometimes imperceptible differences for a child to be ostracized at school. The combination of an odd voice, a poor family background which results in her being dressed less-than-fashionably, and a lack of social skills marked Erica several years ago when she first enrolled. An object of constant teasing, she had abandoned the idea of ever having friends at school. She sought out adults to satisfy her social needs and would be found assisting teachers with bulletin boards and paper-grading during her recess periods. Her father had abandoned her family years ago and Erica and her mother lived in a reconstructed school bus in a trailer park.

One day, Erica was invited by me to have lunch in my office. She was also told to invite another classmate to join us. Erica agonized over whom to invite. She was sure that there was not a soul in the class who would join us for lunch. I assured her that many students would enjoy a respite from the din of the cafeteria to have lunch with the counselor. A nervous Erica appeared at my door at lunchtime with a classmate in tow. We sat and ate and I facilitated the conversation between the girls. Erica had the opportunity to interact socially with a peer. I continued this program with Erica. Each week she would have a new person accompany her to my office for lunch. She reported that students were asking her if they could join her. Over the course of a couple of months, there were a few girls who accompanied Erica regularly for lunch. The conversation got easier and more relaxed. I was soon an observer; my presence seemed extraneous. Erica still gets teased at school, but she is now one of a group of four girls who hang around together. Given the opportunity, she was able to develop her social skills and form friendships to make her days at school more enjoyable.

WORLD ISSUES WITH LOCAL APPLICATIONS

Peace, equality, and development are world issues and certainly the crucial personal issues which permeate the days of an elementary school counselor. The creation of a peaceful environment is critical for student learning to occur. The skills to make peaceful choices when in a confrontational situation can be a determinant of success or failure in one's school career regardless of one's intellectual capabilities. The matter of equality is confronted multivariately. From a broad perspective, the concern is focused on equal opportunities and expectations for all students, irrespective of sex or cultural heritage. From the personal view, the inquiry concentrates on the equality of individual worth. Development of the whole child is the essence of the counseling program. As I work with students ranging in age from five to thirteen, developmental issues are at the core of my sessions. Individual, family, friendship and school concerns merge as the girls quickly pass through these elementary school years.

The school counseling program is based on an eclectic mix of psychological and learning theories. It is an educational model which assumes wellness and normalcy. Problems arise because there is a lack of information, not because of an illness. The principles which guide the program include a holistic view of the child, a respect for self and others as social equals who all have value, and a belief that all behavior is goal oriented.

The primary responsibilities of the school counselor are the following: teaching students to take responsibility for their actions; training students in basic life management skills: communication, decision making, and problem solving; developing self esteem with the belief that students who feel good about themselves and have healthy relationships with others achieve more and are more personally available and ready to do the work for success.

COMMUNICATION SKILLS AS A VEHICLE FOR PEACE

A conflict management program was implemented at our school this year to help promote a peaceful environment. Twenty-six students were selected by their classmates to be trained as Peer Mediators. The students participated in a two week program to prepare them to facilitate the resolution of conflicts that occur on the playground during lunchtime. They do not presume to be capable of breaking up fights, but many of the conflicts are resolved at an early stage, preventing an escalation of the situation. The students are trained in active listening skills, brainstorming techniques, conflict resolution styles, and assertiveness skills as they master the entire mediation process.

Angela and Jennifer, two of the sixth-grade mediators, were surrounded by a bevy of second graders in the hall recently. A conflict had developed between two seven-year-old girls. It seemed as if every girl in that particular classroom had witnessed the precipitating event, and each was determined to contribute to the investigation. It was with great pleasure that I kept my distance and remained an observer. I heard Carla firmly tell the girls that she appreciated their concern and interest and that if she needed to speak with any of them later she would seek them out, but right now she needed to speak only with the two primary disputants. It was a clear, respectful communication. I was impressed with Carla's judgment and her assertiveness. Maintaining appropriate boundaries and allowing the involved students to take responsibility for her behavior in the disruptive situation allowed a peaceful solution to be found in a reasonable period of time. Soon the girls were back on the playground playing joyfully with their friends. It seems that the allowance of expression of feelings and perspectives empowers the children to be accepting of a peaceful resolution.

Participating in the training for Peer Mediation can have a great effect on the extended school community. Parents have reported that mediators have initiated the process in their homes when a conflict has arisen between siblings. Students who have been frequent participants in the process and have experienced satisfactory solutions have independently sought out a mediator to find a peaceful alternative when trouble is brewing with a peer. Hopefully, the skills will remain with these students throughout their lives and will contribute to increased peace in family life.

ANGER MANAGEMENT SKILLS

Teresa sits sullenly in front of me. She has just finished a time out, in a classroom other than her own, for being disruptive. She admits to me that she has a problem controlling her temper. Teresa feels no internal locus of control over her behavior and describes herself as succumbing to the mercy of outer influences. She says she, "Can't help it. When I get mad, I scream or kick whatever is near me." Further probing reveals that her mother is not currently living at the home. Her father has moved into the grandmother's house with Teresa and her brother. Teresa reports that her father also has a violent temper and that she "has seen a lot of violence" in her home. She did not report physical abuse, but stated that her father throws things when he gets angry. Teresa has no sense of control over her emotional state of being at any time.

There were two other girls who also had a very difficult time controlling their emotions, especially their anger. It was tough on them. It was trying for the people around them. I brought these girls together and after a brief discussion we decided to meet one day a week. The purpose of the group was to learn constructive ways of handling anger.

Over the course of the next two months, the girls identified situations that typically started a negative chain of events. Techniques, such as counting to ten or taking out a journal and writing about the situation, were suggested to immediately reduce the emotional negativity. As the weeks progressed, the students learned how to assess their liability in a stressful environment and to use drawing, working with clay and relaxation techniques to manage their anger. The benefits of aerobic exercise in stress management have been well documented. Breathing techniques were demonstrated and practiced. Safe measures were identified at home and at school if a girl thought she was going to explode. Students were encouraged to go and "run it off" instead of destroying property around them which resulted in tarnished friendships and poor student-teacher relationships. As an educational counselor, I focused on using the accountability of the group's members to improve the targeted behavior. The interactive, two-way flow between behavior and emotions became clear to the girls as the weeks progressed. The possession of this information has broken the tie they had to their former behavior patterns. The girls continue to meet regularly to discuss current issues in their lives.

GENDER EQUALITY

The track season has begun. Eleven-year-old Susan is feeling "sad and angry" because although her sixth-grade brother has permission to participate, she has to go home after school to help out with the housework. She understands that her mother, who works full-time, needs her at home, but she is resentful of the fact that she is being treated so differently than her brother. She explains that this pattern has been going on for years and that even though she is really mad, she believes that nothing will change. I encourage her to write down what she would like to say to her mother using the "I MESSAGE" formula we learned in classroom guidance lessons:

I FEEL *(name the feeling)*
WHEN YOU *(name the behavior that is causing the feeling)*
BECAUSE I WANT OR NEED *(state what it is you desire)*

After only a brief conversation, Susan writes, "I feel mad and sad when you make me come home from school and do not let me join the track team because I am a good runner and I want a chance on the team." We role-play what it is her mother might say in response and Susan offers alternative solutions to her mother's possible concerns. I elicit from her the time and place that would be best for approaching her mother. She leaves my office unsure that this will have any positive effect.

I realize that within this family, as with any family, there are generations of deeply embedded expectations and traditions. I do not presume to override any of these. My role in the educational system is to assist in the instruction of communication skills that will enhance a girl's chance for equality in any arena, be it at school or at home or in the workplace as she enters adulthood. The ability to express herself, to state her needs, and to focus on problematic behavior rather than personality issues is a powerful stance to hold. To practice focusing on the issue at hand, rather than dredging up old business, is beneficial to all involved parties.

Equality is an outcome of quality relationships which flourish when there is outstanding communication among all parties. To develop interpersonal communication skills among school age girls is developing the potential for enhanced relationships in their lives. Achieving one's maximum potential is to a great degree determined by the relationships one maintains with others.

Susan stopped by my office the other day. She had approached her mother and had shared her feelings and her needs with her. They negotiated a solution that would allow Susan to join the track team for this season. Susan was quite surprised that her mother had reacted in a positive manner. We discussed that when concerns are presented in a nonthreatening way, people are able to listen and respond more readily. She still feels that more is required of her than her brother at their home, but she did get what she wanted: an opportunity to participate in track. Most importantly, she learned that it is okay to ask for what you want in a family situation.

EMPOWERMENT IS DEVELOPMENT THROUGH INITIATIVE

An eight-year-old girl is crouched down next to the water fountain in the hall. She is crying and her head is turned stiffly into the wall. Only a slight bit of coaxing is needed to urge her out of the school hallway and into my office. Her fist is clenched tightly; in it she has a note from her teacher. It reads:

> The students have been complaining that Laura smells. Can you please speak to her about this? I, too, have noticed it and find it uncomfortable to be around her.

A brief conversation with her reveals that her family was evicted from their apartment and that her family had to move in with her aunt. At night, she shares a bed with her 18-month-old sister who still wets the bed. In the morning, she needs to travel across town by city bus to attend school. She has no opportunity to shower or bathe each morning and consequently arrives with the smell of urine emanating from her body each day. This results in her being the object of derision and rejection in her third-grade classroom. Unfortunately, this pattern may well determine the relationship she has with her peers over the next six years.

The school nurse and I meet with Laura. We explain to her the importance of good hygiene and speak to her quite frankly about the reaction of her classmates and of our concern for her. Together we develop strategies to help Laura cope with the situation she is in. Discovering that she does have access to a sink and washcloth in the morning, we teach her how to give herself a "stand-up bath" before she comes to school in the morning. Laura is encouraged to lay out her school clothes the night before so she is certain to have clean clothes to wear each day. Initiative is one of the many life skills developed in the school counseling program.

KEEPING SAFE AND OUT OF TROUBLE

When the girls enter grades five and six, their peer group becomes very important to them. Hairstyles, lipstick color, and acclaimed musical taste fall into a narrow range of acceptance. Under the influence of peer pressure, many girls are led to behave in ways unimaginable only twelve months prior. From copying homework to stealing from the neighborhood convenience market, the girls are challenged regularly to master the blend of tasks of keeping friends and staying out of trouble. With the risks of misbehavior more dangerous now than in years past, all students need to develop their ability of staying out of trouble. Refusal skills are taught in the classroom environment to assist in the development of these skills.

In the refusal skills model, we acknowledge the things that kids want:

1. To keep their friends.
2. To stay out of trouble.
3. To have fun.

Specific steps are presented to the students to help the girls achieve their goals. For example, twelve-year-old Mary is enticing Melinda to leave school and go to the park with her after they eat lunch. The steps that Melinda would need to follow to achieve her goals are the following:

1. Ask specific question: Who is going? When are we going to leave? How are we going to get there? What are we going to do there?

2. Name the trouble: "That's ditching!"
3. Name the consequences: "My mom would be furious and I'll get grounded. We might get suspended from school. Our teacher will be angry with us."
4. Suggest an alternative: "Let's go play basketball during lunch and we can go to the park this weekend."
5. Leave the door open: If the friend insists on going, Mary will leave the door open by saying, "I don't want to get grounded. I'll be on the basketball courts if you decide you want to play."

The strategy of using specific refusal skills has proven to be invaluable for many students. It has allowed them a way to maintain friendships and stay out of trouble. Possessing the tools to face miscreant influences is vital if a girl is to have a successful school career. Girls experience relief as they discover that they do not need to give into their friends to keep them. It is my hope that this feeling of empowerment goes with them as they progress through their adolescent and teenage years.

THE PEACEFUL ENVIRONMENT: ORGANIZING FOR SUCCESS

Coleen's mother called me on the phone. Midterm reports had gone home the day prior and Coleen's grades were horrible. She was receiving F's in nearly every subject. The teacher had commented that Coleen's grades were due to the fact that she had turned in few assignments. A quick glance at her attendance record indicated that she had been tardy over 50 percent of the school days. I know that this is a reflection of the family's lifestyle and attitudes. I touched base with Coleen at lunchtime and shared with her the concern of her teacher. It became immediately apparent that Coleen was totally overwhelmed and unorganized. She had no method of keeping track of assignments, she had no idea what her homework was for that day, and she admitted readily that her desk was an utter mess. I agreed to meet with her the next day.

After school the next day, I met Coleen in her classroom. Her desk was so full of papers she had gathered during the year that the desk did not even close completely. Together we sorted through each piece of paper and placed them in appropriately marked folders: work to be completed, work that needs to be checked by teacher, work that can be taken home, and so on. Over the course of the next two weeks, I worked very closely with Coleen in developing her organizational skills. She began to use the assignment book provided by her classroom teacher on a regular basis, and she developed a strategy for maintaining a clean and orderly desk. By the end of the quarter, Coleen had made substantial gains in her organizational abilities. I continue to check in with her to make sure that she does not fall prey to the "Mess Monster."

Girls in school are a clear reflection of their homes. When a child hails from a home that may be very loving and supportive, but where disorganization reigns supreme, the child has to make many adjustments to find success in the school environment. Planning and arranging materials and implementing work assignments are skills that very often have to be taught to the developing young girl. The girl then requires support and feedback to integrate these new behaviors into her life. Support provided at the elementary level can have lasting consequences on their school careers and the work environment.

MOVING TOWARD AN INNER PEACE: STRESS MANAGEMENT

A small group discussion on stress is revealing. Causes of student stress can basically be divided into three areas: home, school and friends. All of the girls in the support group agreed that the greatest stressor occurs at home. Witnessing or hearing their parents fight produces the most tension in the lives of these girls. Interestingly, children whose parents are divorced concur that parental fighting is the number one cause of stress in their lives. Stress at home is also caused by parents yelling at the child, by not being listened to, by parents asking too many questions and by being asked by their parents to do too many things at once.

At school, stress occurs by teachers yelling at the class, by teachers talking too much and not letting the students work and by having too much school work to do. Among friends, stress results when a student is seemingly forced to choose between groups of friends, when a friend is not speaking to her and when a friend is putting pressure on you to do something wrong.

Students associated the following physical symptoms with stress: headaches, inexplicable fatigue, stomach pains, crying easily, biting fingernails, sweating profusely, inability to concentrate, and feeling afraid. Techniques to handle stressful responses are presented within the context of the small group. Students are taught how to get a handle on stress. Breathing techniques are practiced and students are encouraged to engage in physical activities. Talking with a friend or caring adult is promoted, as is making sure that the student maintains a balance in her life between work and play. Ensuring that the girl gets a full night's sleep is encouraged, along with instruction in the importance of a well-balanced diet. It is also recommended to the girls that they do something for someone else who may be in a needier position at the time; this charitableness often puts things in a proper perspective for the girl.

As a school counselor, I offer my students a variety of choices from which they can select. The process of growing up and reaching maturity, of becoming self-actualized is a life-long endeavor. The greater the selection of tools and techniques the student has to embrace, the greater the chance of a healthy response to a stressful situation.

EMOTIONAL SELF-CARE

Annalis came to see me in my office recently. She was in an absolute dither. Some boys in her sixth-grade class were calling her "Annal is." Mica stopped by later that day totally upset because a few of the girls in her class had bestowed upon her a less-than-flattering nickname. A short time later Melody had a similar complaint. All three girls were allowing other people to control their emotional states. It took a lot of time for them to believe and understand that they could separate themselves from what others said. Admittedly, it is difficult to ignore, but the reaction of the girls was satisfying the harassers.

We role-played a variety of ways of confronting the situation. Giving an "I Message," ignoring it altogether, or saying something surprising, like "thank you" were some of the options the girls now had. Mica reported back in a few days that saying "thank you" was so startling that the other students had backed off. Annalis continues to find it very difficult to let go of the fervor produced by the name calling. Her locus of control is predominantly external. I need to spend more time with her helping her discover the resources and strength she has within.

THE CIRCLE IS COMPLETED: DEVELOPMENT CONTINUES

It has been only three decades since I attended elementary school. In terms of role expectations and planning for a future career, much has changed for the girl child in our country. Yet, everyday, as I work with elementary school girls I am reminded that much has remained the same.

The ability to communicate clearly needs to be continually developed as a vehicle for interpersonal peace in relationships. Awareness of gender inequality must remain a part of the conversation about school age girls. The development of personal power and autonomy must be a focal point of the girl's life in school. The emergence of an external locus of control is to be celebrated. Organization and stress management are tools that will facilitate a girl's success, both in school and in the work place. Having a method to keep herself out of harm's way is a step toward keeping her on a productive path. Through continuing conversation, the issues of peace, equality and development will be the impetus for the cultivation of valued cognitive growth in the school age girl.

38

Mentoring Toward a Longed for Life

Lynne Nelson

Caged Bird*

A free bird leaps
on the back of the wind
and floats downstream
till the current ends
and dips his wing
in the orange sun rays
and dares to claim the sky.

Grateful acknowledgment is made to the Robert Wood Johnson Foundation, Inc. and the BARD Foundation.
* Reprinted with permission of Random House. Copyright 1994 in *The Complete Collected Works of Maya Angelou.*

But a bird that stalks
down his narrow cage
can seldom see through
his bars of rage
his wings are clipped and
his feet are tied
so he opens his throat to sing.

The caged bird sings
with a fearful trill
of things unknown
but longed for still
and his tune is heard
on the distant hill
for the caged bird
sings of freedom.

The free bird thinks of another breeze
and the trade winds soft through the sighing trees
and the fat worms waiting on a dawn-bright lawn
and he names the sky his own.

But a caged bird stands on the grave of dreams
his shadow shouts on a nightmare scream
his wings are clipped and his feet are tied
so he opens his throat to sing.

The caged bird sings
with a fearful trill
of things unknown but longed for still
and his tune is heard
on a distant hill
for the caged bird
sings of freedom.   *Maya Angelou*

HEARING THE SONG

The theme of freedom permeates our existence in the world in varied and elusive patterns. The image it conveys is unique for each woman and is influenced by the sum of her life's experience. Freedom in this situational context speaks to the woman's ability and power to pursue her individual and her community's common good. Freedom is a process of becoming, creating, and self-development, rather than an abstract ideal.

It is the active forging of harmony with truth, within the woman and without. Freedom is a change of vision, a growth from a narrow caged existence to an existence which soars on, *"on the back of the wind."*

Freedom is achieved within the privacy of the individual heart as surely as it is gained in the global arena. Freedom connotes the process of redressing wrongs, of setting things right. It is based on the premise that each human being is endowed with equal worth. Freedom is an overarching need of humankind. Without freedom, there can be no peace.

This view of freedom is congruent with and fundamental to those themes that provide the framework of this conference: peace, equality and development. Equality and freedom are closely related in forming the fabric that adorns the body of a peaceful world. Freedom is the weaving and equality becomes the garment. Freedom is the process and equality becomes its fruit. Development occurs within the person, as it does within the economic realm of a society. It is descriptive of a process of becoming which enables individuals and societies to soar toward the highest potential possible, to *"sing of freedom."*

Education is a vehicle and power for the development of a common good; it is the tool for the forging of harmony; and the blueprint for development. Education is an enabling mechanism; it opens the cage door to the opportunities and rewards of the world. To educate is to lead; to map the skies; to chart the winds of life's potential for opportunity and freedom. Freedom, at last, for the caged bird.

Education enables each woman to discover and to use her intellectual life, that is, her intellectual equality, to communicate with the men of her society. Sometimes, however, education can be inaccessible to a woman because of her financial limitations, inadequate academic preparation and/or self-limiting perceptions. Some women, minority women in particular, have limited access to and limited success rates in quality educational programs. Success in quality educational programs could open the career doors of their dreams for minority women.

Professional nursing is often named as a career choice for minority women. Nursing has a rigorous, demanding educational preparation. Complex course content must be mastered quickly and applied in the clinical patient care settings. Procedures and interpersonal skills must be learned and refined. The registered nurse is prepared for an active, life-long educational life to meet the on-going demands of a scientific practice.

There is a nationally felt, acute need for larger numbers of minority registered nurses. African-American and hispanic nurses are needed for the general population of patients, as well as, for those African-American and hispanic communities who have dramatic health needs.

Minority registered nurses infuse the practice of nursing with the rich perspectives of their cultural heritages. Such perspectives are needed as new solutions to intractable health issues are sought.

Attrition rates are high among minority students in early nursing program courses. Only 5 percent of minority registered nurses complete the bachelors degree in nursing and less than one percent complete the masters level of preparation. Overall, while there are increasing numbers of minority nursing students enrolled in nursing programs, the number of graduating minority students is on the decline.

FEARFUL TRILLS

A nursing education can be a valuable asset to the minority woman. The successful completion of a nursing education ensures a middle class life for herself and her family. Her position as a registered nurse enables that minority woman to raise the health care standards in her community. Both the individual woman and the community benefit from her education.

For the African-American woman, the educational transition into nursing has familiar components. It offers her challenges and gives her an opportunity to nurture others. The minority woman is familiar with challenges and nurturing. Many of these African-American women students soar in their development as nurses.

For many minority women, however, the educational program is not experienced as a supportive, nurturing process. For these students, the educational process is experienced as oppressive and foreign; its pathway is inscrutable. They struggle with feelings of loneliness, feelings of not belonging, feelings of perceived discrimination, feelings of actual discrimination, and feelings of confusion about expectations. Their prior experiences limit their perceived boundaries. These experiences reflect a summation of the real life as it has been lived within a society marked by an underclass.

For these African-American women, life experiences have included an economic dislocation from the larger society. In addition, some of the women have lacked the experience of a nurturing family during their formative years. Some of the women have experienced personal, as well as, institutional racism and oppression. The theme of freedom which emerges from Angelou's poem seems distant and out of the reach of what has become the normal existence of these women.

Both an actual and a perceived lack of freedom creates a discordant sound in the woman's innermost self which mirrors the experience of her external world. When the barriers that bar her way to a longed-for life have been lowered, the woman may not know the way through the door, so deep is her experience of caged imprisonment. She has internalized the external perception and it becomes her reality. Then the realities which close her in, or tie her down, actually come from within her. Her perceptions include mistrust, fear, and a sense of alienation. The emotions which bind her include anger and even rage towards herself, toward others, and toward the institutions in her immediate environment. These internalized feelings cooperate with the feelings of oppression and of the actual frustrations of the world in depriving her further from being able to claim or create a life of freedom within her own sphere.

OPENING THE CAGE DOOR: THE MENTOR'S SONG

As an African-American woman myself, and a mentor/role model in a school of nursing, I meet many minority women and have witnessed the caged bird's cry. Many of my relationships with students include women who view the educational experience from a framework of fear and mistrust.

After having considerable success in improving retention rates of minority women, I can state that minority mentors are dramatically needed at all levels of education. Mentoring assists in the socialization of the student as a learner and enables the development of self-confidence. In addition, mentoring assists the student to unlock the bars of internal or external prejudice when it exists. Mentoring encourages the minority woman to develop behaviors which help her to view her educational setting realistically. The faculty may view the student as less qualified than her non-minority counterparts. Mentors can validate the strengths of the minority woman and serve as a liaison in problem solving.

The minority mentor is in a position to identify and clarify the goals and dreams of the minority students in deeply personal ways. This role of the mentor/role model, and the terms are used interchangeably here, is especially pertinent for undergraduate education because students are socialized not only into the academic setting but into professional behaviors and beliefs also.

As a minority mentor/role model, I am able to assess the capacity of the student for success and to assist the student to believe in herself, in her own ability for rigorous study and for the beginning acquisition of professional skills. The mentor models the application of concepts, critical thinking and long-range goal setting. The mentor/role model creates a safe environment in which the student may explore her own perceptions regarding professional development. The student is permitted to reason out loud without criticism, and can make mistakes without the loss of confidence or self-esteem.

My view of mentoring uses the feminist perspectives of reciprocity and empowerment. The minority mentor/role model uses these concepts with African-American students who exhibit various degrees of alienation. Reciprocity is experienced in the mentor relationship as a gift exchange in which the value lies in the personhood of each participant. Empowerment, which has various meanings within the mentoring role, can be experienced as an internal awakening in which a trusted mentor acts as a person who encourages the revelation of previously untapped abilities.

For the African-American student who struggles with actual and perceived oppression, the validation of dreams may include assisting the student in the continued ongoing creation and refinement of her goals and dreams.

CLAIMING THE SKY

Many students describe their dreams of becoming a nurse as the act of getting into the nursing program. These students do not consider what it will be like to go through the process of being successful in school, course by course, semester by semester. Without an image of herself as moving successfully through the process of the entire education, these minority students are undermined by unexpected set backs. Their world view becomes defined by incidental events rather than an internal vision and personal drive.

The ability to dream is a mark of freedom. In our educational program, the student is taught to create her goals and dreams based on continuous, incremental progress. As a mentor/role model, I assist the student to understand and to act on the fact that freedom is possible in an imperfect world. Unlocking the chains of anger and rage assists the minority student to be able to begin to walk through the doors to freedom within herself, as well as, within her educational setting. This process, however, can increase the student's sense of vulnerability in an imperfect environment. It exacts a tremendous emotional cost which some students are not willing to pay. As a mentor, I assist the student to direct her anger in a manner that is not destructive to herself or others. The anger can be channeled toward achieving her dreams and goals, and toward the development of a passionate advocacy for the well-being of her patients.

Mentoring is the development of a relationship of trust in which the mentor validates the experiences of the student, and interprets the corporate culture of the educational environment. Strategies for effective study habits are taught to the student. These student strategies move the student to independent action and academic success.

I have learned, day by day, that mentoring a student who demonstrates alienation serves to free that student from her fear. The student is encouraged to reconstruct her concept of self from a person in isolation to a person who is in partnership with the mentor. As a dyad, we explore the environment and its signs and signals. The mentor assists the student to step away from her *"grave of dreams and to open her throat to sing."* The singing metaphor is captured in the personal caring component within the mentor-student relationship. Such a relationship teaches the learner to have an increased understanding of and tolerance for the culture of the educational environment.

The student develops a growing concept of self as a part of the learning environment. I never ask the student to abandon her own culture. I invite her to become bicultural. The minority woman is assisted to incorporate the attitudes and values of the educational setting. The best situation affirms that part of her background, values, and experiences which are unique to whom she is and wishes to be. The minority student sets new goals and has new dreams. Her world opens up. As her vision is stretched she experiences pain, and loss. As the minority mentor, I am there to understand and support her. Each woman must preserve her subversive memory, that is, her attempt to stay in tune with the best of her history and values while incorporating new concepts. Prisoners, once freed, have to remember that now the locks are gone, *"his wings are clipped and his feet are tied."*

THELMA'S CAGE

Thelma sat in my office on a clear cold day filling the small space with her anger. The roads were icy and the tires on her car were bald. She had needed to drive slowly, had needed to avoid certain routes, had skidded a few times, had driven with her heart in her throat, had underestimated the time needed to arrive at school given the weather, and so had been late for her clinical assignment. Tears stood in her eyes, but did not flow. It seemed as though her whole body was drawn into a fist. "What you need to do," I said, "is to apologize to your clinical instructor. Ask if there is some way you might make up for any lost clinical time. Assure her that you will make every effort not to be late again." I knew Thelma fairly well, and had served as her mentor for over a year. Thelma could not afford new tires and had hoped that the winter would be a mild one. She had planned to work full time on her school vacation and replace the tires with some used ones in better condition.

Thelma lives in a one-room rental, supported herself and lived frugally. Thelma was angry. Her life had no room for the slightest thing to go wrong. There was not enough money. There was no emotional reserve to tolerate one more thing. Thelma used anger to cope in life, to survive and probably had done so for some time. Her life had been marked by poverty, the early deaths of her parents, being raised by several relatives and in foster homes.

Thelma had a sense that growing up as an African American meant that the world was against her. Most of her experiences outside of her own cultural environment were described as ranging from unpleasant to oppressive. Thelma saw a racist under every bush. At thirty years old, the available financial support for college presented the first open door to break the pattern of the poverty of her life.

Thelma's life-long dream was to be a nurse. Because Thelma was very intelligent and caring, her dream was a real possibility. The door was opened, but like the caged bird, she *"stalked her narrow cage,"* looking at the world through her, *"bars of rage,"* feeling clipped and tied. She was unfamiliar with the things which would give her the freedom to open her *"throat to sing."*

Thelma had to learn, with my assistance as her mentor, that part of the prison she now experienced was of her own making. It had been forged by years of habitual response to real racism and pain, to actual imagined oppression, and by an unfamiliarity with the things that make for freedom.

There was a long silence before Thelma spoke, "I think it's a waste of time to apologize," she said, her voice a barely controlled whisper. "My instructor has been waiting for something so she could get me. She is just going to give me a clinical warning and begin to try to get rid of me."

A NIGHTMARE SCREAM

"What we need to get clear," I said, "is that what happens in this situation is mostly in your control and depends upon your behavior as a professional. Decide upon the outcome that you want and then let's role play the interaction that you will have with your instructor. I'll pretend to be you."

By the end of our time together, Thelma had seen her way clear to a point of considering apologizing to her instructor. Through the role playing, Thelma saw that there were many possible outcomes to the situation. How a difficult interaction is approached can influence the outcome. Role playing gave Thelma an increased awareness of her negative expectations of herself and of others. "Not everyone is out to get you," I said. "There are people here who really are hoping for you to succeed. The faculty are here to help you to become a nurse. I am one of them." I hoped that Thelma would feel less alienated, but she remained wary. She was aware that there were many students who did not succeed in the nursing program. Many of those students were African American. I suggested that Thelma see a psychologist to get some help with her anger. Her wariness seemed to deepen. She visibly pulled away. It had seemed at some point in our conversation that she had advanced a little in her responses. She did take steps which would assist her to begin to problem solve.

As she left my office that day, the anger had begun to dissipate, but only some of it and only for a while.

Thelma continued to exhibit signs of mistrust of the school environment as well as our mentor relationship. She struggled with the academic material. By mid-semester she was maintaining a B average in the Medical Surgical course, one of the most difficult courses for the students to master. She had few, if any, friends among her peers. She continued a combative relationship with her clinical instructor.

After not seeing Thelma for a while, I called her home. Her phone was disconnected. I asked her instructor how she was progressing on the clinical unit and she told me that Thelma had withdrawn from the nursing program after an explosive encounter with the instructor.

Thelma had maintained the B average, but it had snowed a lot that winter. The roads were always snow covered and icy.

MAE STRUGGLES, THEN LEAPS ON THE WIND

Mae worked full time as a nursing assistant in a convalescent home. In addition, she held a part-time weekend job caring for a housebound elderly man. She attended college in a full time evening program. She had failed her second Medical Surgical nursing examination. She sat in my office attempting to review the study strategies which I had taught her. If she used them, these techniques could have improved her possibilities of success.

Her arms were folded and her head was tilted to one side. We opened her notes from class on the little round table students like to use to spread out their work and to take notes. Mae's arms were folded and so, she wrote nothing down. "Tell me how you studied for this exam and how you think that I might be able to help you," I said. "I have no idea how you can help me," she replied, "You are the expert." I knew Mae's work schedule. She had four children at home under ten years of age. She was a single mother. Her home had been without heat the previous week. Her mother helped out with the children, but I could not imagine that she had been able to take sufficient time to study. Depth of concentration was needed to have done well on the exam. "Mae, I really believe that part of what is going on is that you need to spend more time on your studies than you have been." I paused thinking that what I was about to suggest was going to create a lot of tension. I could see no other solution if she was going to have any chance of success. I wondered how to go about approaching her on the subject of her working hours.

I decided to use a blunt honesty in outlining the course of study that was needed. We opened her textbook, her class notes and journal articles and we began to work together.

"This is what you needed to know for this exam," I said. "This is the level of understanding you need in order to apply it." I took the endocrine system step by step and included the normal functioning, the pathophysiology, the signs and symptoms of deviations in health status, and then all of the complex nursing material needed to care for the very ill patient.

Her silence was thick with something which felt like grief. "Is there any way that you can modify your work schedule, even if just for this semester?" I questioned. "Only if I modify my family's intake of food and other things like that," she said. "You know that this is ridiculous," she continued, "there is just too much work in this course." Another silence crept into the room and I struggled to let it happen. I hoped that some ray of hope would come with it. Mae looked off in the distance, out of the window, and up at the sky. "I have to do this," she said at last, "I have to." "All right Mae," I said, "continue to bring me your notes so that I can check your strategies. I believe that sometimes determination in the face of insurmountable odds can create the most amazing things." I saw Mae periodically for the rest of the semester. *"The caged bird opened her throat to sing."* Most of the time both of us were frustrated.

I became frustrated because she seldom was able to apply the strategies I suggested. And she was frustrated because she continued to seek a way to make the whole process easier and more manageable given her time constraints.

In the end, Mae failed the course. The next semester she was back to repeat the course. She never came to me for assistance or mentoring the entire semester and I only heard of her progress through her instructors. "How's Mae doing?" I would ask when I learned of a particularly difficult exam. "Mae," her instructor would reply with amazed humor, "received a ninety, the highest grade in the class."

Sometimes, I would see Mae in the hallways. She always seemed to avoid me. I thought she was angry with me. Perhaps it was because I could not prevent her first failure. Another semester came and went and Mae was still doing well.

Recently, she was honored along with her classmates in a pinning ceremony signifying the move into the second level of the nursing program. "Mae," I said as I approached her at the reception later, "I want you to know how glad I was to see you pinned. How very proud I am of you and of your persistence in nursing." Her face opened up in the warmest of smiles. "You reached a hand out to me," she said, "and you gave me hope." And the free bird *"dip(ped her) wing in the orange sun rays and dare(d) to claim the sky."*

JILL AND KISHA STAND ON THEIR GRAVE OF DREAMS

Jill and Kisha were from the same neighborhood and had known each other all of their teenage years. It was an area of poor struggling families, overpriced grocery stores and some boarded-up buildings. If you walked down the street you would notice an assortment of paradoxical activities and sights that are a microcosm of inner city life. Some of the most beautiful red roses to grace this earth grow in the well-tended dirt yard of a picket fenced house on the corner. Half of the pickets are missing. From the house next door, you can hear someone practicing scales on a piano with much skill. Men gather to drink wine in one of the alleys. Their heads tip back under brown paper bags. Their eyes glaze over with forgotten dreams.

Jill and Kisha live here. Now in their twenties, they attended college together. They were in the first clinical nursing course, Fundamentals of Nursing. They were not doing well. Because they were friends and study partners, they came together to see me. I usually encourage students to study together in groups, not only for the reinforcement of subject matter, but because studying together fosters the affiliation necessary for most students to succeed.

Together we assessed their time management and study skills. They shared notes. Since Kisha seemed to be able to record the lecture content in greater depth, the notes were mostly hers. They seemed to agree about the nature of their problems in the school. There was too much content.

The lecturers talked too fast in class. The instructors tended to embarrass them on the clinical unit by constantly quizzing them about the rationale for their actions. The test questions were difficult and even in some cases, unfair.

We agreed to schedule meetings in which I would teach them study strategies to address their problems with the nature and extent of the course content. I also began to share with them some of the culture of learning which exists in a traditional class, and how to negotiate the educational system. Most of our time together was spent assisting Jill with the strategies and content. It became clear that any suggestions that I recommended were accomplished by Kisha. Kisha was the one who took the notes. Kisha integrated the material from the text book with the lecture notes. It was Kisha who developed sample nursing care plans, and who increasingly was able to relate the course content to the clinical care of patients. Soon, I was spending time in our meetings trying to get Jill to respond more in our sessions together. "I'm doing better," she would state, "I really am beginning to understand the material." "We are really doing better," Kisha would say, "I think that we will be prepared for the next exam, and will at least pass. We have been studying a lot and using some of the strategies. We also are thinking about becoming involved in the student government association. We are beginning to feel like we belong here." Kisha looked over to Jill. Was it for her affirmation, for her approval?

On the next examination, Kisha did do better. She received a passing score of seventy-eight. Jill failed. She had only improved her grade from the last exam by five points. Both students were still in danger of failing the course. I felt that it would be best to see each woman separately so that I could discover what was going on with Jill.

I saw Kisha protected Jill from any chance of exposure of her difficulties. This action made both students very hostile toward me. It was as if they were asking, "What the hell did I think I was doing? Couldn't I see that they were good study partners and supported one another in being students in the school? What did I think I would accomplish by seeing them individually?" They wouldn't come to our sessions. They did not return for a while. Shortly before the next exam, Jill and Kisha made an appointment to see me individually. Jill came and shared her notes (which I think were actually copies of Kisha's notes) with me and we began to look at the content. She seemed able to recall isolated facts from the course content but could not integrate the concepts. She could not apply any of the basic knowledge to a particular example. Finally, we looked at some test questions together. I asked Jill to reason out loud with me why an answer might be the correct one. She seemed to have difficulty understanding objective questions. "I always have had trouble with understanding what I read." she said. I asked her to explain the content in her own words. She was able to do this only if I cued her. "How did you manage in your basic courses?" I asked her. "I pretty much memorized what I needed to know." She looked at me sadly and said, "I never was a great student. I mostly just made it through the other courses." "Have you thought about going to another, less demanding program?" I asked. I was not sure how she would respond to this. "Does that mean that you think I won't make it here? I'm not smart enough?" Her manner shifted and her sadness was covered by a thin veneer of anger. "I do not think that you are stupid." I said. "I just think that this program may be too fast-paced for you. Your talents and abilities might emerge better in another program." The look she gave me then said, "Sell out!" Finally she spoke. "Thank you for your opinion. I'll think about it." Jill was quick to rise and leave the room.

Later, Kisha came in to see me and we reviewed her notes and content for the next exam. She seemed angry but did not directly express it. I was rigorous with Kisha in reviewing the subject material and in the end she thanked me for my time.

Jill failed the next exam and withdrew from the school. Kisha received an eighty-five and came to see me the next week. "I am withdrawing from this school," she said. "I think that it is impossible for me to succeed here." She had not shown up for clinical and had not called her instructor. I was able to talk her out of making such a move. She agreed to call her clinical instructor and apologize for her behavior and to get her uniform on and go to the unit. "You are doing this because of Jill and it's not going to help her or you if you quit." "You're right," Kisha said, "I know you're right." That day Kisha went on to give excellent care to her patient and contributed in the post care conference with her fellow students and instructor.

By the end of the week Kisha, with a B average, had withdrawn from the school. I phoned Kisha at home. "I just did not belong there." she said, "I wonder if I even belong in nursing." "That is something you will have to decide for yourself," I said, "But, I think that you are throwing away a wonderful opportunity. Get in touch with me if I can do anything to assist you in the future."

The following semester I saw Kisha's name on the list of students who were returning to the course. "This really is my dream," she said when I saw her. "The thing about dreams is that sometimes you might be willing to let them go, but they won't leave you alone. In my sleep I would dream that I was back here working my tail off. I just couldn't get away from this place. So, I'm coming back."

And, with those words, the space between us grew heavy with hope, and with the unspoken recognition of the winds of freedom. *"A free bird leaps on the back of the wind . . ."*

WHAT IS THE COST OF "ANOTHER BREEZE"?

Freedom is the building block of dreams. Many African American women experience those dreams from a closed place, a cage, in which the goodness of the world exists only on the outside and not available to her. *". . . his wings are clipped and his feet are tied . . ."*

As an African American, a nurse, and a mentor of students from diverse cultures, I find that making the dreams emerge lies not only in the economic opportunity of a professional career, but in the inner work necessary for the individual to become a citizen in a number of "worlds and cultures." For the minority person, education is a process of becoming a multicultural learner with an ability to negotiate a number of spheres of educational and professional realities. This occurs but not without cost.

An African-American woman's insights regarding life is a very creative power which she can use for personal peace, equality and self-development and socially for the good of her community.

African-American women who are agents of a new knowledge experience a marginality. She is an outsider within her own community. There is a constant pressure on her to either reject her culture, or to dichotomous behavior, thereby becoming two people, each with different social status and behaviors. The woman becomes bi/multi-cultural.

If she rejects the dominant culture, her self-interest and profession are compromised. If she rejects her traditional social culture, her personal life and feelings of belonging are at risk. Her self-interest is compromised.

A possible and perhaps desirable alternative is for the minority woman to inhabit both cultural contexts, an outsider within her greater world. She then becomes a source of creative ideas and insights made possible from this unique perspective. Being an outsider within, however, comes at a great cost. The cost is the risk of personal loneliness. It is neither peaceful nor equal—but it does support development.

As an African-American woman who is mentor and role model to African American students, I have learned the importance of preparing the women for knowledge of this potential loneliness. The loneliness, in some degree, will await her as she moves toward success.

Mentoring the African-American woman includes assisting her to understand the source and meaning of the song she sings for freedom. It includes offering her the means and way to that freedom. And mentoring her means weaving in the cost of joy along freedom's way.

Mentoring the African-American student includes imparting an understanding that the caged bird will always be an integral part of who she is as long as she remains part of the collective consciousness of all people who long for freedom.

The singing bird will remind her that creating freedom and developing herself is a process that continues to permeate the whole of her life with its constant winds. But, in the end, there is the reward.

"The free bird thinks of another breeze
and the trade winds soft through the sighing trees
and fat worms waiting on the dawn-bright lawn
and he names the sky his own."

REFERENCES

Angelou, M. (1994). The caged bird. In The Complete Collected Poems of Maya Angelou. New York: Random House.

Collins, P. H. (1990). Black feminist thought: Knowledge consciousness and the politics of empowerment: Perspectives of gender. (Vol. 2). New York: Routeledge.

DeMarco, R. (1993). Mentorship: A feminist critique of current research. *Journal of Advanced Nursing, 18*, 1242-1250.

Hansberry, L. (1969). To be young, gifted and black. New York: Signal.

Hooks, B., & West, C. (1992). Breaking bread. Boston: South End.

National League for Nursing. (1994).

Weekes, D. P. (1989). Mentor-protegy relationship: A critical element in affirmative action. *Nursing Outlook, 37*(4), 156-157.

39

Struggle, Commitment, and Determination: An African-American Woman's Journey to Self-Development

Betty W. Barber

Where there is no struggle, there is no progress. Power concedes nothing without a demand, it never has and never will.

—Frederick Douglass

I am an African-American woman. From a historical perspective, it seems paradoxical, but nevertheless true, that the history of women and the history of African-Americans are quite parallel with regard to their struggle for equality, dignity, and respect. The words of Frederick Douglass, "Where there is no struggle, there is no progress . . ." invoke a powerful response every time I read or hear them. The statement is a philosophy of self-determination, perseverance and hope. Such a philosophy was instilled in me during my youth, and has served as a driving force in my life.

When I reflect over my life, beginning with early childhood to the present, I am reminded of a history that is replete with example after example of struggle against racism, sexism, discrimination and injustice.

The following selected anecdotal experiences over the course of my life that portray not only struggle, but the faith, hope, and determination of my family and significant others who supported and encouraged me to persevere and to keep moving forward toward a brighter future.

THE STRENGTH OF FAMILY

Both of my parents were born and reared in Rock Hill, South Carolina. My father, Maso Witherspoon, proudly tells of how he met and fell in love with my mother, Refula Smalls. He says it was love at first sight and after a short courtship they were married in 1932, in the midst of the Depression. Shortly thereafter, they moved to Charlotte, North Carolina, and that is when I was born, the fourth of ten children.

My parents were hard-working Christian folk. Although, as children growing up, we had very few material things, we were grateful to have wonderful, loving, caring parents who nurtured us in a Christian home. We were members of a church that held church services every night of the week and all day on Sundays. Our church had very strict rules regarding social activities, and Mama, in particular, was a rigid enforcer of the rules, especially for myself and my sister. Except for school and church activities, our social life was pretty much restricted. My brothers, however, enjoyed a little more flexibility socially.

Second only to religion was the importance placed on education. Neither of my parents had a college education. Actually, Papa, who had not gotten beyond second grade, was illiterate. Mama had finished high school, but during those days high school only went to seventh or eighth grade. Perhaps their strong desire for us to get college educations was based on the difficulty they had in finding decent employment with limited education.

For many years, Papa worked as a cook for the Southern Railroad Company. This meant that he was gone for long periods of time. Mama worked as a domestic for White families.

EDUCATION: THE SEGREGATED
SCHOOL SYSTEM

I enrolled in first grade at Meyers Street Elementary School in the Fall of 1944. At that time, education was structured under the so called "separate but equal" policy. Policy or not, the segregated southern schools were anything but equal in comparison to White children's schools.

Both the elementary school and the high school which I attended were located in an urban, run-down, over-populated community. I had to walk five or six blocks to my elementary school. The neighborhood was not safe for children to travel alone. I walked to and from school with groups of other children in the neighborhood and we were always chaperoned by a parent or older high school student.

The classrooms were crowded, the desks shabby, the books old with pages torn, but we were blessed with wonderful teachers. They were strong disciplinarians concerned not only with our education but with our overall well-being as children. I have fond memories of many of my elementary school teachers, in particular, my fifth grade mathematics teacher, Mrs. Sarah Alston.

Mathematics was one of my favorite subjects and Mrs. Alston was a very good teacher. She was one of those "no-nonsense" types who did not cut any of us any slack. The homework assignments were due on time and no excuses were accepted. I knew that a late assignment would result in punishment not only from Mrs. Alston, but from my Mama as well when I returned home.

One morning while sitting in class waiting for the tardy bell to ring, a group of us were talking about the "ragged" books we had to use. It was a well-known rumor that the books we used were "hand me downs" from the White schools. We were not aware that Mrs. Alston was listening to our conversation, but we were soon to find out.

When the tardy bell rang, Mrs. Alston called me and my classmates, who were involved in that discussion, to the front of the classroom. She proceeded to tell the class that my classmates and I were complaining about the "ragged" books we were using. And for the next few minutes (which seemed like an eternity) she lectured us about the evil of being ungrateful. She reminded us that things could be much worse; that our ancestors had much less, yet became great people. We had a history lesson right there in the midst of our mathematics class. As I stood there confused and humiliated, it was as if the words coming from Mrs. Alston were an echo from my parents. Mama always gave thanks to God for the little things in life. One of Papa's favorite sayings was "You take what you got and make the best of it."

No, I will never forget Mrs. Alston. At the time I did not understand nor did I appreciate her reaction to what seemed to be an innocent conversation with my classmates. However, as an adult I realized what a valuable lesson she taught me and it has served me well.

A WOUNDED SENSE OF SELF

The White family Mama worked for had a daughter, Betsy. Betsy and I were of the same age and in the same grade, fifth, when she began taking me to work with her on a regular basis. Aunt Mary, called "Aunt" by the kids in the neighborhood, had taken ill and informed my mother that she could no longer come to our home to take care of us while my mother was at work. My sister, then a junior high school student, had a part-time job after school. Unable to find a replacement for Aunt Mary, my Mama arranged with her employer to adjust her work schedule. She stayed home until I got out of school, then took me to work with her. My brothers were allowed to stay home with my older brother, Bill, in charge.

At first, I was very excited about going to work with Mama. Betsy and I got along very well together. She seemed to enjoy having me there to play with after school. However, we had to abide by the rule of completing our homework before going out to play. It seemed that Betsy always finished her homework first. Initially, she would wait patiently for me to complete my homework, but gradually she began to insist on helping me finish the assignment so we could have more time to play. Her impatience took its toll. Soon she was practically telling me the steps and answers to my mathematics problems before I had time to read and understand what I was doing. I did not consider myself to be a bad math student, I just needed more time to read and understand the concepts. I wanted to tell Betsy to stop and leave me alone but I was afraid that if Betsy and I did not get along with each other, it would make things hard for Mama. Gradually, I began to feel that Betsy was much smarter than I. "Why was it so much easier for her to understand everything?" I thought to myself. I wished that I was as smart as Betsy and I wondered if she thought I was dumb. This was a very difficult time for me. I suffered quietly. My sense of self was temporarily diminished.

In Sullivan's view, self-development comes through conscious and unconscious perceptions of personal experiences, including achievements, failures, conflicts, and embarrassments. The self is constantly reinforced by feedback received from significant persons in the environment. When the message received is a positive appraisal, the part of the self reinforced is the "good me." When the message received is negative appraisal, the part of the self reinforced is the "bad me."

HIGH SCHOOL

Second Ward High School was one block up the street from the elementary school I attended. For years, I had gazed up the street at the high school with excitement and anticipation. Finally, I was there, in the freshman class.

There were only two Black high schools in the city of Charlotte. West Charlotte High School was the other school and it was located on the West side of the city where the more affluent Black families lived. The two schools were very competitive, especially in sports.

Second Ward High School was a focal point for the social and cultural events in the Black community. Although the building itself was very old and lacked many of the more modern state-of-the-arts resources and facilities, it was a source of pride to the community. The year before I went there, the construction of the new gymnasium was completed and extensive renovations were done on the auditorium.

The Drama Club traditionally gave two major performances a year which were open to the public. A small admission fee was required, but there was always a sell-out audience. Other activities open to the general public were the arts festival, talent shows, Spring festival, and the student debating team.

I did not participate very much in extracurricular activities. With academic interests presiding, I spent most of my time reading and studying. As a sophomore, I had become extremely competitive academically. My desire to succeed was almost overbearing, perhaps even slightly unhealthy. My classmates often teased me about being a bookworm, but that did not distract me.

LIBRARY RESOURCES

One incident in my junior year of high school stands out vividly in my mind. A major part of the final grade during the junior year was based on a term paper. Being the competitive student I had become, I set myself to earn an "A."

The collection of books in our school library was very poor. The Black public library was not much better. Blacks were not allowed in the library for Whites. Nonetheless, I wanted to write on "Euthanasia." Between the two libraries available to me, I was not able to find, I believe, more than one or two sources. Very frustrated, even in tears, I told Mama of my dilemma. A few days later, much to my surprise, my mother had managed to get several books on this topic from the library. She had shared the problem I had finding books for my term paper with her employer, who in turn went to the library for Whites and checked the books out for me to use. I was overcome with joy.

For the next few weeks I worked diligently, reading these books and writing my paper. The day after I turned my paper in, my English teacher sent a note to my homeroom teacher that she needed to speak with me after class. I just knew she was going to compliment me on my paper. But that was not the case. Much to my dismay she had read my paper and concluded that I had cheated. She asked me, "Where did you copy this paper?" pointing to the bibliography. Knowing that I could not have gotten those references from our school library or the Black public library, she was convinced that the term paper was not my work. I was devastated. My mother had to come to school to speak with my teacher and the principal to explain how I got the books, and she was very disturbed. I finally got a "B" on the paper, but at that point the grade was no longer important to me.

UNSETTLING WORK EXPERIENCE

The work ethic in our family was a strong influence, not only because it was considered a good form of discipline, but because it was necessary for each family member to contribute to the finances of the family, if possible. My brother, Bill, was the first of the children to find a full-time job. He dropped out of high school in tenth grade, against the wishes of my parents, and started working at a local clothing store. He alter got his diploma by passing the General Equivalency Diploma (GED), and volunteered for military service. At age sixteen, my sister, Martha, began a part-time job after school in the cafeteria of Charlotte Memorial Hospital.

It was during my Junior year in high school that I submitted an application for part-time work at the hospital where my sister was now working full-time. I was placed on the waiting list. While I was waiting to be called, Mama told me her employer knew a woman that needed help in her home. I really did not want to do domestic work, but I was afraid Mama would be insulted if I said this to her. After all, working in the home of White folk was an honest living and the only type of work I had ever known Mama to do. This would also be a means to an end. I wanted to earn money to help pay for my college tuition. With a college degree, I reasoned, I would be able to get a respectable job paying a decent salary so that I could help my family.

Mama gave me the telephone number of the woman who wanted help—I will call her Mrs. X. I made arrangements to begin working for her the following week. Mrs. X was legally blind and perhaps between 65 and 70 years old. She lived alone but was very independent and capable of moving about in her home. I found her to be very pleasant. She seemed to be pleased with my work, too—why shouldn't she have been? Mama had trained me well. I knew I was competent, respectful, dependable, an excellent housekeeper, even capable of assisting her in preparing meals.

I had been working for Mrs. X for about six months and things were going quite well. One day, however, she seemed upset. She informed me that she needed to go into town to do some shopping but the person who usually accompanied her could not come that day. She told me that I would have to go with her on the bus into town. This was extremely unsettling for me. You see, at age sixteen, I had never been downtown alone. I was always accompanied by my older sister or brother, my mother, or another adult. My perception of "downtown" was that it was not a friendly place for Blacks. Mama had very strict rules about what to do and what not to do. She always said to me, "Don't wander away from the adult person, don't touch anything unless you are going to buy it, and so forth." There was always a feeling that the White salesperson was following you around or staring you down to assure that you didn't steal something. Then, too, this was during the "Jim Crow" period in the South when Blacks had to be seated at the back of the bus and could not eat at the lunch counters in the stores.

Well, I felt that I had no choice but to go with her, and so I did. We proceeded to the bus stop and when the bus pulled up, my worst fear became a reality. Mrs. X got on the bus and sat in the very first seat. What was I to do? This legally blind woman who I was accompanying to town took a seat in the front of the bus. She told the bus driver to call out her stop but said nothing about the fact that I was with her for assistance. I was afraid to even think about sitting or standing in the front of the bus. I slowly walked to the back of the bus and sat in a position that allowed me to observe Mrs. X. When the bus driver called out her stop, I walked to the front and assisted her off the bus. At that moment, my fear turned to anger. I thought about leaving her to find her own way. But I realized I did not know how to go home from there. I felt so trapped, realizing that I was as dependent upon her as she was upon me.

As if the bus incident wasn't enough, even more happened during that trip. We went into the "5 & 10¢" store which had a lunch counter, where she sat down and ordered something to drink. Since Blacks were not allowed to sit at the lunch counter, I was left to wander the isles in the store, remembering not to touch anything, until she was finished.

That was the last day I worked for Mrs. X. When I finally got home and told Mama what had happened, she listened sympathetically then calmly told me to call Mrs. X and tell her that I could not work for her anymore. I was somewhat disappointed that my mother did not protest more strongly. But then I should have known that such behavior would have been out of character for Mama. Although growing up in the South and keenly aware of and exposed to the evils of segregation and racism, we were taught never to hate anyone. The reality of racism was rarely spoken about in our home, which was a place of peace. Even to this day, when experiencing stressful situations, I can reflect and meditate on my childhood experiences and enjoy a certain calm.

DeJoie's 1992 book, *African-American Women: Overcoming Disabling Factors,* addresses the point that while "engulfed daily with overt and subtle references which infer inferiority, more racial than gender, the African-American woman must tap into internal fortitude to initially maintain and subsequently reinforce a positive self-concept."

During my formative years, I was exposed to a social and political climate which challenged my personal sense of value as a human being. I was fortunate, however, to have the support of wise parents who instilled in me the faith that, "When God allows a burden to be upon you, He will put His arm underneath you to help." I truly believe that the disabling barriers which I experienced during my youth and teenage years empowered me to deal more effectively with the next stage of my adult life. Adversity builds character, and I am encouraged by Carlyle's words, "Out of the lowest depths there is a path to the loftiest height."

EDUCATION CONTINUED: THE COLLEGE EXPERIENCE

After graduating high school, I felt I was now an adult. I was eighteen years old and ready to take on the world—or so I thought!

In the Fall of 1956, I began my freshman year at North Carolina Agricultural and Technical (A&T) College, now North Carolina A&T State University, one of the historical Black colleges.

I was the first in my family to go to college. My parents were so proud. Majoring in nursing was an easy decision. Without the benefit of advice from high school guidance counselors (who were non-existent in my high school), the only other profession I knew about was teaching. Of the two choices, nursing appealed most to me. As there would always be sick people, as a nurse I would always have the security of employment. I would go to college, study hard, become independent and continue to help my family. Perhaps I'd also meet a nice young man, marry and bear a few children. The college climate was both challenging and intellectually stimulating. I was inspired by the interaction that occurred in the classroom between the nursing professors and the students. My sense of pride loomed in the presence of so many role models to look up to.

THE CLINICAL EXPERIENCE: A STRUGGLE WITH PATERNALISTIC SEXISM

As a student nurse, I had my first experience with clinical practice in my sophomore year. I had looked forward to this phase of my curriculum with high expectations. Finally, I would be taking care of real patients! During my first week of clinical practice at L. Richardson Hospital, I realized, however, that I was not as prepared as I thought. My first assignment was on an overcrowded hospital ward with wall-to-wall patients. It was obvious that there were not enough nurses to provide adequate care for so many very sick patients and the head nurse had a real "attitude" problem. In retrospect, I suppose she was responding to being understaffed and over-worked. Student nurses played a major role in the provision of patient care. The nursing staff relied heavily on our contributions and looked forward to our arrival each day.

By the end of the semester, I had observed situations that caused me to question my choice of nursing as a profession. I was disillusioned to witness scenes where the nurses, no matter how busy they were, stopped what they were doing and stood when a physician walked into their station. They would rush to bring him a patient's chart or anything else he demanded. They allowed rude and disrespectful behavior from the physicians, not all that rare, to go unchallenged. Right before my eyes were classic examples of patriarchal control.

I found this behavior to be in conflict with the concepts, values and beliefs I was being taught, at least theoretically, regarding nursing as a profession. Professional socialization is the process whereby the values and norms of the profession are internalized into an individual's own behavior and concept of self. Yet, between my intellectual knowledge of what professional nursing was and the reality of what I was witnessing nursing to be, a struggle ensued. I was faced with the reality that nursing throughout history has been confronted with societal forces which have determined the behavior of nursing in practice. Women constitute the majority in nursing, and women, like Blacks, Jews and others, have been considered to be an oppressed group. Witnessing oppression and feeling the cognitive dissonance disturbed me deeply.

Toward the end of my sophomore year, I began to sink into depression. Knowing the sacrifice my family was making for me to have the opportunity to go to college, how could I call home and tell Mama that I had changed my mind about wanting to be a nurse?

At the end of the year, during the evaluation period, I spoke very openly with Professor H. Brown, the coordinator for Medical/Surgical

Nursing. I shared with her the dilemma I was experiencing as a student nurse regarding the status and image of nursing as a profession.

It was the wise counsel and advice of my professor which led me to the conclusion that it was my challenge as a student nurse to complete my education and become an advocate for professional nursing. At that moment, I made a commitment to accept this challenge and resolved that as a graduate professional nurse I would become a strong advocate for the values and beliefs of professional nursing.

MY RICHARD

It was a beautiful spring night and I was all caught up in the excitement of my upcoming graduation which was about a month away. Richard and I had been dating for about two years and we were going to the end-of-year gala dance. We were having our final dance before the evening was to come to an end, the song "For Your Love I Would Do Anything" was playing, when Richard asked me if I would marry him and slipped an engagement ring on my finger. I said yes and the rest is history. I graduated cum laude in the class of 1961, and a year later, when Richard graduated, we were married. Richard was in the A&T Reserve Officers Training Corp (R.O.T.C.) and was commissioned as a 2nd Lieutenant in the U.S. Army upon graduation.

OUR EUROPEAN EXPERIENCE: A PIECE OF HISTORY

After the initial three months Basic Training period at Aberdeen Proving Grounds in Maryland and at a military base in New Mexico, Richard received orders for the Zweibrucken, Germany United States Army Post. I was very happy when he informed me that I would be going with him to Europe.

We arrived in Bremerhaven, Germany, by ship in March 1963. Socializing into the military culture as a civilian woman was both exciting and challenging. As a new bride, relatively new in my professional career of nursing, I now had to adjust to the role of being the wife of a military officer.

Additionally, I had to deal with the beliefs regarding the role of women. There were and remain many views regarding the role of women in society which stem back to the mid-nineteenth century. During that period women led very circumscribed lives. Legally, a woman was considered a ward of her father or husband. She had no independent rights, since common law held that the husband and wife were one, and that *one* was the husband. It was not considered proper for respectable women to have careers or even to be educated. Fortunately, Richard did not subscribe to these Victorian standards, and was one of the strongest supporters of my career aspirations.

As the wife of a military officer, there were certain expectations and protocols required. My life had suddenly taken on new dimensions. Role identification became a central force to reckon with. The three key tasks confronting me were: (1) my continued personal growth as an individual; (2) my career aspirations; and (3) my role as wife of a military officer. I felt that redefining and affirming my role as a woman was perhaps the most significant ingredient necessary for me to integrate these three elements into a homogeneous life.

I became socialized into the Officers' Wives Club almost immediately. We were a very diverse group, and met monthly at each other's homes, on a rotational basis. It was a very relaxed social environment and provided strong support for each of us.

We had been in Germany for about a year when we experienced, with the rest of the world, two very tragic events which occurred back home in the States. The first was the senseless and shameful bombing of the Sixteenth Street Baptist Church in Birmingham, Alabama on September 15, 1963. The life of four precious Black girls were snuffed out by a dynamite blast while they were sitting in a Sunday School class. Richard remembered with deep sadness, the morning after the bombing when his platoon sergeant, Sgt. Robert Jackson, came into his office and informed him that Denise McNair, one of those little angels, was his niece. Both men sat and wept.

Two months later, November 23, 1963, I was sitting alone in my living room when a news flash came over the radio that President Kennedy had been assassinated. I remember feeling so alone, so far away from home, so isolated. What was happening to my country?

While I enjoyed and valued the company of the Officers' Wives Club, I missed the professional stimulation of working as a registered nurse. I began to explore opportunities for employment at the military institutions in the area.

The availability of nursing positions for civilian nurses was limited. I submitted my application to both the U.S. Army Hospital in Landstuhl, Germany, and the Royal Canadian Air Force Hospital. I was placed on the waiting list at both institutions.

As the Royal Canadian Air Force Hospital had a volunteer nurse program and provided transportation to and from the hospital, I decided to work as a volunteer. Within three months, a regular salaried position became available and my status was changed from volunteer to part-time regular status. Most of the patients, as well as the nursing staff, were French. The opportunity to observe and participate in the delivery of health care to individuals of a different culture was invaluable.

I had been working for about six months at the Royal Canadian Air Force Hospital (RCAFH) when I got the call from the U.S. Army Hospital offering me a full-time position. With ambivalent feelings, I submitted my letter of resignation to the RCAF Hospital and accepted the full-time position at the U.S. Army Hospital.

A few months after beginning my new job, I began experiencing morning sickness along with a few other tell-tale signs. Yes, my pregnancy test came back positive! This was not a planned pregnancy. We had talked about waiting for another year or so before starting our family. We wanted to tour some parts of Europe first. Oh, but the joy of anticipating our first child was far greater than any regrets of having to delay or modify our plans to tour Europe.

MOTHERHOOD

Our beautiful daughter, Victoria Lynette, was born June 25, 1964. I wanted so much to have my mother come for those first few weeks, to see her first grandchild, but I knew that we could not afford to send for her. Without Mama to assist and give me advice, I found Dr. Spock's book the next best thing. So it was myself, my baby and Dr. Spock.

When Vicky was four months old, I decided to go back to work. This was not an easy decision. There was a part of me that wanted to stay at home with my baby and take leave from my nursing career until we returned to the States. Yet, we knew that this was a good opportunity for us to tour Europe. To do so, however, we needed both of our salaries.

With the help of the Post Chaplain for our military base, we were blessed to find a very fine German woman to provide child care. The chaplain shared a mutual relationship with a German priest named Father Kueblic. Father Kueblic spoke perfect English, and it was he that recommended Fraulein Giesler to us for child care.

Fraulein Giesler was obviously very fond of the baby, and gave very good care. There was one slight problem, she could not speak English and I could not speak German. However, Richard was fairly fluent in German and occasionally Father Kueblic would come to visit and serve as an interpreter.

Richard received his orders to return to the States in August of 1966. Fraulein Giesler had remained with us all this time and had become very

much like extended family. Vicky was now two years old and very attached to Fraulein Giesler. Also, she had developed about as much German vocabulary as English. At age two, my baby was apparently bilingual.
German and English—how is that for cultural shock for a Black woman
from North Carolina!

When the day finally arrived for us to leave, it was all bitter-sweet. We
were excited about going home, but we were painfully aware that we
were going to miss Fraulein Giesler's care.

HOME AGAIN: CONTINUING THE JOURNEY

Less than a year after we returned to the States Richard received an honorable discharge from the Army as a Captain. We relocated to Pittsburgh,
Pennsylvania, where he accepted employment as an executive with West-
inghouse Electric Corporation.

I worked as a staff nurse at the Oakland Veterans' Administration Hospital. Although I had a degree in Nursing and more than five years' experience, I realized that in order to advance to leadership and managerial
positions I would have to obtain an advanced degree.

A dominant national force at this time was the women's movement in
education. It galvanized women into action to overcome discrimination,
stimulated research, and opened a whole new field of inquiry: feminism.
Actually, the movement had two separate, yet overlapping, objectives: to
end discrimination and improve women's access to educational opportunity and power within the institution and to add to the knowledge of
women through research, writing, and the creation of new courses and
programs.

It was during that period of time the new Masters of Science Program
to prepare Clinical Nurse Specialists was implemented at the University
of Pittsburgh. In the Fall of 1970, I became the first African-American student to be admitted to this program.

Vicky was now a very active first grader and our second child, Richard
Jr., was one year old. Adjusting to the responsibilities of wife, mother, and
full-time graduate student was quite a challenge. Just as challenging was
the reality of being the only Black student in my class and one of a few
Blacks among the entire student population at the university. All of my
prior formal education, you see, had occurred at all-Black institutions.

A Black student who enters college without prior experience with
other cultures experiences culture shock the first few weeks on campus.

That student is immersed with individuals and groups of different races, cultures, sexual orientations, and beliefs. I was fortunate that my coping skill, which I had developed over years of exposure to adverse situations, served me well here. As an adult learner, I also had a fair command of my sense of self and was confident that with a commitment to hard work I could succeed. A person's skin color, ethnic identity and/or gender may loom large in achieving success. However, as important as these overt characteristics may be, they are seldom, if ever, the sole determining factor in achieving success. Family and earlier educational and religious influences, socioeconomic status, self-awareness, self-confidence, personal values, and aspirations are also significant contributors. I held fast to my belief that much of self-respect involves self-reliance—knowing that I am a person of value and that I have within myself the potential to achieve.

After completing my Master's degree in Clinical Specialization in Neurological Nursing, I accepted a teaching position in the Undergraduate School of Nursing at the University of Pittsburgh.

THE ACADEMIC EXPERIENCE

My teaching experience at the University of Pittsburgh was intellectually stimulating. As a faculty member, I followed the nine-month academic year calendar, which allowed me to have my summers free to spend more time with our children.

The university had a very generous tuition reimbursement program for the faculty, so I began taking graduate courses in education to enhance my teaching skills. Eventually, I submitted a formal application to the Ph.D. Program in Higher Education and was accepted. I continued to work full-time as a nursing professor and took my course work on a part-time basis. After the birth of our third child, a beautiful angel, Sharon Elizabeth, I requested an educational leave from the university to complete my degree.

With my husband and three children proudly looking on, I was conferred the Ph.D. in Higher Education by the University of Pittsburgh in June of 1979. This was one of the most exciting days of my life. From the great granddaughter of a slave to a university doctorate.

We relocated to Somerset, New Jersey. Dr. Benjamin Hooks, the Executive Director of the NAACP appointed Richard to be his Deputy Executive Director. The Headquarters for the NAACP was in Manhattan, New York which was a reasonable commute from New Jersey. I remained in academia as a professor of Nursing and later Assistant Dean of Nursing at Rutgers, the State University of New Jersey, for seven years. Currently, I am at Kean College of New Jersey, the Dean of the School of Natural Sciences, Nursing and Mathematics with academic rank as a Full Professor in the Department of Nursing.

REFERENCES

Leddy, S., & Pepper, J. (1985). Conceptual bases of professional nursing. Philadelphia: Lippincott Co.
Smith, C. (1992). Education for the 21st century. National Association for Equal Opportunity in Higher Education.
Wandersee, W. D. (1988). On the move: American women in the 1970s. Boston: Twayne Publishers.

40

Planning for Success

Elaine L. Cohen

Success can take on many perspectives and of itself means different things. One can also move along life's path and never take the occasion to reflect upon achievements which could leave success unacknowledged and unrewarded. So it is within the context of recognition of accomplishments, self-development, and personal strength that I will share some pointers on attaining career success.

THE PLANNING PROCESS

Early in my career, I methodically planned and calculated the steps I would need to become professionally successful. The planning process plays an important part in my success because it provides a sense of focus and direction. It also gives me the general perspective and resourcefulness needed to hunt down and take advantage of opportunities that might not have been obvious to the uninitiated. These career steps include both service and academic options.

Acquiring practice experience gives me the confidence as well as a strong clinical base and people skills necessary in a leadership role. The academic exposure taught me critical thinking and provided the stimulus and competence to embrace lifelong research interests.

Invariably, much of my self-worth is tied to my drive to succeed and to my professional, educational, and scholarly achievements. I had made the decision to contribute professionally to my chosen career and have since been committed to that goal. I have also been described by one of my professors as an architect of the profession and have endeavored to live up to that characterization in my writings and philosophy. My interests lay in developing the overall framework and foundation for professional practice.

THINGS CAN GO AWRY

For all of my planning, commitment, and drive, sometimes things do not go as scheduled. It is during those times when I am experiencing a professional setback and not feeling very successful that it takes incredible reserve and strength to continue along my career path.

There have been occasions when I have not been astute enough to recognize danger signals even though they were flashing in my face. One memorable situation occurred when I accepted a position without thoroughly investigating the options involved. I arrived on the job totally enamored with myself and all the wonderful things I was going to accomplish. Little did I know that I was being set up to fail.

The political scene was a vicious one with different administrative players vying for the top position. My talents and ideas were being used by one individual (my boss) who I had initially trusted. I became expendable as soon as my organizational plan was developed. Fortunately, I became aware of this individual's motives midway in my tenure at this institution and I collected all the reserve I could muster to go and confront her.

She was quite surprised, shocked, I should say, that I called her out. I remember declaring how disappointed I was and that if she could not provide the basic support and backup that I expected to receive, I would resign. Of course, I knew ahead of time that this individual had much vested interest in the game she was playing and that I would inevitably be forced to leave. Either way, I was very happy that I resumed control over my destiny.

What I have learned from these types of situations is that those "down" periods can challenge me to be at my most creative. In fact, this "off" time allows me the opportunity to reflect, regroup, and redirect myself. Often, to my surprise, what arises from this juncture is something that is very successful. My best published work comes from these intervals.

LEARNING FROM OTHERS

Another important aspect of my success comes from my ability to listen and learn from other successful individuals. I have been greatly influenced by other women who have taken a personal interest in me and provided necessary and most needed support. Some have helped redirect my energies, others have been visionary and inspirational in their approach. All have helped in reaffirming my competence, strength, and courage to succeed.

STAYING FLEXIBLE

One of the important factors to success is taking advantage of an opportunity even if it means changing your course midway. Maintaining flexibility can work wonders for your career. An example will help illustrate my point. I have always taken the time to get to know my professors; to share my ideas and learn about their views and interests.

Consequently, after one of my meetings, I was recommended to serve as a research assistant on a major, nationally funded project. This meant switching my own research focus and completely rewriting my Master's thesis to fit the project's objectives and goals. I remember vividly spending that summer in the library reading and writing the research topic. Needless to say I would have preferred to spend my summer elsewhere.

As it turned out, this project led to some national exposure for me and job offers at prestigious institutions. It also literally opened doors where I thought none had existed. I have become keenly aware of hidden opportunities and have learned to juggle my priorities to take advantage of these choices and situations.

DEVELOPING SUPPORT SYSTEMS

Another element that has led to my success and continues to do so is establishing strong support systems. I am very fortunate to have a very supportive spouse as well as some wonderful friends and mentors. All have played an integral part in encouraging me and providing love and understanding. I have also learned not to take myself too seriously and, when necessary, "let go" of preconceived ideas.

I have been allowed to fail and offered the support to get back on my feet and start again. I have since learned that failing gives you the opportunity to "regroup" and appreciate the effort involved and things that need to be done for the future.

THE NAY-SAYERS

The best way to deal with negative people is to ignore them! In the course of my career, I have come across those who were either jealous of my accomplishments or just had it out for me. Some have even come under the guise of so-called friends. What I have found in my experiences is that these individuals are too exhausting to deal with. They zap all your energy and reserve.

I have made a conscious effort to be polite, but do not allow myself to be persuaded too much by what they say. In fact, I use their negativity to my benefit. When someone tells me that I am only kidding myself or states that something is impossible to accomplish, I dare myself to take on the challenge. Ninety-nine percent of the time things work out. Those are the kind of odds I can live with!

HELPING OTHERS

It is a professional obligation to mentor and assist other individuals in attaining their career goals. I maintain this philosophy because of the help I have received along the way. I attempt to be vigilant of my staff's and colleague's interests and concerns and offer my talents when appropriate.

I am often approached to provide assistance in writing and publishing. I also schedule time to help other women who are in the process of returning to school and require guidance and support. Sometimes I am invited to just "shoot the breeze." It is amazing what can be learned. I have found that those efforts can be extremely rewarding and lead to continuous self-exploration and satisfaction.

SUMMARY

I consider myself a very successful woman. Success, however, can be elusive in nature and at times very personal. To quote a dear and wise friend of mine "being successful doesn't mean you have all successes." It is within this framework that success can be most meaningful.

Although I lead a very hectic life, I do take time out to enjoy long walks with my husband and just plain "hang out." I also savor quiet time with friends. Writing and publishing have become a passion and a means to make a contribution to my profession.

41

Notes Toward the Valorization of a Cultural Image

Allan Graubard

AN INTRODUCTION? PERHAPS . . .

This essay is the result of a very generous suggestion by Dr. Munhall that I participate in the present discussion. As a poet, I approached this willingly, but with inclinations perhaps unique to myself. I do not, by that, seek any sort of justification beyond my presumptions, which should make themselves known to you in the succeeding, few pages. On the other hand, I do hope to clarify a relationship that is, by its nature, somewhat obscure—at least when depicted against any background formed about codes of "objective truth." I emphasize this simply because, to me, it is a notion within a universe of other notions, some old, some new. It is neither a goal nor a penchant. Beyond that, or before if not beside and within it, is an image or series of images: women who have become a measure of their time—our time—both through their acceptance of imposed limitations and as a source of transgression and renewal. For these women are more imaginary only as they tend to become real . . .

THE SETTING

World War II becomes an open door, a passage. With men inducted into the armed services, women stream into the workforce as never before. They take over jobs reserved previously for their husbands, lovers, uncles, cousins, sons, or male friends. Jobs they were told—how recently? how long ago?—they were not suitable for are now open to them because there is no one else, because they must pitch in, because war production depends on them, because the freedom they have still yet to possess completely is at stake or made to seem at stake: to work, at least; to strive openly and equally for whatever it is they desire; this freedom so long rationalized for them, denied to them, costumed for them as men wanted it or agreed to it when pushed, when pushed to the brink. They work the assembly line, manage other workers, sit on planning boards, assuming the dictates of a power they rarely considered appropriate or possible for themselves before—the appropriate, the possible itself, being defined, catalogued, exemplified for them by those who now inveighed a destruction heretofore unseen on this earth. They know this and they accept it. Most champion it. It's a fait accomplis.

Yet the great historical trauma opens a wound between men and women that has yet to heal. And with ever greater consciousness of its effects, origins, patterns, ruses, gambits, constraints, capacities, women come to realize just how much they've been had. They see the roles they were forced to play by "circumstance," "society," "expectations," by "femininity," by their "irrational" nature. They see them more clearly now than ever before. They see them, and even as they assume them, they subvert them, one woman at a time.

How?

Their phantoms are projected onto a large silver screen: the ring, the field, the garden, the hell, the play pen where they embrace, for all to see, the myths they accept, sometimes create and suffer, dispel and critique, laugh at and cry over, forget and rush back to because nothing seems the same afterward, or so much of the same. Because adulation is a prize of great value. Because popular art is the medium of the times. Because the power that emanates from an image is equal, even superior, to that which burns from the bore of a gun. Because in their haste to comprehend who they are, they forget where they've come from. Because their amnesia is a device that can please them and those who connive to keep them fit for sex, child rearing, the common pleasures and subtle brutalities of family and corporate life. Because it doesn't matter all that much—or does it?—

that here, in a dark theatre, in rows of seats, they can fix a persona sufficient to their needs, and through which they can recover something of who they are or what they have lost in seeking themselves.

And suddenly, between the image before them and the reality that awaits them, a simulacrum forms, a space of conjuration, where one can just as easily be taken for the other, where distinctions evaporate, and where the risk of dispossession grows as imminent as the image is ephemeral. And a taste of ash spots their lips, a dream of burned flesh lingers subtly about them.

Who?

Ida Lupino, Gene Tierney, Ava Gardner . . .

THE CHARACTER/THE WOMAN

They're no longer so innocent. They've lived through class conflicts, the struggle for unionization, prohibition, the frenzy of the twenties, the depression, the Hollywood code, the specter of world revolution, the fascist reaction, and so much more. They've been through the mill. They know the gamut. They've been hurt, victimized by men, by work, by society, by family, by other women. Perhaps they've struck back, perhaps they haven't. Perhaps they've already paid the price either way. Perhaps they've gotten off free, or felt they have by the skin of their teeth. Perhaps they're on the rebound searching for love, for success, for a thrill. Perhaps they can't wait to find their man, the man they've been told to expect. Perhaps they don't expect much at all, so they take who they can get. They put on lipstick, powder their faces, splash perfume over their bodies so they won't have to smell the odor of their hurt, their loneliness, or their fear. They slip on tight, attractive dresses, the kind that reveal just enough to entice a man's attentions. They measure themselves in mirrors where desirability and grit commingle with power and guilt. They're as tough as nails and as sweet as honey—an unbeatable combination, and don't they know it! And they'd just as soon push a knife in your back as fall victim to another illusion.

They're confused, angry, too beautiful for words, too sexy to take. They string men to their wishes and shake them loose whenever they've a mind to. They're volatile and open, practical and passionate, and more than cunning. They use their vulnerabilities the best way they know how: as a lure, a seduction. It works for them, usually. They get just enough to realize that they could compete with men, even on men's terms, and win more times than not. They know this but don't flaunt it. It's not in their best interests.

You can take a man for a chump and get away with it, but do it quietly and don't gloat. Their "sweetness" is their final trump. They know just how foolish men can be. They also know they're not in the driver's seat, that they sit beside "him," that the wind blows through their hair as "he" shifts gears; that "he" turns the wheel, determines the direction and the speed, to say nothing of an industrial complex that built the car and works, quite well, to keep men on top, in the board room as well as the bedroom.

Ida Lupino, Gene Tierney, Ava Gardner tell us as much. They also know that if everything doesn't happen because of their men, it happens in relation to them; that their power as women is proportional to their attractiveness to them; and that their men set the standards, sanctify the rituals, even if it means accommodating, now and then, to something seemingly foreign to them: conception, pregnancy, birthing, caring; even if it means formalizing their own ignorance in matters of love. Men are "blinded by passion," "undone by romance," the best of them steer clear; women, like black widows, set the snares and exact their payments. The irony doesn't surprise them: men forge the set up, then suffer their willingness to gratify themselves at "her" expense. In the end, the sexual fix stands, the rules are set. Their men have only to wear one or another mask to fulfill their roles and everything else falls into place.* The future is bright, too! After the debacle of millions of deaths, how could it not be? Remember, remember and clench your teeth, Ladies. Quiet! Don't say a word, just stand there and shimmer. It's a man's world, not a woman's, and when it all comes down to it, when the final judgments are made, men will come through—haven't they always?—armed with indifference, narcissism, scientific objectivity, and their self-celebrated, "courage" to separate from their emotions, to "see things as *they* are," or so they presume.

Yet these women appeal to us long after they have passed, long after others have taken their place. And those that remain—Angelica Huston, Kathleen Turner—carry something of them, some precious bit of what made them tick. The lineage is immediate; the generation preserved. There's something in them that reminds us of our own peculiar timeless and timely uncertainty. Look, they play for keeps. They never take no for an answer. They've staked men at their word and beat them in doing so. Now and then they even come out on top, knowing all the while that it doesn't mean so much, in this labyrinth where shadows of beings shift about and duel for preeminence, in the theatre as well as the street.

---

*A strange but true situation. Men give over to women a power to command them while, at the same time, managing the affair to their purposes. Of course, that is men's belief. We are lucky that women have always been so much other than men imagine them to be.

Afterward, of course, they gather their things, slip on their coats and head out, satisfied for the moment or seeking something else to distract them from their boredom—the film being just enough and never enough. But are *they* ever bored? Do these women we follow decade after decade ever confess to being bored? They don't. They can't allow themselves to be seen being bored. Boredom itself would spell their undoing.* Or it would once again, framed just so, allow them to traffic in allure. They wear enough cosmetics as it is. Add on another layer? They'd grow angry, and not just with the smoldering pith of a despair that they use to touch up, with perfect hand, the customary sultriness men expect of them. Their anger would build. Perhaps they'd look around, take stock, and realize something more than what they had before. They might even refuse the predictable hysterias "common to their sex" and by which men have kept them, to a large degree, to an ever smaller degree, as men would wish.

They'd learn something, or learn how to use something they have not, could not, would not before: their boredom. They'd recognize perhaps that they didn't need men at all. That they had themselves, their silence and their "passivity" distinct from how men framed them. That they had risen to the occasion anyway as many times on their own as not. That they were perfectly able to resist the fickle phenomenon of their "beauty," as men saw it, protected it, promoted it, priced it. Perhaps they'd come to see that their power extended far beyond their sex, and the pleasures men dreamed or that they dreamed men dreamed in them, found in them, choreographed for them, danced to with them. And a touch of freedom would reanimate a vision of life that men did not prescribe; women's lives, carefully rescued from what remained uniquely theirs and incompletely his; the tatters unwound, respooled, rewoven. And then done again, and again.

This vision would root, it would feed on their sweat, their labor, their greed, their tenderness, their concern, their duplicity. It would return to women something more fundamental than any face lift against the tides of aging. It would, at the same time, accentuate their humanity beyond the moral and aesthetic strictures they had come to adopt as their own, but which never were to begin with. It could, drawing from the gutsy intelligence of these heroines of cinema noir, turn women's heads backward and forward at the same time: to the earliest covens where healers met to commune with nature—and whose murderous fate at the hands of the Church we know all too well—to fin de siecle struggles for suffrage,

---

*The subject of boredom is immensely important in the determination of an individual self. The race to keep boredom at bay through obsessive distraction does not, for all that, delay the encounter. It can render it virtually useless, however.

to the conflicts of gender politics, to the most stunning celebrations of subversive imagination.

Ida Lupino, Gene Tierney, Ava Gardner tell us as much. Their struggles remain. For the destiny of too many women, dare I say the majority of women, their passions strike home, one way or another.

OTHER COMMENTS

Clearly though, because women still abide in contradiction with a culture they have no means to deny for being a voice of, they have assumed a becoming that reveals both with equal or unequal concern. Their capacity here to straddle the two worlds—the one they were born into, the one dimly or more clearly seen and still to come—keeps them, and the men they choose to take with them, in suspense. It is this suspense—by way of anticipation, a sense of immanence, certainly a despair that yet may coil in the heart of love—that will enable women to see more and farther than they have before. Their strength, too, is here: rooted in the struggle to preserve their independence, however it is expressed, given the present conditions of life across the globe.

And yet one essential aspect is also, and because of women's struggles, that much more prescient: distinction by gender alone is as baseless a generalization as any other that allows us to overlook the obscurity of an individual existence for an idea, however seemingly transparent or compelling it is. To abuse one for the other turns the tables, all right, but does so within a context that allows for little more. It is the same game, a game we have all but exhausted in our efforts to satisfy it during these last decades of the 20th century. But it is a game that continues and in whose trajectory passion finds itself lost more times than not . . . Clearly, the comments I have offered are equal parts fantasy and deliberation. Nor do I believe it is a matter of convincing. These sets of circumstances certainly exist. I feel them as others do, as perhaps you have or have not. Even your possible refusal to admit to this does little to dissuade me from continuing.

SOMETHING MORE?

Today these women appear to us as real as they are excessive. Circulating within a world defined particularly by men, by machismo, they offer a way out, even in the acceptance of their fatality to that world. Perhaps it is their sense of compassion, revealed in a glance, a smile, but revealed surreptitiously or passively, and which they rarely allowed themselves to assent to so openly. That they use their compassion as a source of strength, even allure, in contradistinction to men, does not prevent their men from turning to them for just that either. The attraction is real enough, the attracted needful. Yet, for me, these women are and are not as they appear. But that is also unique to their characterization, or at least their characterization makes them available to: their certain or uncertain *recreation* in other eyes, mine as yours. As their men need them for what they lack, we need them for what they incompletely reveal, usually suffer, but certainly speak to. It is in this recreation that their capacity as metaphor lies, and not only for what they defined for their time and ours, at least in terms of sociocultural representation, but for what they allow us to see anew. And that is why I have chose them as subjects for this brief, if aleatory, essay.

They recreate themselves perpetually. It occurs with each thought, each risk, each compromise, each repudiation or agreement they make. It occurs even with each bosomy breath. It is desire, their desire, reconforming to its own devices the situations they encounter and then seek their satisfactions or frustrations in. It is decisive then that their desire be understood and that the freedom desire seeks generally, for them as for us, not be camouflaged as it is so often both in the words we/they use to express it and the actions with which we/they chart by its light. Neither can exist without the other, neither can propel itself toward those successive limits that, at first glance, seem justifiably prohibitive—but which, because of that, are all that more fit to contest. To accept any other sort of momentum would, for them as for us, condemn all to the kind of perpetual victimization that we have grown used to, culture wide, worldwide, however much it angers us. In a sense, this victimization carries the history of our culture to its present conflictive limits. And it is a history that understanding alone cannot prevent us from returning to. It is a history that begins in a war that opened up to women what they did not possess so completely before, and which still continues in a plethora of guises.

These heroines of the cinema noir offer us a grounding and a possibility. The aura of recognition that they exemplify meets our own need to remake them in an image perhaps more suited to the immediacy of our passions and of our historical moment—but which, at the same time, does not disfigure the grandeur of their practicality. Between the two, as the terms of any metaphor that bridges the silence between thought and the body, desire and realization, inhibition and scandal, we find ourselves.

MORE AGAIN?

(They say less than they mean and do more than they say. Their appearance now takes on the demeanor of a possibility that echoes within each of us.)

We know them, a thousand times over we know them: victimized women who strike back as they know, as they can. Yet the violence of their desire to be free of the forces that restrain them also clouds their vision. For the men they seek, the men who "hold the cards," so to speak, appeal to them in proportion to how well they satisfy the charms they string about their own guilt in the effort: both from knowing that these are the only men they can deal with and that these men appear so much less, or so much more, than their desire. It is also a reciprocal relation that men suffer but from an apparently more powerful vantage. Nonetheless, they suffer it, too.

To leave this as it is though would fail to recognize the imaginative license taken in its execution, even as men wrote them in film after film, even as I write them here. So I have done little but confound that license with my own view and extend it. Certainly, realism has no place here just as it has no place within the pantheon of the cinema noir. Nor am I satisfied with any sort of patina or routine that projects an appearance all too easily accepted as the "way things are." For we know—how well? how little?—that things are never the way they appear to be, or rather, are that way only to the point of their own transgression.

Finally, let me be clear about the reason why I have chosen to begin with what could rightly be called the caricature of a woman, a caricature initially created by men to accompany them perhaps within the solitude necessary to create it. No doubt, all this is true. Equally true is the fact that it was precisely this sort of woman that women as men came to adore, a woman who could meet men on their turf and offer something neither could accept or reveal on their own. No matter how they were masked by their many seductive poses, which they executed exquisitely, they still express possibilities for something more—for a type of love that could only be unconditional and reciprocal. They still carry within them this great yearning, this tear in the fabric of being, for which men also hunger for whether they admit it to themselves, to others, or not—and which, in this context, reveals something decisive about the cultural origins of WWII and its succeeding contexts, most equally tragic in regard to love. Through it all, the desire for embrace with an other, with *the* other if possible, remains paramount.* The women of noir, with a most caustic but appreciable sense of reality, do not at the same time relieve themselves of this wondrous cause. For me, that was enough to set my mind

---

* Nor is this embrace final, a romantic apotheosis. On the contrary, it is, so to speak, an embrace of recognition, an initial if rapturous moment within a rapport whose future depends upon the clarity of dialogue each partner sustains within it.

racing. And if I have succeeded here in offering just another caricature of a woman from whom I have still much to learn, at the very least I have done so via an inescapable sense of necessity: of being free to aspire beyond the given order of perception and events; of being free enough to choose a body and a means of desiring that that body be as much itself as other, of being coincident with and impregnated by thought rather than servile to it.*

---

*For a more definitive explication of the relationship of thought to the body, I refer you to Annie Le Brun's introduction to the complete works of the Marquis de Sade, *Sade, A Sudden Abyss,* published in 1993 by City Lights Books, San Francisco.

42

Powers

Barbara Stevens Barnum

When Dr. Patricia Munhall asked me to contribute to this book on and by powerful women, I told her that I wasn't certain I qualified. I didn't think of myself as a powerful woman. Not that I thought of myself as lacking power; power just wasn't something I really thought about.

Yes, I'd written a bit about it in my books on nursing management. I'd even made a few speeches about it, but only when it was an assigned topic. It simply wasn't one of my major interests, and it certainly had never produced any self-introspection. Power was a "removed" concept of intellectual interest somewhere between other concepts like delegation and networking, all of which—while perfectly valid notions—lacked any particular fascination for me.

Pat assured me that I qualified—and could not escape writing this piece on that account. Hence, I have been led to ruminate on power as a personal concept. Once forced to the task, I admit the concept held some innate fascination: Was I or wasn't I powerful? I had no idea. I soon discovered that I was uncomfortable with the connotations of *powerful* while quite willing to admit that I had certain *powers.* I suspect they are powers we all share to varying degrees, but I'll make them more personal here. Perhaps I'll end up with a general taxonomy of powers, perhaps not.

PARADOXICAL POWER

I'm going to label the first power *paradoxical.* For me, this is the most important power, and we'll never know to what extent we possess it. It's the power to make a difference in someone else's life. I prefer to think of it as the ability to make a *positive* difference. On the day Pat gave me this assignment, someone whom I regarded with great esteem told me I had made a positive difference in her life. The reasons don't matter here, but I was both humbled and amazed. It would never have occurred to me that I was anything more than a colleague.

The incident recalled an earlier event when a young woman, whom I'll confess I didn't even recognize, came up and thanked me for helping her on a matter of major importance in her life. I have no memory of the advice I gave (although what she reported sounded like something I would say) or of contacting the people involved on her behalf (although they were people I could have, hence probably did, call on).

In essence, I visualize the incident as follows (based on the woman's accounting—which I still don't remember): bright potential student drops by my office for advice; she wants to do something everyone tells her can't be done; I say she can do it if she's willing to pay the price; she says she's willing; I put her in contact with the people who can arrange it. As unusual act on my part? Hardly. So benign, in fact, that I have no memory of it. And yet, surprise, this small act had the power to enhance someone's life.

The point is that the most important power we have is the ability to open doors for others, and most of the time we'll never know when we open a major one. It's just part of the job, part of a busy day. Whether those doors are contacts, role modeling, or just advice that proves worthwhile, this paradoxical power can be very potent. The interesting thing is our state of relative ignorance about the process, for the identical act, done for another person, might have little importance—in other words, hold no paradoxical potency.

If there's a celestial scorecard somewhere, it would be interesting to know a life's batting average in relation to paradoxical power. During our lifetimes, however, none of us will know how powerful we actually are and that's probably for the best.

THE POWER TO ESCAPE TRAPS

In trying to identify my particular powers, I decided that I'm pretty good at escaping traps. What I mean by that is the power to avoid being hoist on the petard of one's own successes. I realize that one can be trapped by personal failures as well, but frankly, I suspect that most people reading this book are more vulnerable to being victims of their successes.

For me, an important internal measure of success is being faithful to the natural flow of one's life. In my case, sometimes that meant leaving behind external measures of success for lesser or no signals of success at all. I was reminded of this power yesterday when someone told me she was staying in a job she had grown to hate because she could retire with a full pension in five years. Perhaps her power is fortitude in the face of adversity; for me that decision would have been falling for a trap.

I was rather old when I learned to appreciate the power to escape traps, namely, when I left a named chair and division directorship at Teachers College, Columbia University. I can't tell you how many people asked me how I could leave such a prestigious position for, well, nothing. When I explained to the first couple of people that "it was time," they simply gave me uncomprehending stares. I gave up groping for an explanation. Until then I had naively assumed that when people ran out of steam for one project, one job, one life, they changed it for another.

I think, perhaps, I was protected from the urge to be trapped by achieved status because of family attitudes. In growing up, one of my children was very disturbed by a woman who was rather full of herself and her status. The three year old solemnly labeled her a "hufty lady." Thereafter, when anyone called you a hufty lady in my family, you knew it was time to let the wind out of your sails.

THE POWER TO CREATE

When a job or a life feels uncreative, it's time to change it. In this respect, I will always be grateful to nursing. It has allowed me to be a vagabond within the trappings of a single profession. I have been practicing nurse, educator, administrator (in both education and service), editor, consultant, and writer. For me, a new job is new power: power to grow, to learn, to succeed or fail. Please don't think I'm offering the nomadic life as an ideal model. The truth is that I stand in awe of those people who can be creative in the same role for a lifetime. They are amazing. There are also those who stay in place after every vestige of creativity has been sucked dry.

As I've aged, I've had to add different creativities to my plate. For me, a skill once achieved becomes a competency and it no longer *feels* creative. Today, I write fiction—weird fiction (too weird my agent tells me)—but that's where my creativity takes me. I've been at fiction a while, and I'm pretty good at it. Fortunately, I still have enough to learn to keep me at it longer. Some day—if you like really weird stuff—you'll be buying one of my novels. When writing fiction starts to feel routine, I'll probably learn to decorate hats or brew herbs.

I'm not sure how creativity feels for other people, but I know it can be expressed in a million different ways. I think the power to be creative is an absolute life essential—like the ability to breathe. We are born creators; to squelch that power, or to let others squelch it, is a major circuit failure.

THE POWER TO FAIL

One of the most important powers that I have (or think I have) is the power to fail and admit it. The truth is that I do some things exceptionally well, others with mediocre talent, and others I simply flub. Only hufty ladies refuse to admit when they fail. Refusal to recognize failure cuts off something important in me, something human. For me, refusal to admit an inadequacy (or worse, a miserable mistake) instills fear. Fear of being found out? I'm not sure. But I do know I'd rather live with failure than fear—hands down. Perhaps it's enough to admit a failure to oneself, but I think it's a mark of power to be able to admit it to others as well.

Besides, it's sort of nice to be wrong now and then. Infallibility is boring, not to mention impossible. To my way of thinking, not trying is a greater sin than failure. (I know that's a cliche, but it's true nonetheless.)

I would list my failures for you, but I don't dwell on them. I try to recognize them, admit them, and move on. A word of advice: Don't ever clump your failures together or they start to form a category that you don't want in your life.

THE POWER TO STAY WITH ONE'S JOY

With the exceptions of figuring out income taxes and walking the dog, I mostly do things I enjoy in life. Some would say that's a flaw rather than a power, but it *feels* like a power. Once I almost stayed in a job too long for the sake of someone else. But I didn't, and my leaving turned out to be the best thing that could have happened to that person. Sacrifice is a dirty word; act from joy.

Notice that joy is different from self-interest. I don't think anyone gets real joy from making someone else miserable. Joy is too big for that; joy corrects for the pettiness that may circle self-interest like a waiting wolf.

AVOIDING UNNECESSARY FRUSTRATIONS

What makes people think in terms of power? If I had to form a hypothesis, I'd predict that the degree to which one focuses on power is a function of the degree of frustration one experiences at the hands of others.

In that respect I have a serious power: the ability to avoid unnecessary frustrations. For example, I have accepted that a geriatric dog has accidents. My way to avoid frustration is to buy very cheap rugs, wash and replace them frequently.

When I think about it, I spent much of my life avoiding things that frustrate others. On a theory that everyone develops bladder control before they're 21, I refused to cope with potty training children. On a theory that no one in my family was allergic, I finished a doctorate with dust resting amiably under every bed.

And I've learned that if a colleague objects to by behavior, my clothes, my ideas, well, it's his baggage, not mine. Somehow nursing creates a lot of judgmental people; trying to please them all is guaranteed to produce frustration at best. Yet in honesty, I'll also admit to a good bit of luck in my career. I've been blessed with jobs that allowed for maximum creativity, minimal shackles.

This is not to say that I avoid all frustration—just unnecessary frustration. I can get as irate as anyone else when the telephone repairman fails to show on the day you stayed home from work to let him in.

CONCLUSIONS AND RUMINATIONS

If I am powerful (and I'm still not certain the word applies), the powers I've discussed are the ones I'll claim. I began this paper thinking I might arrive at a taxonomy of powers, but now I'm not so certain. It occurs to me that we all may have different sets of powers. Let me know if your list differs from mine.

How does one recognize power? I'm not certain, but for me it doesn't always relate to the more obvious signs and signals. I know people in high positions who are miserable and feel hamstrung and powerless. Yet others inhale power from high position, no matter what frustrations accompany the role. Of course, there are times when the signs and signals do relate. Between the millionaire and beachcomber, I think the former has a pretty obvious power advantage.

I'm certain that power doesn't depend on how many subordinates are subject to your will. Sometimes executive decision making is more a burden than a power. For me, nothing is worse than the agony of deciding whether or not to fire someone or discharge someone from a program. What will it do to them? What will it do to others? To this day I fret over the first student I dismissed from a nursing education program. Would she really have been a danger to patients? What did removal from the program do to her life? Responsibility for decisions such as this is not power but stewardship—the hardest part of stewardship.

At the end of this deliberation, I'm left mostly with a lot of questions about power. Do the people who seem to crave it have more lofty, more difficult goals? Do those who lack it obsess over it for that reason? Why do some people simply glory in exercising it? And how on earth can you measure one man's power against another's?

Perhaps the best signal of power is how one feels about the sort of life one's powers produce. I like my life pretty much the way it is—give or take the fact that part of any life is luck and part design. On the whole, my design suits me, so perhaps I'm powerful after all.

Will these ruminations make me feel any more powerful? I doubt it. I can be brought down fast by that telephone repairman or a kid whispering under her breath, "hufty."

Index

411